Meeting Psychosocial Needs of Women with Breast Cancer

National Cancer Policy Board

Maria Hewitt, Roger Herdman, and
Joseph Simone, *Editors*

INSTITUTE OF MEDICINE
NATIONAL RESEARCH COUNCIL
OF THE NATIONAL ACADEMIES

THE NATIONAL ACADEMIES PRESS
Washington, D.C.
www.nap.edu

THE NATIONAL ACADEMIES PRESS 500 Fifth Street, N.W. Washington, DC 20001

NOTICE: The project that is the subject of this report was approved by the Governing Board of the National Research Council, whose members are drawn from the councils of the National Academy of Sciences, the National Academy of Engineering, and the Institute of Medicine. The members of the committee responsible for the report were chosen for their special competences and with regard for appropriate balance.

This study was supported by Contract/Grant No. N02-CO-01029 between the National Academy of Sciences and the National Cancer Institute, and a grant from the Longaberger Company through the American Cancer Society. Any opinions, findings, conclusions, or recommendations expressed in this publication are those of the author(s) and do not necessarily reflect the views of the organizations or agencies that provided support for the project.

Library of Congress Cataloging-in-Publication Data

Additional copies of this report are available from the National Academies Press, 500 Fifth Street, N.W., Lockbox 285, Washington, DC 20055; (800) 624-6242 or (202) 334-3313 (in the Washington metropolitan area); Internet, http://www.nap.edu.

THE NATIONAL ACADEMIES
Advisers to the Nation on Science, Engineering, and Medicine

The **National Academy of Sciences** is a private, nonprofit, self-perpetuating society of distinguished scholars engaged in scientific and engineering research, dedicated to the furtherance of science and technology and to their use for the general welfare. Upon the authority of the charter granted to it by the Congress in 1863, the Academy has a mandate that requires it to advise the federal government on scientific and technical matters. Dr. Bruce M. Alberts is president of the National Academy of Sciences.

The **National Academy of Engineering** was established in 1964, under the charter of the National Academy of Sciences, as a parallel organization of outstanding engineers. It is autonomous in its administration and in the selection of its members, sharing with the National Academy of Sciences the responsibility for advising the federal government. The National Academy of Engineering also sponsors engineering programs aimed at meeting national needs, encourages education and research, and recognizes the superior achievements of engineers. Dr. Wm. A. Wulf is president of the National Academy of Engineering.

The **Institute of Medicine** was established in 1970 by the National Academy of Sciences to secure the services of eminent members of appropriate professions in the examination of policy matters pertaining to the health of the public. The Institute acts under the responsibility given to the National Academy of Sciences by its congressional charter to be an adviser to the federal government and, upon its own initiative, to identify issues of medical care, research, and education. Dr. Harvey V. Fineberg is president of the Institute of Medicine.

The **National Research Council** was organized by the National Academy of Sciences in 1916 to associate the broad community of science and technology with the Academy's purposes of furthering knowledge and advising the federal government. Functioning in accordance with general policies determined by the Academy, the Council has become the principal operating agency of both the National Academy of Sciences and the National Academy of Engineering in providing services to the government, the public, and the scientific and engineering communities. The Council is administered jointly by both Academies and the Institute of Medicine. Dr. Bruce M. Alberts and Dr. Wm. A. Wulf are chair and vice chair, respectively, of the National Research Council.

www.national-academies.org

THOMAS J. SMITH, Professor, Virginia Commonwealth University, Richmond, VA

EDWARD WAGNER, Director W.A. (Sandy) MacColl Institute for Healthcare Innovation, Group Health Cooperative, Seattle, WA (as of May 1, 2003)

SUSAN WEINER, President, The Children's Cause, Silver Spring, MD (until April 30, 2003)

ROBERT C. YOUNG, President, American Cancer Society and the Fox Chase Cancer Center, Philadelphia, PA

Consultants

Patricia A. Ganz, MD, Jonsson Comprehensive Cancer Center, UCLA Schools of Medicine and Public Health, Los Angeles, CA

Pamela J. Goodwin, MD, MSc, FRCPC, Marvelle Koffler Breast Centre, Department of Medicine, Division of Epidemiology, Samuel Lunenfeld Research Institute, Mount Sinai Hospital, University of Toronto

Study Staff

Maria Hewitt, Study Director (until April 18, 2003)
Roger Herdman, Study Director (as of April 19, 2003)
Gelsey Lynn, Research Assistant
Timothy Brennan, Research Assistant
James Ryan, Ph.D., Editor

NCPB Staff

Roger Herdman, Director, National Cancer Policy Board
Anike Johnson, Administrator
Rosa Pommier, Financial Associate

Reviewers

This report has been reviewed in draft form by individuals chosen for their diverse perspectives and technical expertise, in accordance with procedures approved by the National Research Council's Report Review Committee. The purpose of this independent review is to provide candid and critical comments that will assist the institution in making its published report as sound as possible and to ensure that the report meets institutional standards for objectivity, evidence, and responsiveness to the study charge. The review comments and draft manuscript remain confidential to protect the integrity of the deliberative process. We wish to thank the following individuals for their review of this report:

Joan R. Bloom
University of California, Berkeley
Joanna Cain
Oregon Health & Science University
Michele Dabrowski
University of Utah
Betty Ferrell
City of Hope National Medical Center
Stewart B. Fleishman
Beth Israel Cancer Center
Donna Greenberg
Massachusetts General Hospital
Richard P. McQuellon
Wake Forest University Baptist Medical Center
Anne Moore
Cornell University
Edward Perrin
University of Washington
Sally Redman
Institute for Health Research, Australia
Lee N. Robins
Washington University School of Medicine
Lidia Schapira
Massachusetts General Hospital
Selma R. Schimmel
Vital Options International

Although the reviewers listed above have provided many constructive comments and suggestions, they were not asked to endorse the conclusions or recommendations, nor did they see the final draft of the report before its

release. The review of this report was overseen by **Merwyn Greenlick**, Oregon Health & Science University, and **Enriqueta Bond,**
Burroughs Wellcome Fund. Appointed by the National Research Council and the Institute of Medicine, they were responsible for making certain that an independent examination of this report was carried out in accordance with institutional procedures and that all review comments were carefully considered. Responsibility for the final content of this report rests entirely with the authoring committee and the institution.

Contents

EXECUTIVE SUMMARY   1

1. INTRODUCTION   11

2. EPIDEMIOLOGY OF BREAST CANCER   15
    INCIDENCE AND MORTALITY, 15
    PREVALENCE, 16
    STAGE AT DIAGNOSIS,16
    RISK FACTORS ASSOCIATED WITH BREAST CANCER,17
    SUMMARY,20

3. PSYCHOSOCIAL NEEDS OF WOMEN WITH
       BREAST CANCER   21
    PSYCHOSOCIAL NEEDS OF WOMEN BY PHASE
       OF CARE, 22
    PREVALENCE OF PSYCHOSOCIAL DISTRESS, 31
    RISK FACTORS ASSOCIATED WITH PSYCHOSOCIAL
       DISTRESS, 58
    SUMMARY, 61

4. PSYCHOSOCIAL SERVICES AND PROVIDERS   70
    PSYCHOSOCIAL SERVICES, 70
    PROVIDERS OF PSYCHOSOCIAL CARE, 78
    SUMMARY AND RECOMMENDATIONS, 90

5. THE EFFECTIVENESS OF PSYCHOSOCIAL
   INTERVENTIONS FOR WOMEN WITH BREAST
   CANCER   95
   HISTORY OF PSYCHOSOCIAL INTERVENTION
       RESEARCH, 96
   METHODOLOGIC ISSUES, 99
   REVIEW OF THE LITERATURE, 105
   SUMMARY, 129

6. DELIVERING PSYCHOSOCIAL SERVICES   133
   THE EVOLUTION OF BREAST CANCER CARE AND ITS
       IMPLICATIONS FOR THE PROVISION OF
       PSYCHOSOCIAL SERVICES, 133
   THE STRUCTURE AND DELIVERY OF PSYCHOSOCIAL
       SERVICES TO WOMEN WITH BREAST CANCER, 136
   PSYCHOSOCIAL SERVICE USE, 140
   SUMMARY, 161

7. BARRIERS TO APPROPRIATE USE OF
   PSYCHOSOCIAL SERVICES   165
   ACCESS TO CARE, 165
   SUMMARY AND RECOMMENDATIONS, 193

8. RESEARCH   199
   STATUS OF BREAST CANCER-RELATED RESEARCH, 200
   RESEARCH PRIORITIES, 219
   FINDINGS AND RECOMMENDATIONS, 225

APPENDIXES   229
A. WORKSHOP AGENDA AND PARTICIPANT LIST, 229
B. TABLES AND BOXES SUMMARIZING EVIDENCE
   FROM CLINICAL TRIALS, 234

Executive Summary

More than 250,000 women in the United States will hear the diagnosis of breast cancer every year. Most women will be cured by surgery, which no longer means a mastectomy in many cases. Additional treatment, designed to prevent a recurrence in the breast or spread of the cancer to other areas of the body, may be recommended at the time of diagnosis. This may include radiation therapy, chemotherapy, and hormonal therapy. More than 25 percent of women with breast cancer will die because the disease has spread beyond the breast and lymph nodes. Whereas, breast cancer is curable when it is confined to the breast and regional lymph nodes, metastatic breast cancer is not curable. Women with breast cancer suffer psychologically not only from the diagnosis and initial therapy (with the resultant side effects) but also from the fear of recurrence and of dying of the disease.

This report on meeting the psychosocial needs of women with breast cancer was prepared by the Institute of Medicine (IOM) and National Research Council National Cancer Policy Board (the Board) and is based in part on a comprehensive workshop held at the IOM, October 28 and 29, 2002 (see Appendix A). The report is one of a three-part series from the Board on cancer survivorship, and it follows and builds on the Board's 1999 report, "Ensuring Quality Cancer Care," in which the Board concluded that psychosocial support services were an essential component of quality cancer care. The present report is intended to speak to stakeholders and policy makers in cancer care, to women with or concerned about breast cancer, and the interested general public.

It is a timely communication since cancer treatment in general, and breast cancer treatment in particular, has moved from being delivered

1

mostly in the hospital to the present situation in which treatments are given almost exclusively in the ambulatory care setting. Psychosocial services for women, which in the past, if available, were also largely hospital-based, have not been made available to the same extent in the new outpatient treatment areas. Consequently, a reassessment of the present accessibility, extent, and efficacy of psychosocial services for women with breast cancer is imperative. Breast cancer differs from many other cancers in that it is essentially limited to women, and it also has high incidence, good survival, and well-defined risk factors and screening technologies. Nevertheless, given the crosscutting nature of psychosocial distress in cancer, as defined below, the Board believes that much of the information gleaned from the study of breast cancer patients is also applicable to other cancer patient groups treated now in clinic settings.

This report outlines the status of psychosocial interventions in general and suggests directions for research, delivery, and policy that may be appropriate to other sites of cancer as well as to breast cancer. Specifically, the report means to understand the impact of a diagnosis of breast cancer on a woman, her family and community, the psychosocial needs of such women, and the opportunities to provide support to them along the disease trajectory.

The report addresses 5 questions:

1. What is psychosocial distress, and how frequently does it occur among women with breast cancer at each stage?

2. What interventions are available to treat psychosocial distress at all stages of disease, and how effective are they?

3. What is the status of the delivery of psychosocial interventions and care to women with breast cancer?

4. What barriers prevent women with breast cancer from getting psychosocial interventions and appropriate psychosocial care?

5. What can be done to improve psychosocial care for women with breast cancer?

What is psychosocial distress and how frequently does it occur?

Distress in cancer has been defined as an unpleasant emotional experience that may be psychological, social, or spiritual in nature. Distress exists on a continuum beginning with the "normal" and expected feelings of fear, worries, sadness, and vulnerability in coping with cancer and its treatment. However, these normal feelings may extend to become more severe, even disabling, symptoms of anxiety or a formal diagnosis of major depression. Severe distress may relate to the illness or its treatment, a severe social problem, or a family problem, or it also may result from a spiritual or existential crisis created by confronting a threat to life (NCCN, 1999)[1] or from the complications of treatment. Psychosocial issues and distress are logically likely mostly cancer site non-specific, but they have been most extensively studied among women with breast cancer. In particular, women with breast cancer have been examined for the impact on psychological function at each stage of disease and during survivorship.

The studies show highest distress at transition points in treatment: at the time of diagnosis, awaiting treatment, during and on completion of treatment, at follow-up visits, at time of recurrence, and at time of treatment failure. Taken overall, around 30 percent of women show significant distress at some point during the illness, and the number is greater in women with recurrent disease whose family members are also distressed (see Chapter 3).

What interventions are available to treat psychosocial problems and distress at all stages of disease and how effective are they?

Interventions to address psychosocial problems and distress begin with basic information about the disease and treatment options from the breast cancer care clinician (often a medical oncologist). This clinician, regardless of medical specialty, should express support, encourage patients to voice their fears and concerns, encourage coping, and provide medication when needed to control symptoms like insomnia and anxiety. Psychosocial services should be provided by oncology caregivers as a part of total medical care, but referrals to specialists in psycho-oncology, social work, pastoral counselors, and other professionals may be necessary where the level of distress is high. The frequency of visits to a psycho-oncology professional may vary from a single encounter to several, and the timing and duration may also vary from very brief to extending over months or, at times, even years. Today, there are many community-based services available to women with breast cancer at no charge. Evidence from 31 randomized clinical trials, meta-analyses, and non-randomized studies supports the inclusion of psychosocial interventions in routine clinical care. This body of research

---

[1]The National Comprehensive Cancer Network (NCCN) is a not for profit, tax-exempt corporation that is an alliance of the world's leading cancer centers. Established in 1995 to enhance the leadership role of member institutions in the evolving managed care environment, the NCCN seeks to support and strengthen the mission of member institutions in three basic areas:

1. To provide state-of-the-art cancer care to the greatest number of patients in need;

2. To advance the state of the art in cancer prevention, screening, diagnosis and treatment through excellence in basic and clinical research;

3. To enhance the effectiveness and efficiency of cancer care delivery through the ongoing collection, synthesis and analysis of outcomes data.

documents that several psychosocial interventions reduce psychosocial problems and distress among women with breast cancer. Psychosocial factors and interventions are also related to other aspects of cancer such as pain and other side effects, as is discussed later in this report.

What is the status of psychosocial care delivery?

A number of cancer centers, institutions, and organizations (see below) have noted the importance of addressing cancer-related psychosocial concerns in the context of total care and explicitly recommend provision of adequate psychosocial services: However, the degree to which these recommendations are carried out is highly variable, and they are not monitored in any way to determine the quality of care in this area.

- National Cancer Institute (NCI)-designated comprehensive cancer centers;
- Institutions approved by the American College of Surgeons' Commission on Cancer;
- Institutions belonging to the Association of Community Cancer Centers; and
- National Comprehensive Cancer Network members (standards of care and guidelines direct the management of psychosocial distress in patients with cancer).

As discussed in Chapter 6, estimates are imprecise, but surveys suggest that perhaps 10 percent and at the most 30 percent of women with breast cancer have used psychosocial services (often of a relatively informal nature), although two-thirds of significantly distressed women indicate that they would accept services if they were routinely offered. Many women with breast cancer rely solely on family, friends, and clergy for social support. Some may find information and support on the Internet, for example, young survivors coalition, cancerandcareers.org, or the American Society of Clinical Oncology's "People living with Cancer." Other women, however, do not have social supports built into their lives. They may also lack access to psychosocial services, either because care providers do not refer them to the available services or because of other barriers (e.g., no health insurance or no reimbursement for services).

What barriers prevent women with breast cancer from getting appropriate psychosocial interventions and care?

Several barriers impede appropriate care. The dramatic shift in the delivery of almost all cancer care from inpatient hospital to outpatient settings has not included a similar shift in the outpatient psychosocial services to the outpatient clinics and private oncology office practices. Increased complexity of care has limited access even further. Women with breast cancer usually see multiple specialists (e.g., surgeons, radiation oncologists, medical oncologists), and care is often not well coordinated. Fragmentation of care is an added psychological burden; the patient is not given care by a single, trusted physician. In addition, the outpatient offices and clinics are extremely busy; the length of time doctors can spend with patients is often limited, and the opportunity to bring up psychosocial problems may be lost. Receiving adequate information and the ability to ask questions in a comfortable way are basic needs for addressing psychosocial concerns. Breast cancer care occurs primarily in private office-based practices that routinely do not employ psychosocial professionals.

Another barrier is the lack or inadequacy of health insurance coverage. An estimated 8 percent of women with breast cancer are uninsured, or, if patients are insured, there is coverage of mental health services with lower reimbursement levels or placement of mental health services in behavioral health contracts, separate from medical coverage. Still other barriers are the reluctance to discuss psychosocial concerns with the busy oncologist provider; the stigma associated with seeking or using mental health services; physicians' failure to ask patients about distressing emotional symptoms; and the lack of simple, rapid instruments for screening for psychosocial distress (see Chapter 3). All are barriers to the symptoms receiving appropriate recognition, diagnosis and treatment by supportive and psychosocial services.

Also, primary oncology teams in outpatient offices are often not familiar with clinical practice guidelines for managing psychosocial distress; they often work in environments that do not provide psychosocial services onsite; and they often are not aware of the psychosocial resources in their local communities. The situation is complicated additionally by the paucity in many communities of identified professionals with skills in managing psychosocial and mental health issues in patients with cancer. As part of a new initiative to help locate appropriate professionals, the American Psychosocial Oncology Society (APOS) now provides a Directory online (www.apossociety.org) and through a toll-free help line for patients and families (1-866-APOS-4-HELP).

Overcoming barriers to appropriate use of psychosocial services will require advocacy, monitoring of psychosocial services through quality assurance programs to ensure compliance with standards of care, physician education, training in communication skills, and research relative to identifying and overcoming barriers. The Board understands that, in addition to these listed actions, appropriate use means that determinations of eligibility for psychosocial interventions ensure that women with breast cancer who neither want nor need these interventions are not subjected to them. Attending unnecessary sessions can be difficult for patients, a waste of time for both patients and therapists, and uneconomical.

What can be done to improve psychosocial care for women with breast cancer?

Board Recommendations

The Board intends that the information contained in this report will be instructive in improving care for women with breast cancer in the ambulatory setting and will enhance understanding of psychosocial, psychiatric, and quality of life issues, the barriers to their appropriate management and routine inclusion in total care, and the range of interventions that are available to relieve distress. In addition, the Board hopes that the information will be helpful to women with breast cancer and to the public. Many of the psychosocial issues reviewed are likely relevant and applicable to other sites of cancer.

The Board also has formulated some recommendations to be considered by policymakers and stakeholders responsible for breast cancer care. These are steps to improve the delivery of care, the knowledge and training of providers of care, and the research base that will lead to the development of a better understanding of psychosocial needs and better ways of addressing them.

To improve clinical practice:

Breast cancer care clinicians, such as oncologists and other medical professionals, responsible for the care of women with breast cancer should incorporate planning for psychosocial management as an integral part of treatment. They should routinely assess and address psychosocial distress as a part of total medical care. Validated assessment instruments are available to screen for distress, anxiety, depression, and quality of life. Quality of life instruments also can be used to identify function (psychological, social, physical, sexual) and to facilitate discussion of patient concerns, and serve as a basis for referral. Financial considerations may dictate that in most instances screening is carried out using simple, rapid tools such as the Distress Thermometer or Hospital Anxiety and Depression Scale (HADS).

Providers of cancer care should meet the standards of psychosocial care developed by the American College of Surgeons' Commission on Cancer and follow the National Comprehensive Cancer Network's (NCCN) Clinical Practice Guidelines for the Management of Distress. Education about psychosocial needs and services should be undertaken through collaboration between professional organizations and advocacy groups.

The NCI, the American Cancer Society (ACS), and professional organizations (e.g., American Society of Clinical Oncology, American College of Surgeons, American Association of Colleges of Nursing, American Psychosocial Oncology Society, American Society of Social Work, American Society for Therapeutic Radiology and Oncology, Oncology Nursing Society) need to partner with advocacy groups (e.g., National Breast Cancer Coalition, National Alliance of Breast Cancer Organizations,Wellness Community, NCCS) to focus attention on psychosocial needs of patients and resources that provide psychosocial services in local communities and nationally.

Organizations with effective outreach to cancer constituencies should be assisted in making resource directories available to providers and patients; these directories would identify the range of supportive services, from the free services of advocacy groups to services provided by mental health professionals.

To improve professional education and training opportunities:
Sponsors of professional education and training programs (e.g., NCI, ACS, ASCO, ONS, AOSW, ACS-CoC, APOS) should support continuing education programs by designing, recommending, or funding them at a level that recognizes their importance in psycho-oncology for oncologists, those in training programs, and nurses and for further development of programs similar to the ASCO program to improve clinicians' communication skills; and

Graduate education programs for oncology clinicians, primary care practitioners, nurses, social workers, and psychologists should evaluate their capacity to incorporate a core curriculum in psycho-oncology in their overall curriculum taught by an adequately trained faculty in psycho-oncology and to include relevant questions in examination requirements.

There is a great need for continuing education and graduate education for clinicians and researchers in psycho-oncology. Research training in psychosocial oncology is needed to ensure the highest quality of clinical investigations. It is important to encourage graduates into the field by providing training opportunities such as postdoctoral fellowships. Additional clinical training programs are also needed to address the shortage of well-trained psychosocial clinicians. Nurses play a central role in providing cancer care and currently have limited oncology training. Psychosocial content could usefully be integrated into basic nursing education.

To improve research opportunities:
Research sponsors (e.g., NCI, ACS) and professional organizations (e.g., American Society of Clinical Oncology, American College of Surgeons,

American Association of Colleges of Nursing, American Psychosocial Oncology Society, American Society of Social Work, American Society of Therapeutic Radiology and Oncology, Oncology Nursing Society) need to support efforts in collaboration with advocacy groups (e.g., National Breast Cancer Coalition; National Alliance of Breast Cancer Organizations) to enhance practice environments to promote coordinated, comprehensive, and compassionate care. Rigorous evaluations of the cost and effectiveness of delivery models that show promise in improving access to psychosocial support services are needed. These might include:

• Collaborative practices in which a psychologist or other mental health provider forms a partnership with an office-based oncology provider to make psychosocial services available within the oncology practice;
• Comprehensive breast cancer centers that generally integrate supportive care into a "one-stop-shopping" model of clinical practice;
• Breast cancer nurse managers who provide case management, education, and supportive care within oncology practices;
• Novel models of psychosocial services, such as ICAN project, in phase 2 demonstration, which utilizes master's level counselors who receive a core curriculum in psychosocial oncology;
• Demonstration projects to test the effectiveness of clinical practice guidelines on the management of psychosocial distress in improving psychosocial outcomes;
• Development of measures of quality of cancer care that pertain to supportive care (including psychosocial services). Measures might include provider assessment of psychosocial concerns, the provision of information regarding community supportive care resources, and satisfaction with care.

In general, investigators working in this field should recognize that studies in the past would in many cases have been stronger if they had been conducted using other than selected patients mostly in tertiary settings, or if the studies had not been unblinded, with small sample size, of insufficient power, of short duration, and other methodological shortcomings. Future study designs should try to minimize such weaknesses.

Research sponsors (e.g., NCI, ACS) should continue to support basic and applied psycho-oncology research. This might include:

• Further development of simple, rapid screening tools for identifying the patient with distress in outpatient offices and training of primary oncology teams in diagnosis of distress that exceeds the "expected" and when referral to supportive services should be made;

- Studies that assess the relative effectiveness of various psychosocial interventions, using population-based patient samples of adequate size, the timing and duration of interventions, and innovative and inexpensive modes of administration (e.g., internet-based approaches);
- A consensus conference to develop a battery of standard instruments for outcome measures to permit comparison of data from studies carried out by different research groups;
- Organization of a psychosocial clinical trials group in which a network of researchers could address key questions in multi-center studies that would allow access to large, population-based samples;
- Clinical trials of psychosocial interventions that are conducted within routine breast cancer care in which cost and quality of life are outcome measures;
- A registry of ongoing psychosocial research/trials to assist researchers in identifying and tracking new areas of study.

The NCI should support a special study to ascertain the use of, and unmet need for, cancer-related supportive care services (including psychosocial services) in the United States. The results of such a study could provide benchmarks against which care can be measured and performance monitored. Such a study would document existing disparities in service use by age, race/ethnicity, geography, and insurance coverage.

1

Introduction

An estimated 251,200 women were diagnosed with invasive and in situ breast cancer in 2002 (American Cancer Society, 2002). For most of these women, initial feelings of shock, disbelief, and distress were followed by physical recovery and a return to good psychological health. A small group of women, however, had lingering and sometimes disabling psychological problems following their diagnosis. Most of these women lived to join the more than 2 million survivors of breast cancer, but may experience episodic or persistent distress. Nearly 40,000 women died of breast cancer in 2002, some of whom experienced poor coping, with inadequate support at the end of life. Of course, the number of people affected by these psychological problems is much greater than the number diagnosed and includes family, friends, and others in the community.

The recognition and study of the psychological consequences of the cancer experience is the subject of the discipline of psycho-oncology, a field that emerged as a distinct discipline in the mid 1970s. For the first time, cancer, once a taboo topic, could be discussed openly, and more patients became willing to share their feelings and experience and participate in studies. Breast cancer has been the most extensively studied cancer from the standpoint of psychosocial sequelae, dating back to the mid-twentieth century, and remains the paradigm for the field (Shapiro et al., 2001).

In this report, the National Cancer Policy Board reviews the now-extensive psycho-oncology literature to inform policy decisions regarding the delivery of compassionate breast cancer care. The purpose of this report is to:

- characterize the psychosocial consequences of a diagnosis of breast cancer,
- evaluate the effectiveness of services to alleviate psychosocial distress,
- assess the status of psychosocial interventions in the context of contemporary breast cancer care,
- assess the status of professional education and training and applied clinical and health services research, and
- propose policies to improve the quality of care and quality of life for women with breast cancer and their families.[1]

Individuals with cancer may have cancer-specific concerns, such as fear of cancer recurrence, and generalized symptoms such as worry, trouble sleeping, fatigue, and anxiety about going to the doctor. Underlying mental illness may also be exacerbated by the experience of being diagnosed with cancer or living with the disease. To capture the broad range of concerns of individuals with cancer, the Board, in this report, has relied on the definition of "psychosocial distress" from the National Comprehensive Cancer Network. "We have defined 'distress' as it applies to cancer, as follows. Distress is an unpleasant experience of an emotional, psychological, social, or spiritual nature that interferes with the ability to cope with cancer treatment. It extends along a continuum, from common normal feelings of vulnerability, sadness, and fears to problems that are disabling, such as true depression, anxiety, panic, and feeling isolated or in a spiritual crisis" (NCCN, 1999: 114).

ROLE OF THE NATIONAL CANCER POLICY BOARD

The National Cancer Policy Board (the Board) was established in March 1997 at the Institute of Medicine (IOM) and National Research Council with core support from the NCI and CDC to address issues that arise in the prevention, control, diagnosis, treatment, and palliation of cancer. The 20-member board includes health-care consumers, providers, and investigators in several disciplines (see membership roster). This report is one of three reports that comprise a Board initiative to address issues of concern for cancer survivors, with an emphasis on what happens following the primary treatment of cancer. The first report in that series, "Childhood Cancer Sur-

---

[1]Excluded from this review are the small number of men with breast cancer and healthy women who are at high-risk for breast cancer because of their genetic makeup or family history. The Board recognizes that each of these groups have unique health and psychosocial needs, but elected not to cover them in this report. The Board hopes in future reports to examine issues related to genetic testing and cancer.

vivorship: Improving Care and Quality of Life," was published in 2003, and the final report on adult survivorship is expected in 2004. These reports (and others) follow and build on the Board's 1999 report, "Ensuring Quality Cancer Care," which recommended strategies to promote evidenced-based, comprehensive, compassionate, and coordinated care throughout the cancer care trajectory. In that report, the Board recommended that individuals have access to psychosocial support services; the report's focus, however, was on primary treatment, and it did not extensively address issues related to the psychosocial needs of individuals with cancer (Institute of Medicine, 1999).

Like its predecessors, this report speaks to stakeholders and policy makers in cancer care, to women with or concerned about breast cancer, and to the interested general public. This in-depth examination of cancer-related psychosocial issues is based, in part, on a 2-day IOM workshop held October 28–29, 2002, "Meeting Psychosocial Needs of Women With Breast Cancer" (see the workshop agenda in Appendix A). In addition to the Board's core support, the workshop and this report were made possible by a generous grant from the Longaberger Company through the American Cancer Society. Two papers commissioned for the workshop were essential to this report, one by Dr. Patricia A. Ganz, on the assessment of psychosocial distress in clinical practice, and the other by Dr. Pamela J. Goodwin, a review of literature on the effectiveness of psychosocial intervention for women with breast cancer.[2]

The Board decided to focus on breast cancer largely because of the robust literature and extensive experience in this area. The Board, however, considers breast cancer a paradigm and suggests that the policy recommendations in this report are applicable to the psychosocial care provided generally to individuals with cancer.

FRAMEWORK OF THE REPORT

The report consists of several background chapters (Chapters 2–8) that summarize evidence that the Board used in formulating its recommendations, presented and discussed in the Executive Summary and Chapters 4, 7, and 8.

Chapter 2 reviews the epidemiology of breast cancer to characterize the group of women at risk for psychosocial distress.

Chapter 3 characterizes the psychological and social consequences of a diagnosis of breast cancer, the frequency of psychosocial distress, and the availability of assessments tools to help health-care providers identify women who may benefit from psychosocial interventions.

---

[2]These papers are available at www.IOM.edu/ncpb.

Chapter 4 presents a brief description of the range of psychosocial interventions that are available, the sites in which they are offered, the providers who offer them, and psycho-oncology education and training opportunities for health-care providers.

Chapter 5 reviews the effectiveness of psychosocial interventions with an emphasis on evidence from randomized clinical trials. The chapter concludes with a discussion of outstanding research issues that need to be addressed.

Chapter 6 characterizes the delivery of psychosocial services in the context of contemporary breast cancer care, describes a number of service programs, and presents evidence regarding use of psychosocial services by women with breast cancer.

Chapter 7 examines barriers to the receipt of psychosocial services, including issues related to access to care and limitations of systems of care.

Chapter 8 surveys ongoing clinical and health services research aimed at improving psychosocial care and outlines research priorities to improve services to women with breast cancer.

REFERENCES

American Cancer Society. 2002. *Cancer Facts & Figures 2002*. Atlanta: American Cancer Society.

Institute of Medicine. 1999. *Ensuring Quality Cancer Care*. Washington DC: National Academy Press.

Institute of Medicine. 2001. *Improving Palliative Care for Cancer*. Washington DC: National Academy Press.

National Comprehensive Cancer Network. 1999. NCCN practice guidelines for the management of psychosocial distress. National Comprehensive Cancer Network. *Oncology (Huntingt)* 13(5A):113–147.

Shapiro SL, Lopez AM, Schwartz GE, Bootzin R, Figueredo AJ, Braden CJ, Kurker SF. 2001. Quality of life and breast cancer: Relationship to psychosocial variables. *J Clin Psychol* 57(4):501–519.

2

Epidemiology of Breast Cancer

This chapter presents a brief overview of the epidemiology of female breast cancer to provide estimates of the size and characteristics of the population at potential risk for cancer-related psychosocial distress. The characteristics of the population, such as cancer stage, a woman's age at diagnosis, or her race and ethnicity, significantly affect disease prognosis, insurance status, and other circumstances, as well as emotional responses to breast cancer.

INCIDENCE AND MORTALITY

At birth, females face a one in eight chance that breast cancer will develop over a lifetime (American Cancer Society, 2002). In 2002, there were an estimated 203,500 new cases of invasive breast cancer (and 47,700 cases of ductal in situ cancer) among women (American Cancer Society, 2002). Excluding cancers of the skin, breast cancer is the most common cancer among American women, accounting for nearly one of every three cancers diagnosed. In 2002, there were an estimated 39,600 deaths from breast cancer. Only lung cancer causes more cancer deaths in women. Women believe they are more likely to get breast cancer than suffer a heart attack or develop diabetes (Avon Breast Cancer Foundation, 2002), despite the higher risk of these other conditions. To put the burden of breast cancer into perspective, 32 million women are living with cardiovascular disease and 513,000 women died of cardiovascular disease in 1999 (American Heart Association, 2002).

15

PREVALENCE

In 1999, there were an estimated 2 million women with a history of breast cancer, representing 41 percent of the nearly 5 million female cancer survivors or 23 percent of 8.9 million total cancer survivors (Table 2-1). Among women with a history of breast cancer, 35 percent had been living with their diagnosis for less than 5 years, while 16 percent were survivors of 20 or more years.

STAGE AT DIAGNOSIS

The prognosis of invasive breast cancer is strongly influenced by the stage of the disease, or how far the cancer has spread when it is first diagnosed. Local stage describes cancer confined to the breast, regional stage tumors have spread to the lymph nodes, and distant stage cancers have metastasized (spread to distant sites) (American Cancer Society, 2001). As shown in Figure 2-1, the 5-year survival rate is highest for early stage cancer (96.4 percent), and lower for regional stage (77.7 percent) and distant stage (21.1 percent) cancer (American Cancer Society, 2001).

Most breast cancer (63 percent) is localized at diagnosis, but this varies by race (see discussion below). Fewer women are diagnosed with regional (28 percent) or distant (6 percent) disease. Other women are diagnosed with noninvasive cancer that has not spread beyond its site of origin. These so-called *in situ* breast cancers are either lobular (originating in the breast

TABLE 2-1 Estimated Cancer Prevalence, United States, January 1, 1999

	Number	Percent
Total	8,928,059	100.0
Sex		
Male	3,929,515	44.0
Female	4,998,544	56.0
Site		
Breast	2,051,280	23.0
Other	6,876,779	77.0
Years since breast cancer diagnosis		
Total	2,051,280	100.0
0 to 4	724,510	35.3
5 to 9	495,499	24.2
10 to14	326,501	15.9
15 to 19	173,627	8.5
20+	331,143	16.1

SOURCE: Ries et al., 2002.

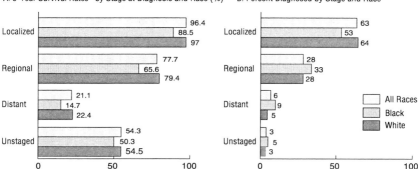

A. 5-Year Survival Rates* by Stage at Diagnosis and Race (%)   B. Percent Diagnosed by Stage and Race

FIGURE 2-1 Female breast cancer, United States, 1992–1997.
*Survival rates are based on follow-up of patients through 1997. American Cancer Society, Surveillance Research, 2001.
DATA SOURCE: NCI Surveillance, Epidemiology, and End Results Program, 2001.

tissue made up of glands for milk production) or ductal (originating in the ducts that connect lobules to the nipple). *In situ* breast cancers affect

approximately 54,300 women (47,700 ductal carcinoma *in situ*) each year in addition to the 203,500 invasive breast cancer cases diagnosed (American Cancer Society, 2002). The majority of these tumors will not become invasive. Most oncologists believe that lobular carcinoma *in situ* is not a true cancer, but is instead a marker of increased risk for developing future invasive cancer (American Cancer Society, 2001).

SOME RISK FACTORS ASSOCIATED WITH BREAST CANCER

Age

The risk of breast cancer and death from breast cancer increases sharply with age for both white and African American women (Figure 2-2) (American Cancer Society, 2001). Breast cancer is predominantly a disease of older women, with 45 percent of incident cases and 59 percent of breast cancer deaths occurring among women age 65 and older (see Figure 2-3 below; Ries et al., 2002).

Race and Ethnicity

The incidence of breast cancer is higher among white as compared to African American women. By age, the rates among white and African

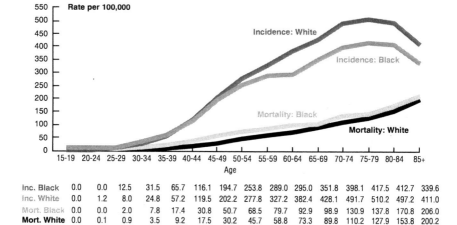

	15-19	20-24	25-29	30-34	35-39	40-44	45-49	50-54	55-59	60-64	65-69	70-74	75-79	80-84	85+
Inc. Black	0.0	0.0	12.5	31.5	65.7	116.1	194.7	253.8	289.0	295.0	351.8	398.1	417.5	412.7	339.6
Inc. White	0.0	1.2	8.0	24.8	57.2	119.5	202.2	277.8	327.2	382.4	428.1	491.7	510.2	497.2	411.0
Mort. Black	0.0	0.0	2.0	7.8	17.4	30.8	50.7	68.5	79.7	92.9	98.9	130.9	137.8	170.8	206.0
Mort. White	0.0	0.1	0.9	3.5	9.2	17.5	30.2	45.7	58.8	73.3	89.8	110.2	127.9	153.8	200.2

FIGURE 2-2 Female breast cancer. age-specific incidence and death rates, by race, United States, 1994–1998. American Cancer Society, Surveillance Research, 2001.
DATA SOURCES: NCI Surveillance, Epidemiology, and End Results Program, 2001, and National Center for Health Statistics, 2001.

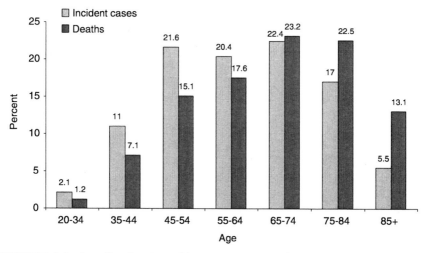

FIGURE 2-3 Age distribution of breast cancer incident cases and deaths, 1995-1999.
SOURCE: Ries et al., 2002.

American women are similar until age 50 and then begin to diverge (Figure 2-2). The breast cancer mortality rate is higher among African American as compared to white women (Figure 2-4). The incidence and mortality rates for breast cancer are generally lower among women of other racial and ethnic groups (i.e., Asian and Pacific Islanders, American Indians, Hispanics) as compared to white and African American women (Figure 2-4) (American Cancer Society, 2001). When analyzed by race, survival is more favorable at each stage for white as compared to African American women (Figure 2-1). African American women are more likely than white women to be diagnosed when their cancer is at an advanced stage (e.g., 9 versus 6 percent with distant stage cancers). This later stage at diagnosis, in part, explains the overall poorer survival of African American as compared to white women with breast cancer (72.0 versus 87.0 percent surviving 5 years). Just over half of the survival difference can be attributed to the later stage at detection and tumors that are more aggressive and less responsive to treatment. The presence of additional illnesses and various sociodemographic factors (e.g., lack of health insurance) also contribute to the observed differences in survival between African Americans and whites

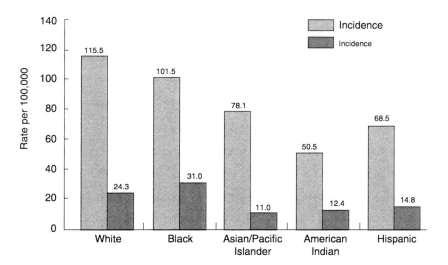

FIGURE 2-4 Female breast cancer incidence and mortality rates,[a] by race and ethnicity, United States, 1992–1998. American Cancer Society, Surveillance Research, 2001.
DATA SOURCES: NCI Surveillance, Epidemiology, and End Results Program, 2001, and National Center for Health Statistics, 2001.

[a]Rates are age-adjusted to the 1970 US standard population.
†Persons of Hispanic origin may be of any race.

(American Cancer Society, 2001). A recent literature review of clinical trials and retrospective studies in the United States that compared survival between white women and African American women with breast cancer found that socioeconomic status replaces race as a predictor of worse outcome in many studies (Cross et al., 2002). According to this review, relative to white women, African American women were more likely to be diagnosed at a younger age and with more advanced disease that appeared to be more aggressive biologically.

SUMMARY

Breast cancer represents a significant health burden to American women. In 2002 there were an estimated 203,500 diagnoses of invasive breast cancer and 39,600 deaths. There are over 2 million women alive with a history of breast cancer. Age is a key risk factor associated with breast cancer, with 45 percent of new cases and 59 percent of deaths occurring among women age 65 and older. Most women (63 percent) are diagnosed with localized breast cancer that has a very favorable prognosis. Their 5-year survival was 96 percent, although some of these same women will eventually develop or have already developed recurrences. Although African American women are less likely to be diagnosed with breast cancer, when they are diagnosed, they are more likely to be diagnosed with regional or distant disease that has a less favorable prognosis. Other racial and ethnic groups (i.e., Asian and Pacific Islanders, American Indians, and Hispanics) have both lower breast cancer incidence and mortality rates.

REFERENCES

American Cancer Society. 2001. *Breast Cancer Facts & Figures 2001–2002*. Atlanta: American Cancer Society.

American Cancer Society. 2002. *Cancer Facts & Figures 2002*. Atlanta: American Cancer Society.

American Heart Association. 2001. *2002 Heart and Stroke Statistical Update*. Dallas: American Heart Association.

Avon Breast Cancer Foundation. 2002. *Women's Health Index 37*.

Cross CK, Harris J, Recht A. 2002. Race, socioeconomic status, and breast carcinoma in the U.S: What have we learned from clinical studies. *Cancer* 95(9):1988–1999.

Ries LAG, Eisner MP, Kosary CL, Hankey BF, Miller BA, Clegg L, Edwards BK, eds. 2002. *SEER Cancer Statistics Review, 1973–1999*. Bethesda, MD: National Cancer Institute.

3

Psychosocial Needs of Women
with Breast Cancer

Most women experience at least some psychosocial distress during the course of their breast cancer diagnosis and treatment. The level of distress varies from woman to woman and, within an individual, over the course of diagnosis and treatment. Cancer-related distress can be expected to dissipate with time for the majority of individuals diagnosed with cancer. For others, however, such distress may interfere substantially with comfort, quality of life, and the ability to make appropriate treatment decisions and adhere to treatment (Irvine et al., 1991; Massie and Holland, 1991). Psychosocial distress can be related to physical problems like illness or disability, psychological problems, and family issues and social concerns such as those related to employment, insurance, and supportive care access.

The frequency and patterns of psychosocial distress that occur among women with breast cancer depend greatly on which concerns are included in the operational definition of distress and how it is measured. However, most of the literature on the psychosocial aspects of breast cancer suggests that the vast majority of women adjust well to the diagnosis of breast cancer and manage the complex and sometimes aggressive treatments associated with primary treatment and recurrent disease (Bloom et al., 1987; Frost et al., 2000; Ganz et al., 1996, 1998a, 2002; Maunsell et al., 1992; Schag et al., 1993). Recent studies that have examined quality of life and depression among disease-free breast cancer survivors using standardized instruments with norms available from the general population suggest high levels of functioning in the early and later years after primary treatment (Dorval et al., 1998; Ganz et al., 1996, 1998a, 2002). Even for women with recurrence of breast cancer, psychological well-being is often maintained (Bull et

21

al., 1999; Frost et al., 2000; Ganz et al., 2002). For a minority of women however, a diagnosis of breast cancer contributes to significant psychosocial distress that can interfere with functioning and well-being. Assessing the factors that contribute to resilience, effective coping with cancer, and positive psychological outcomes associated with the cancer experience is of increasing interest to researchers (Brennan, 2001; Cordova et al., 2001; Justice, 1999; Petrie et al., 1999; Tomich and Helgeson, 2002), and some of these studies show reductions in the need for medical visits with benefit finding (Stanton et al., 2002) (see section on Measuring Psychosocial Distress). This chapter reviews some of the psychosocial concerns that have been described among women at various points along the disease continuum.[1] Estimates of the prevalence of psychosocial distress are then presented. The chapter concludes with a discussion of risk factors associated with psychosocial distress and methods that are available to identify women who are distressed and who may benefit from intervention.

PSYCHOSOCIAL NEEDS OF WOMEN BY PHASE OF CARE

Some of the most common psychosocial concerns reported by women with breast cancer include:

- Fear of recurrence,
- Physical symptoms such as fatigue, trouble sleeping, or pain,
- Body image disruption,
- Sexual dysfunction,
- Treatment-related anxieties,
- Intrusive thoughts about illness/persistent anxiety,
- Marital/partner communication,
- Feelings of vulnerability, and
- Existential concerns[2] regarding mortality.

To some degree, these concerns are expected and are experienced by all women at some point after their diagnosis and treatment for breast cancer. There is variation, however, in the extent to which women accept these concerns, cope with them, and adapt to living with a degree of uncertainty about the future. Some women live in a state of persistent rumination about the illness and are overwhelmed with concerns about the inability to control what will happen. Effective strategies for enhancing coping are actively being stud-

---

[1]Much of this chapter was drawn from a background paper by Patricia A. Ganz, "Psychosocial Services for Women with Breast Cancer: Needs Assessment in Clinical Practice," commissioned by the National Cancer Policy Board.

[2]Fear of dying.

ied by many research groups. For most women with breast cancer, coping strategies focusing on realistic expectations can facilitate the adaptation to the illness that occurs over time. For certain women, however, adaptation and coping may be extremely difficult and intervention may be needed.

The breast cancer experience has several distinct phases, each characterized by a unique set of psychosocial concerns. These phases coincide with aspects of the clinical course of the illness and related treatments. What follows is a review of the distinctive psychosocial needs associated with diagnosis, primary treatment, the special issues related to non-invasive breast cancer, completing treatment and re-entry to usual living, survivorship, recurrence, and palliation for advanced cancer. Oncology and primary care practitioners must be prepared for the range of psychosocial issues that may arise among their patients who are at various points along the breast cancer treatment continuum. The psychosocial impact of breast cancer must also be understood in the context of other issues that affect women's coping, quality of life, and well being, such as socio-economic factors and cultural factors, the availability of social support, access to health care, and the presence of other chronic illness or life crises.

Diagnosis

Although women clearly vary in their responses, most who are told that they have a diagnosis of breast cancer acutely experience fear and disbelief. Prior to being diagnosed with cancer, most do not perceive themselves to be at higher than usual risk for the disease, in part, because most often (about 75 to 80 percent of cases) there is no family history of breast cancer. Although unprepared for this event, once the diagnosis has been made they nevertheless face an array of medical consultants and the necessity to make crucial treatment decisions. The first few days and weeks after a biopsy will involve further evaluation to determine the stage of the disease and the prognosis, largely based on tumor characteristics (e.g., size, histology, hormone receptor status, nodal involvement). The results of these predictive and prognostic factors performed on the primary tumor can be difficult for physicians to interpret and are frequently confusing to patients as well. Decisions about type of surgery (mastectomy, mastectomy with reconstruction, lumpectomy), subsequent adjuvant therapy (standard vs. investigational), and radiation therapy, and even where to have treatments performed (which hospital and which specialists) can be challenging. Suddenly, the woman must deal with vital issues about which she usually has little knowledge and background, and she must choose a medical team to provide and coordinate her care. Second opinions are often helpful during this process (Clauson et al., 2002), and it is inadvisable for a woman to make hasty medical decisions that she might later regret (reviewed in Rowland and Massie, 1998).

However, women do not always share fully in the decision about treatment choices (Chou, 2002). Some women rely on their physicians to make the decision and in some settings, like HMOs, women are not routinely included in the decision-making process. A recent dissertation (Chou, 2002) found that when women did participate in treatment decision making to the extent they wanted, they chose more conservative options (breast-conserving surgery plus radiation therapy) than when they did not participate as fully as they would have liked.

A concern during this phase is information overload for the patient and her support system (spouse, family, and friends). The medical care team often sees the complexities of decision making around breast cancer treatments as being routine, but for the woman, the presentation of treatment options (e.g., mastectomy versus lumpectomy; adjuvant chemotherapy or not) is far from routine. There are two extremes of responses in this situation: she may rush to treatment because of anxiety and concern that the cancer must be taken care of immediately, or she may have difficulty in making a decision, thereby creating a substantial delay while obtaining second, third, and fourth opinions (reviewed in Rowland and Massie, 1998).

Treatment

Primary Treatment

Once the treatment plan is decided, women with breast cancer may experience some relief of anxiety and distress, but new fears may arise in anticipating and receiving the planned treatment. Surgery, particularly lumpectomy and axillary dissection, is often done as an outpatient or short stay procedure. Even the length of hospital stay for mastectomy has been shortened from what it was just a few years ago (see also Chapter 6). This means that someone must be available to assist the woman at home, particularly with household tasks or other activities that require arm mobility) and some nursing care (e.g., management of surgical drains and dressings). Women undergoing mastectomy and immediate reconstruction, especially with soft tissue flaps from the abdomen, will have longer hospitalizations and a more protracted recovery from surgery. A woman needs to be prepared for what to expect with each of these procedures, and such preparation is important for her psychological well-being and recovery (Wickman, 1995). Extensive reviews of the safety of breast implants and specific information for women about this have recently been completed (Bondurant et al., 1999, Griff et al., 2000) and should reassure women that reconstruction is a reasonable, effective, and safe procedure, although not without some local complications. The psychological issues with women and breast implants and their satisfaction with results were extensively reviewed in the report by Bondurant and colleagues (Bondurant et al., 1999).

Similarly, women benefit from being prepared for the experience of radiation therapy. Many women feel anxiety associated with being in the treatment room "all alone," while the therapy is being delivered. They must become accustomed to baring their breast and disrobing among technical staff. In addition, the variation in skin reactions, local symptoms, and fatigue associated with 6 weeks of daily radiation therapy all need to be explained to women, so that they understand what to expect as treatment proceeds. It is important for the medical staff to attend to these symptoms when they arise and to provide reassurance about their normalcy and the expected eventual recovery and successful result. Some women electing breast conservation will experience lingering doubts about the comparable efficacy of this treatment approach to mastectomy, and they may need continued support and reassurance about their treatment choice. Finally, the waiting room of the radiation therapy department is sometimes distressing to breast cancer patients, especially when they see patients who are much sicker and are receiving palliative therapy for advanced cancer. Nursing and physician staff should acknowledge these issues and directly address them when breast cancer patients report their concerns about their own health and mortality.

Adjuvant Therapy

There is a wide range of adjuvant therapies—from tamoxifen as a single agent, to complex chemotherapy regimens with or without tamoxifen, to newer hormonal therapies. As new treatments emerge and the latest results of clinical trials presented at scientific meetings are widely publicized, patients have many questions about whether or not to take the standard, established therapies or to elect to take the newer ones for which there is limited or less robust data. Other decisions may focus on whether or not to enter a clinical trial. Many breast cancer patients compare notes with other patients, and often learn that their treatments are different from those of the other women in their support group or in the office waiting room. It is important to reassure women about the varied prognoses of women with breast cancer and that many different treatment strategies can be used for the same stage of disease. It is advisable for a woman to receive as much information and consultation as necessary before embarking on a course of adjuvant treatment. This helps to ensure that she understands the treatments that are most appropriate for her, given her specific medical, personal, and social situation. The process of gathering information is often stressful, but usually leads to better understanding and acceptance of the treatment plan.

Most adjuvant chemotherapy is well tolerated, and women often continue many of their usual activities (childcare, household activities, paid employment) albeit often on a reduced schedule, especially modified by treatment administration. Hair loss, nausea, and vomiting are among the most distressing side effects, followed by fatigue and changes in body image and weight (Shimozuma et al., 1999). The difficulty here is that adjuvant treatment takes someone who is trying to recover physically and psychologically from a diagnosis of cancer and surgery, and adds additional associated physical symptoms for a period of 4 to 6 months. While perceived by most women as a reasonable "insurance policy" against subsequent breast cancer recurrence, adjuvant treatment significantly decreases quality of life while it is being given. Many women have a love–hate relationship with adjuvant treatment, feeling protected by it and even wanting more intensive therapies, but nevertheless feeling distressed and overwhelmed by some of the physical symptoms that they experience while receiving treatment.

Tamoxifen therapy may be used by itself or in combination with adjuvant chemotherapy in some women. While the medical evidence for its benefits in improving survival and preventing breast cancer recurrence is overwhelming, in the eyes of many women it is still seen as a controversial and potentially toxic therapy. Women may be especially concerned about the risk of endometrial cancer, and physicians must directly address the risks and benefits of tamoxifen therapy with each patient. Other frequent concerns of women about tamoxifen relate to psychological well-being, weight gain, hot flashes, and sexual functioning. Many of these problems are common in breast cancer survivors and are not specifically related to the drug tamoxifen (Day et al., 2001, 1999; Fallowfield et al., 2001). In addition, studies with aromatase inhibitors in advanced or adjuvant settings (or even for prevention) suggest that these agents which block estrogen formation, may be an improvement over tamoxifen for breast cancer treatment. Women may wish to have this more recent information and to discuss its implications (Santen, 2003). There are many possibilities in therapy, and women may wish to explore variations consistent with good practice to fit their needs.

Over 70 percent of women become amenorrheic following breast cancer treatment. For younger women who develop breast cancer, amenorrhea is accompanied by a host of hormonal changes either coming on prematurely or intensifying menopausal symptoms in the more mature. These changes are intimately interwoven with psychosocial and behavioral symptoms: mood, anxiety, cognitive impairment, fatigue, and even weight gain. Serotonin reuptake inhibitors are FDA approved for both autonomic and affective symptoms of "pre-menstrual" disorder (late-luteal phase disorder) and for treatment-related menopausal symptoms. Patients often describe cognitive impairment with hormonal treatment or chemotherapy for breast cancer (described in Warga, 2000).

Much of the distress, after the initial shock of diagnosis and adjustment to treatment, is interwoven with decisions that may impede quality of life, and the need to adjust to such physical and emotional changes. Type of surgery, choice of chemotherapy when more than one choice is acceptable, type of radiation therapy (external beam, brachytherapy), and the decision to forgo hormonal suppression are some of the issues that have emotional consequences because they affect anxiety, mood, and stamina.

Non-Invasive Breast Cancer

With the increasing use of screening mammography, the rate of diagnosis of non-invasive ductal carcinoma *in situ* (DCIS) has increased substantially (see Chapter 2). In some communities, DCIS cases account for as many as 20 percent of the incident cases of breast cancer. Although there are potential benefits of diagnosing an early non-invasive cancer, for many women the anxiety associated with this condition is tremendous. Many women feel confused when they are told that their condition is not serious, yet they receive the same local treatments as women with invasive breast cancer. In spite of the efficacy of local treatment with breast conservation, women with a diagnosis of DCIS face a continuous risk of recurrent disease in the involved breast as well as the contralateral breast. For many younger women, this situation can be very distressing, with the uncertainty and risk labeling which this diagnosis causes. As women with DCIS face menopause, they may struggle, given the results of recent trials of hormone replacement therapy, with whether hormone replacement therapy is safe for menopausal symptom relief given their medical history. This combination of breast cancer risk status and menopausal symptoms can affect quality of life for this unique group of breast cancer patients.

Genetic Risk and Its Psychological Management

An added issue for women with breast cancer is today's high level of awareness of enhanced genetic risk for daughters and sisters. This adds a burden of guilt and immediately raises the issue of whether genetic testing should be done to determine actual gene status. In addition, genetic testing raises questions about who and what to tell about the results, which could affect health and life insurance coverage; how to deal with children who are minors; and how to advise daughters about risk and surveillance (beginning at what age and with what kind of follow-up?). These issues are well addressed with women today in the major cancer centers, where there are genetic counselors who take a careful medical and psychological history, explain the meaning of the tests, their possible inconclusive information, and offer help in how to decide who to tell about the results. In general, women appear to handle the information relatively well, whether they are found to be positive or negative. After an initial response of distress with preoccupation with potential bad news, the impact is generally transient and women regain emotional control. However, those testing positive who carry the burden of added risk or recurrence often describe feeling like "walking time bombs" and psychosocial support groups for these women have been found to be helpful in reducing anxiety and distress.

Additional decisions must be made by the woman who is BRCA 1/2 positive about what surveillance she will undertake to reduce her risk and assure an early diagnosis. Regular clinical breast examinations and mammograms are often the chosen route. Control of anxiety and depressed feelings about the genetic risk is important to assure that they adhere to their surveillance program. For some women, however, the level of anxiety (and their perception of risk) is so high that they consider prophylactic bilateral mastectomies. While many consider it, only a small percentage actually go through with it, largely because of an especially high level of risk or a level of anxiety which is intolerable. In most centers, a psychiatric evaluation is done to assure that the woman has a full understanding of the issues and that psychological factors have been taken into account. At Memorial Hospital in New York, Mary Jane Massie, psychiatrist, is requested to evaluate each women preoperatively, and this evaluation is taken into account as a factor in the decision to proceed with surgery.

Decisions about childbearing, in the face of high risk or actual breast cancer, confront many women, and the emotional toll is very high as they contemplate, with knowledgeable oncologists, what course of action they should take. The need for psychological or psychiatric intervention can be very helpful to control anxiety when weighty decisions must be made that will influence future life. Supportive visits and anti-anxiety medication, if needed, should be available for these women (J. Holland, personal communication, September 18, 2003).

Post Treatment

At the end of primary breast cancer treatment—whether it is at the conclusion of 6 weeks of radiation therapy or after 4–6 months of adjuvant chemotherapy—most women experience a mixture of elation, fear, and uncertainty (reviewed in Rowland and Massie, 1998). Although they have mastered the many aspects of their treatment regimen, they have little preparation and information to guide them in their recovery from treatment. This is coupled with their planned discharge from intensive interaction with the health-care system. No longer do they have daily or periodic visits to the treatment center. In fact, they may not have a scheduled return visit for several months after the completion of therapy. In some managed care settings, a woman is referred back to her primary care physician and may have no further contact with the oncology treatment team. During this transition or re-entry period, women may have questions about their symptoms and their care. Who will she talk to about the non-specific joint pains that are bothering her, or the fatigue and difficulty sleeping she is still experiencing? Could these be signs of recurrence? Why is she still experiencing so much fatigue when her treatments ended several weeks ago? Why is her family not paying as much attention to her, and why do they expect life to go back to normal when for her it has been changed forever? The post-treatment transitional period is a time of considerable psychosocial distress. The paradoxical increase in anxiety has been observed at the end of both radiation and systematic chemotherapy (Holland and Rowland, 1991). Nevertheless, many women find positive meaning and describe posttraumatic growth from the cancer experience (Ganz et al., 1996). Nevertheless, fear of recurrence is frequently a dominant emotion that is difficult to control, especially before or during follow-up visits.

There has been growing interest in the late effects of breast cancer treatment and the quality of life of long-term survivors beyond the acute phase of treatment. Several published studies have compared breast cancer survivors to healthy, age-matched populations of women and have found few differences in their long-term physical or emotional well-being (Andersen et al., 1989; Dorval et al., 1998; Ganz et al., 2002, 1998a). A recent study of long-term adjustment of women 20 years after treatment in a large multicenter clinical trial found cancer worries to be negligible; however, 18 percent of women had posttraumatic stress symptoms, and many reported lymphedema (27 percent) and numbness (20 percent) as persistent problems (Kornblith et al., 2003). There is some evidence that women who receive adjuvant therapy may have more physical disruption than those who receive no further therapy, and that women who receive chemotherapy may have more sexual dysfunction and possibly more cognitive dysfunction than survivors who did not receive similar therapy (Ahles et al., 2002; Brezden et al., 2000; Ganz et al., 1999; Ganz et al., 2002; Meyerowitz et al., 1999; Schagen et al., 1999; van Dam et al., 1998). With the growing number of breast cancer survivors, as well as increased research funding targeting this population, new evidence will be forthcoming regarding these cognitive and psychosocial concerns (Gotay and Muraoka, 1998).

Recurrence

The overall survival for early stage breast cancer is excellent, and many women can anticipate a normal life expectancy. That is why so much of the patient's and the medical team's efforts are invested in primary treatment decisions and the delivery of initial treatment—to ensure the best chance for long-term disease-free survival and optimal quality of life. However, even under the best of circumstances, a significant number (about 30 to 40 percent overall) of women will experience recurrence of breast cancer, and this can occur many years after the initial breast cancer diagnosis. While shock and disbelief are common emotions at diagnosis, hopefulness and a treatment plan that is expected to lead to long-term disease-free survival usually counter these emotions. In contrast, recurrence of breast cancer is experienced as a failure by both the patient and her treatment team. One recent study of 378 long-term breast cancer survivors showed that many women attribute their disease to stress (42 percent) and a lack of recurrence to having a positive attitude (60 percent) (Stewart et al., 2001). This suggests that many women with breast cancer blame themselves for their disease or its recurrence.

Recurrence is almost always associated with clinical symptoms from the cancer—insidious onset of pain, cough, or the development of skin nodules, for example. The clinical symptoms of recurrence provide tangible evidence of the seriousness of the situation, and the emotions that had been elicited at the time of diagnosis tend to recur and are intensified, particularly with respect to depressive symptoms. This is often a challenging time for the patient, her family, and the treatment team. In a recent study, significant impairments in physical, functional, and emotional well-being were found among women with recurrent breast cancer, and family members reported significant impairments in their own emotional well-being (Northouse et al., 2002).

Recurrence can be local, treated with combinations of excision, radiation, and chemotherapy, depending on individual circumstances. Systemic recurrence can be treated to prolong survival and enhance quality of life, but cannot be cured, so treatments with minimal toxicity are preferred. These medical circumstances have psychosocial implications and given the frequency of recurrence deserve continued research attention (NCCN, 2000: 46).

Nevertheless, women who faced initial aggressive treatments are often unwilling to accept less intensive treatments at recurrence. In the 1990s many women sought high-dose chemotherapy programs in spite of insufficient evidence for efficacy. Often this occurred because these women were reluctant to contemplate long-term and unending therapies. They saw intensive, time-limited, "potentially curative" therapies as an alternative. To some extent, this approach fulfilled a psychological need to gain some control over a situation that felt out of control. Physicians often shared in this misconception regarding treatments that were unproven. For many of these women, taking an action, obtaining second opinions, and seeking experimental therapies became the focus of their efforts when they faced metastatic breast cancer. Today, many women are beginning to view recurrent breast cancer as a chronic condition that can be controlled long-term, even if it cannot be cured. The comparison to the control of diabetes is often helpful. Awareness of second- and third-line therapies for recurrent disease makes this concept more plausible. Women may reach their decisions either on the advice of their physician or by sharing in decision making in various ways (Chou, 2003)

Advanced Breast Cancer

Attention to the symptomatic and pain relief needs of the woman with advanced breast cancer is central to her emotional and physical well-being (Massie and Holland, 1992). The management of pain syndromes, including post-mastectomy pain syndrome, was well described in the 1980s by Foley (Foley, 1985). The early study of Spiegel and Bloom (Spiegel and Bloom, 1983) documented interventions to reduce distress and pain in metastatic breast cancer. Breitbart and colleagues (Breitbart et al., 2000) have shown the association of pain and the increase in symptoms of depression and anxiety. A biopsychosocial model, illustrating the interplay of somatic (pain) with psychosocial aspects was outlined by Syrjala and Chapko (Syrjala and Chapko, 1995). In the presence of uncontrolled pain, the woman with breast cancer will function at a lower level and will likely become less able to maintain her usual social role as mother, spouse, worker, or caretaker, although many women continue their normal activities in the face of major functional impairments. Concern for spiritual and existential matters often marks this phase of the illness, as women focus on their legacy to their families and children and engage in planning for their future (Butler et al., 2003, Foley, 2000, McGuire et al., 1989).

PREVALENCE OF PSYCHOSOCIAL DISTRESS

An estimated one-third to one-half of individuals diagnosed with any type of cancer experience significant levels of distress (Derogatis et al., 1983; Zabora et al., 2001a). Distress varies by cancer site. According to one study conducted at the Johns Hopkins Cancer Center, individuals diagnosed with cancers known to be associated with the highest mortality and poorest prognosis (e.g., cancers of the lung, pancreas, and brain) had greater levels of distress than individuals with cancer associated with more favorable prognoses (e.g., cancers of the breast, colon, and prostate) (Zabora et al., 2001a) (study results shown in Table 3-1 below). Other predictors of distress were younger age, fewer social supports, and lower socioeconomic level.

Estimates of the prevalence of psychosocial distress among women with breast cancer depend on how distress is defined and measured. Some estimates are based on a diagnosis of mental disorder as determined by a psy-

TABLE 3-1 Prevalence of Distress By Cancer Diagnosis

Cancer site or type	Prevalence of distress (%)
All cancers	35.1
Lung	43.4
Brain	42.7
Hodgkin's	37.8
Pancreas	36.6
Lymphoma	36.0
Liver	35.4
Head and neck	35.1
Adenocarcinoma (unknown primary)	34.9
Breast	32.8
Leukemia	32.7
Melanoma	32.7
Colon	31.6
Prostate	30.5
Gynecological	29.6

SOURCE: Adapted from Zabora et al., 2001a.

chiatric interview, while others are based on measurement of psychological states using scores from self-administered assessment tools. Many of the prevalence studies of cancer-related psychosocial distress have been conducted among women recruited from cancer centers or major universities, though a minority of cancer patients receive their care in such settings.

A multi-center study published in 1987 by Bloom and colleagues focused on the psychosocial distress of women in the year following breast cancer diagnosis. They were compared to "healthy" women (no present illness), women after cholecystectomy (an operation with less impact on self image), and women who had had a negative breast biopsy. Five cross-sections of women were interviewed at 3-month intervals for the first 12 months post-diagnosis. The earliest cohort was assessed longitudinally. Over 400 women with breast cancer were studied in five centers from 61 hospitals in 11 states. The findings indicated that early distress from breast cancer was dissipated within 1 year following diagnosis so that the group of women with breast cancer did not differ as to distress levels from the women in the other groups. However, among the women who had received adjuvant chemotherapy during the year, levels remained elevated at 1 year (Bloom et al., 1987).

Individuals who agree to participate in research studies may differ from those who choose not to participate. Further complicating estimates of prevalence of cancer-related psychosocial distress is the frequency with which psychiatric problems occur among the general population (Massie and Holland, 1989; Rowland, 1999). A study by Morris and colleagues (Morris et al., 1977) found that women who were depressed prior to breast cancer were depressed in the period following diagnosis. Many studies assess psychosocial distress within a group of cancer patients without examining a control or comparison group. Prevalence estimates also vary by the reference period used. Some studies report psychosocial distress within a year (1-year prevalence), while others report distress at a point in time (point prevalence). Studies of psychosocial distress have usually been conducted among patients with recently diagnosed cancer. Increasingly, however, researchers are beginning to assess the psychosocial adjustment of cancer survivors who have lived with cancer for many years.

This section reviews what is known about the prevalence of psychiatric morbidity in the general population, the definition of cancer-related psychosocial distress, and methods to measure the prevalence of psychosocial distress among individuals with breast cancer.

Prevalence of Psychiatric Morbidity in the General Population

Estimates of the prevalence of mental disorders in the United States come from two large community surveys, the National Institute of Mental Health Epidemiologic Catchment Area Program (ECA) and the National Comorbidity Survey (NCS) (Box 3-1) (Kessler et al., 1994; Regier et al., 1984). Although the studies differed somewhat in methodology, they concluded that overall 1-year mental and addictive disorder prevalence rates in the United States approach 30 percent.[3]

Further analyses of data from these studies, limiting prevalent cases to those whose symptoms were clinically significant, reduced the prevalence of mental or substance use disorder to 18.5 percent (see Table 3-2) (Narrow et al., 2002). Clinically significant cases were symptomatic individuals who: (1) had mentioned their symptoms to a doctor or other professional, (2) had symptoms that interfered with their everyday life, or (3) took medication for symptoms. Of note is the higher prevalence of clinically significant mental and substance use disorders among younger individuals between 18 to 54 years of age. Anxiety, phobia, mood disorder, and depression are among the most common clinically significant mental disorders in the general adult population.

Relatively high rates of psychiatric morbidity, especially depression, have been foud among individuals with chronic medical conditions (Evans et al., 1996–1997; Katon and Ciechanowski, 2002; Katon and Schulberg, 1992; Krishnan et al., 2002; Musselman et al., 1998; Nemeroff et al., 1998). Ac-

---

[3]The 1-year prevalence rate is the proportion of individuals who would be expected to have a mental or addictive disorder anytime in the past year.

BOX 3-1
Studies of the prevalence of mental disorders
in the United States

National Institute of Mental Health Epidemiologic Catchment Area Program (ECA)

The ECA was conducted from 1980 to 1985 in 5 sites, and included 18,571 household and 2,290 institutional residents 18 years and older. Two face-to-face interviews were conducted 12 months apart. Diagnostic and Statistical Manual of Mental Disorder (DSM-III) psychiatric diagnoses were assessed with the Diagnostic Interview Schedule (DIS).

National Comorbidity Survey (NCS)

The NCS was a cross-sectional survey of a nationally representative household sample of 8,098 adolescents and adults aged 15 to 54 years, conducted from 1990 to 1992. The University of Michigan version of the Composite International Diagnostic Interview (UM-CIDI) was used to obtain DSM-III-R diagnoses.

Generalized anxiety disorder and post-traumatic stress disorder were assessed only in the NCS. Obsessive-compulsive disorder, anorexia nervosa, somatization disorder, and cognitive impairment were assessed only in the ECA.

SOURCE: Narrow et al., 2002.

---

cording to one recent review, approximately half of patients with Parkinson's disease or Alzheimer's disease have major depression and one in five patients have depression at the time of diagnostic catheterization following acute myocardial infarction or following stroke (Krishnan et al., 2002).

Prevalence of Psychiatric Morbidity Among Individuals With Cancer

An oncologist or other health-care provider seeing a patient with cancer for the first time should reasonably assume that the patient has the same baseline risk of mental and substance use disorders as an age-sex counterpart in the general population, plus the additional risk introduced by cancer and its treatment. What evidence is there that individuals with cancer have higher rates of mental disorders? One of the first studies reporting relatively high rates of psychiatric disorder among cancer patients was conducted by Derogatis and colleagues (Derogatis et al., 1983). As part of their study, 215 cancer patients, randomly selected from new admissions to three collaborating cancer centers, were evaluated by psychiatrists and psychologists using a formal psychiatric interview along with

TABLE 3-2 Estimates of the 1-year Prevalence Of Mental Disorder in the United States, adjusted for clinical significance.

Disorder	Total	Age 18 to 54	55 and older
Any mental or substance use disorder	18.5	20.9	14.2
Any mental disorder	14.9	16.5	13.2
Any substance use disorder	6.0	7.6	2.1
Any anxiety disorder	11.8	13.3	10.6
Any phobia	7.8	8.0	7.2
Generalized anxiety disorder	—	2.8	—
Panic disorder	1.4	1.7	0.5
Obsessive–compulsive disorder	2.1	2.4	1.5
Posttraumatic stress disorder	—	3.6	—
Any mood disorder	5.1	5.7	3.4
Major depressive episode	4.5	5.2	2.8
Unipolar major depression	4.0	4.5	2.7
Dysthymia	1.6	1.6	1.6
Bipolar I disorder	0.5	0.6	0.1
Bipolar II disorder	0.2	0.3	0.1
Schizophrenia/schizophreniform	1.0	1.2	0.4
Antisocial personality disorder	1.5	2.0	0
Anorexia nervosa	0.1	0.1	0
Somatization	0.2	0.2	0.3
Severe cognitive impairment	0.7	0.2	2.0

NOTE: No data indicates rates not available in ECA or NCS.
SOURCE: Adapted from Narrow et al., 2002.

patient self-report assessments. Patients terminally ill or who were very disabled were excluded from the study. Roughly half of the patients had breast cancer, lung cancer, or lymphoma with the remainder having other types of cancer. Almost half (47 percent) of the patients had psychological symptoms consistent with a psychiatric disorder (Diagnostic and Statistical Manual of Mental Disorder, DSM-III)[4] which was primarily (85 percent) Adjustment Disorder with symptoms of reactive anxiety, depression, or a mix of both. Men and women were equally likely to receive a psychiatric diagnosis. Of note was the variation in prevalence across the three study sites: 24 percent in Baltimore (Johns Hopkins Medical Institution), 46 percent in Rochester (University of Rochester Medical Center), and 69 percent in New York (Memorial Sloan-Kettering Cancer Center). This may reflect differences in interview technique, interpretation of diagnostic

---

[4]A reference work developed by the American Psychiatric Association and designed to provide guidelines for the diagnosis and classification of mental disorders. The DSMIII has been revised several times since the publication of this study and is now the DSM IV-R.

criteria or, more likely, differences in the patients seeking care at each center. In general, patients with an Adjustment Disorder respond to psychological counseling, psychotherapy, and at times, medication, for the control of sleep disturbance, anxiety, and depressive symptoms.

A recent report from the Agency for Healthcare Research and Quality (AHRQ), "Management of Cancer Symptoms: Pain, Depression, and Fatigue," concluded that major depression and depressive symptoms occur frequently in cancer patients. According to their review of the literature, prevalence rates varied from 10 to 25 percent for major depressive disorders, a rate at least four times higher than in the general population (Agency for Healthcare Research and Quality, 2002). The timing of the assessment, concurrent treatment, medical morbidity, pain, gender, and age of subjects contributed to the wide range of estimates. The higher rates are usually seen in patients with more advanced illness and uncontrolled pain or other physical symptoms. Included in this spectrum of depressive disorders among patients with cancer is the DSM-IV diagnosis of Mood Disorder Related to Medical Illness, which is common in patients with severe or uncontrolled physical symptoms, especially pain.

Health-Related Quality of Life

Depressive symptoms that may not reach criteria for a DSM diagnosis, and are thus considered subsyndromal depressive symptoms, are far more prevalent in cancer, but they often represent a significant detriment to quality-of life. Since the Derogatis study was published in the early 1980s, investigators have developed conceptual models to describe the range of impacts that cancer has on psychological and physical health, functional status, symptoms, and other aspects of life such as family relationships and spiritual or existential concerns. A large body of research has been devoted to conceptualizing and measuring health-related quality of life. Instruments that have emerged from this body of science have provided valid tools to measure social, physical, psychological, and sexual function. Some instruments have been developed with a core to measure overall functional areas and include modules that assess functional problems associated with specific sites of cancer. The EORTC-QLQ developed by Aaronson and Cella's FACT quality-of-life are both widely used instruments and have been translated into may languages (Aaronson et al., 1993, Cella, 1995; Mandelblatt and Eisenberg, 1995; Montazeri et al., 1996). Other generic tools have been developed for the assessment of distress, psychological problems, or specific psychiatric disorders (e.g., anxiety, depression) among patients with chronic illness or among the general population.

Nevertheless, quality of life remains a less-explored facet of survivors' lives. Given recent improvement in survival times, this broader concept of psychological health and well being is becoming more important. Most studies show that many survivors continue to experience negative effects of cancer or cancer treatment on their lives after primary therapy. These effects include sexual and psychological functioning concerns. Also, some reports have shown positive coping strategies and enhanced quality of life. Additional quality of life studies are needed to understand the needs of longer term survivors and what kinds of support they want (reviewed in Gotay and Muraoka, 1998).

Definition of Psychosocial Distress

According to the DSM-IV, a mental disorder is "a clinically significant behavioral or psychological syndrome or pattern that occurs in an individual and that is associated with present distress (e.g., a painful symptom) or disability (i.e., impairment in one or more important areas of functioning) or with a significantly increased risk of suffering death, pain, disability, or an important loss of freedom" (American Psychiatric Association, 1994: xxi). Individuals with cancer may experience a mental disorder as a result of cancer or treatment, or they may experience an exacerbation of a prior psychiatric disorder (e.g., recurrent depression). Other concerns range from cancer-specific concerns, such as fear of recurrence, to more generalized symptoms of worry, fear of the future, fear of death, trouble sleeping, fatigue, and trouble concentrating. The term "psychosocial distress" has been coined to reflect this broader set of concerns (National Comprehensive Cancer Network, 1999). As conceived, distress is a "multi-factorial unpleasant emotional experience of a psychological (cognitive, behavioral, emotional), social, and/or spiritual nature that may interfere with the ability to cope effectively with cancer, its physical symptoms, and its treatment. Distress extends along a continuum, ranging from common normal feelings of vulnerability, sadness, and fears to problems that can become disabling, such as depression, anxiety, panic, social isolation, and existential and spiritual crisis" (NCCN, 2003). Distress may be experienced as a reaction to the disease and its treatment and also as a result of the consequences of the disease on employment, health insurance, and social functioning including family relationships (Kornblith, 1998; McEvoy and McCorkle, 1990). Breast cancer may, for example, impose an economic hardship because it affects women's ability to work. In one recent study, the probability of breast cancer survivors working was 10 percentage points less than that for women without breast cancer (Bradley et al., 2002). However, this study found no reduction in hours worked among the women who continued in their jobs.

Measuring Psychosocial Distress

This section describes selected instruments that have been used to measure psychosocial distress in United States women with breast cancer and upon which estimates of the prevalence of psychosocial distress are based.

Among these are two generic instruments (i.e., the Hospital Anxiety and Depression scale (HADS) and the SF-36 of the Medical Outcomes Study) and six cancer-specific instruments:

1. Brief Symptom Inventory (BSI)
2. Cancer Rehabilitation Evaluation System (CARES)
3. Distress Thermometer and Problem List from the National Comprehensive Cancer Network Guidelines for Management of Psychosocial Distress
4. European Organization for Research and Treatment of Cancer (EORTC) Quality of Life Questionnaire (QLQ-C30)
5. Functional Assessment of Cancer Therapy-Breast (FACT-B)
6. Quality of Life Breast Cancer Instrument

Many of the instruments useful in capturing the various dimensions of psychosocial distress among individuals with cancer attempt to measure what is referred to as health-related quality of life (HRQOL) (Cella, 1995; Mandelblatt and Eisenberg, 1995; Montazeri et al., 1996). HRQOL assessments are self-rated subjective evaluations of health and well-being generally in at least four areas: psychological functioning, physical functioning, social functioning, and symptoms and side effects (Figure 3-1). Aspects of

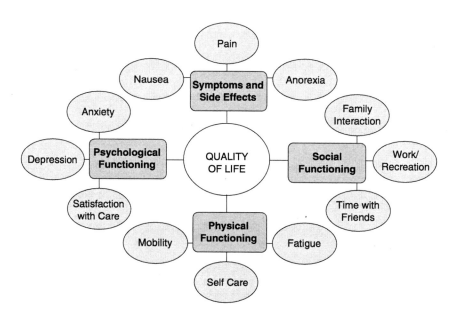

FIGURE 3-1 Quality of life: conceptual model.
SOURCE: Tchekmedyian et al., 1990.

HRQOL life that predominate in the assessment of psychosocial distress are those related to psychological functioning and social functioning. Health-care providers traditionally measure aspects of physical functioning, symptoms, and side effects.

Most of the instruments described in this section were developed for research purposes and were designed to categorize groups of patients as distressed or not. Although the tools meet the needs of researchers, they may not be suitable for use by health-care providers in clinical settings who are interested in evaluating individual patients to determine their need for psychosocial intervention. Instruments developed in research settings need to be carefully evaluated before being used clinically to evaluate patients. An instrument's validity, in this context its ability to correctly identify the presence and absence of distress, needs to be determined as does its reliability, its ability to provide consistent results. These and other important attributes of clinical screening tools are described in Box 3-2.

While it would be desirable to have well-validated instruments to use as screening tools to help health-care providers identify women who may benefit from psychosocial interventions, not all of the instruments that have been used in research settings have psychometric prerequisites for their use in individual patients and should be considered discriminative instruments only for use with groups of patients (McHorney and Tarlov, 1995). Few of these instruments have actually received rigorous testing with breast cancer patients. The National Cancer Institute (NCI) through its HRQOL Intergroup Committee has recently summarized the use of HRQOL instruments in clinical trials (Trimble et al., 2001). While additional research is needed, some of these instruments hold promise as clinical assessment and screening tools for clinical use (see also Chapter 6).

Hospital Anxiety and Depression Scale (HADS)

One of the most widely used instruments to screen for depression, anxiety, or psychosocial distress in cancer patients, especially in Europe, is the Hospital Anxiety and Depression Scale or HADS (Bjelland et al., 2002; Herrmann, 1997; Zigmond and Snaith, 1983). This tool provides separate scores for anxiety and depression, with cutpoints that have been determined to identify possible mood disorder (Carroll et al., 1993) (see Box 3-3). The HADS has the advantage of being brief, and its items do not overlap with somatic complaints (e.g., fatigue) that may be caused by cancer (Zigmond and Snaith, 1983). The HADS has been used to assess depression and anxiety among women with both early and advanced stage breast cancer. In one study of 211 women with advanced breast cancer, 27 percent were categorized as probable cases of anxiety and/or depression. Among the 155 women who completed an assessment 1 to 3 months later, 13 percent were classified

BOX 3-2
Definitions of Screening Test Performance

The performance of a screening test is often defined by its validity, determined by measures of sensitivity and specificity, its reliability or repeatability, and its yield, the amount of previously unrecognized disease that is diagnosed and brought to treatment as a result of the screening.

Validity

The sensitivity (se) of a screening test is the proportion of people with the condition who test positive. Specificity (sp) is the proportion of people without the condition who test negative. A related measure, the positive predictive value, is the portion of individuals with a positive screening test who actually have the condition. If screened individuals are assigned a position in a 2&2 classification scheme based on their health status and test result, values for the three measurements can be defined as follows:

		Actual Health Status	
		+	−
Test Result	+	True Positive (TP)	False Positive (FP)
	−	False Negative (FN)	True Negative (TN)

Measurement: Question Answered:

Sensitivity (se) = $\dfrac{TP}{TP + FN}$ How often does the test correctly identify individuals with the disease?

Specificity (sp) = $\dfrac{TN}{TN + FP}$ How often does the test correctly identify individuals without the disease

Positive predictive value = $\dfrac{TP}{TP + FP}$ Among individuals with an abnormal test, what proportion actually have the disease?

Reliability

A reliable screening test is one that gives consistent results when the test is performed more than once on the same individual under the same conditions. Two major factors affect consistency of results: the variation inherent in the method and observer variation.

Yield

The yield of a screening test depends on the sensitivity of the test and the prevalence of unrecognized disease. When there are many undiagnosed cases in a population, the yield of a screening test will be high.

SOURCE : Mausner et al.,1985.

BOX 3-3
Items Assessed on the Hospital Anxiety
and Depression Scale (HADS)

Doctors are aware that emotions play an important part in most illnesses. If your doctor knows about these feelings he will be able to help you more. This questionnaire is designed to help your doctor to know how you feel. Read each item and underline the reply which comes closest to how you have been feeling in the past week. Don't take too long over your replies; your immediate reaction to each item will probably be more accurate than a long thought out response.

1. I feel tense or "wound up" (anxiety)
   - most of the time (3)
   - a lot of the time (2)
   - from time to time (1)
   - occasionally, not at all (0)

2. I still enjoy the things I used to enjoy (depression)
   - definitely as much (0)
   - not quite so much (1)
   - only a little (2)
   - hardly at all (3)

3. I get a sort of frightened feeling as if something awful is about to happen (anxiety)
   - very definitely and quite badly (3)
   - yes, but not too badly (2)
   - a little, but it doesn't worry me (1)
   - not at all (0)

4. I can laugh and see the funny side of things (depression)
   - as much as I always could (0)
   - not quite so much now (1)
   - definitely not so much now (2)
   - not at all (3)

5. Worrying thoughts go through my mind (anxiety)
- a great deal of the time (3)
- a lot of the time (2)
- from time to time, but not too often (1)
- only occasionally (0)

6. I feel cheerful (depression)
- not at all (3)
- not often (2)
- sometimes (1)
- most of the time (0)

7. I can sit at ease and feel relaxed (anxiety)
- definitely (0)
- usually (1)
- not often (2)
- not at all (3)

8. I feel as if I am slowed down (depression)
- nearly all the time (3)
- very often (2)
- sometimes (1)
- not at all (0)

9. I get a sort of frightened feeling like "butterflies" in the stomach (anxiety)
- not at all (0)
- occasionally (1)
- quite often (2)
- very often (3)

10. I have lost interest in my appearance (depression)
- definitely (3)
- I don't take so much care as I should (2)
- I may not take quite as much care (1)
- I take just as much care as ever (0)

11. I feel restless as if I have to be on the move (anxiety)
- very much indeed (3)
- quite a lot (2)
- not very much (1)
- not at all (0)

12. I look forward with enjoyment to things (depression)
- as much as ever I did (0)
- rather less than I used to (1)
- definitely less than I used to (2)
- hardly at all (3)

13. I get sudden feelings of panic (anxiety)
- very often indeed (3)
- quite often (2)
- not very often (1)
- not at all (0)

14. I can enjoy a good book or radio
    or TV program (depression)
- often (0)
- sometimes (1)
- not often (2)
- very seldom (3)

NOTE: On either the anxiety or depression scale, a score of 7 or less indicates a low probability of mood disorder, scores of 8–10 indicate doubtful mood disorder and scores of 11 or more indicate a probable mood disorder (a total score of 21 is possible on each scale).

SOURCE: Zigmond and Snaith, 1983a.

as being persistently anxious or depressed (Hopwood et al., 1991a). When investigators compared the classification of 81 of these patients with findings from an independent interview by a psychiatrist, the HADS correctly identified 75 percent of women diagnosed by the psychiatrist. The HADS, however, misclassified 26 percent of "normal" patients as having anxiety or depression. The authors concluded that HADS could be used to screen patients with advanced cancer for affective disorders (Hopwood et al., 1991b).

In a more recent study, HADS classified, at the time of diagnosis, 39 percent of 80 women with metastatic breast cancer as having anxiety and 31 percent as being depressed. When monitored every 8 weeks over a 16-month period, no statistically significant difference in mood was detected over time, although there was a trend for mean anxiety and depression to decrease (Fulton, 1998).

Several investigators have raised questions about the usefulness of the HADS. In one recent Danish study, for example, the prevalence of anxiety and depression as measured by HADS was similar among 538 newly diagnosed breast cancer patients at low risk of recurrence and 872 women randomly selected from the general population (Groenvold et al., 1999). The investigators suggest that the HADS may not be suitable for use in the general population, thereby calling into question the validity of their comparisons. Others have suggested that the HADS is not a sensitive enough instrument, noting that in a study of 266 women with early breast cancer HADS, using the recommended cut point of 11 or greater, identified only 24 percent of women with a clinical diagnosis of anxiety and 14 percent of women with a clinical diagnosis of depression. According to clinical interviews, 50 percent of the women were depressed and 37 percent of women had an anxiety disorder (Hall et al., 1999). Similar concerns were raised in a study of 303 women with early stage breast cancer where the HADS identified only 5 percent of women who were determined to be depressed and 8 percent of women with anxiety. Lowering the cut-off scores for the HADS improved identification (Love et al., 2002).

In addition to these assessments of prevalence and of the value of the screening instrument itself, the HADS has been used to monitor outcomes in a number of psychosocial intervention studies of breast cancer patients (Montazeri et al., 2001; Spiegel et al., 1999). There has been limited use of the HADS in North American clinical practice settings, although its brevity and psychometric properties suggest that it may be very useful. Investigators in the United Kingdom have validated automated screening for psychological distress among hospitalized cancer patients (the study was not limited to women with breast cancer). Responses using computer touchscreens based on the HADS instrument were comparable to those obtained by psychiatric interview (Cull et al., 2001; Velikova et al., 1999). The computerized screening system enabled data to be collected, scored, collated, and reported in real time to identify patients who warranted further clinical assessment.

Other Instruments to Assess Depression and Anxiety

Several instruments have been critical to the characterization of the frequency of anxiety and depression among breast cancer patients participating in research studies (van't Spijker et al., 1997), but are not yet recommended for use as assessment and screening tools in the clinical setting. These psychological assessment instruments include the General Health Questionnaire (GHQ), the Profile of Mood States (POMS), and the Center for Epidemiologic Studies Depression Scale (CES-D).[5] Few of these instruments have been used outside the research setting. Some of these instruments have normative values for the general population making comparisons possible between research subjects and the general population. For example, the expected frequency of depression in the general population using the CES-D (with a cut-point equal to or greater than 17) is 21 percent. The CES-D was used to assess depression among 864 disease-free survivors of breast cancer as part of a large cross-sectional study conducted in two metropolitan areas, Los Angeles and Washington, DC. In this sample, CES-D scores in this range among breast cancer survivors (23 percent) were similar to those observed in the general population (Ganz et al., 1998a). The CES-D has been assessed among women with breast cancer and found to be valid and reliable (Hann et al., 1999).

The Medical Outcomes Study SF-36

The Medical Outcomes Study Short Form (SF-36) was designed for use in clinical practice and research, health policy evaluations, and general

---

[5]For information on these instruments, see a meta-analytical review by van't Skijker and colleagues (van't Spijker et al., 1997)

population surveys. The instrument measures eight aspects of functional status, well-being, and self-perceived health (Ware and Sherbourne, 1992):

Functional status
1. Physical functioning (10 items)
2. Social functioning (2 items)
3. Role limitations attributed to physical problems (4 items)
4. Role limitations attributed to emotional problems (3 items)

Well-being
5. Mental health (5 items)
6. Energy and fatigue (4 items)
7. Pain (2 items)

Overall evaluation of health
8. General health perception (5 items)[6]

The SF-36 has been widely used to assess populations with chronic illness (Stewart et al., 1989; Wells et al., 1989), including women with breast cancer and breast cancer survivors (Frost et al., 2000; Ganz et al., 1996; Ganz et al., 1998a). A shorter version, the SF-12, is now available and provides a rapid screen for QoL without providing the greater details from the longer form in terms of the richness of the sub-scale information. The SF-36 was, for example, used as part of the study by Ganz et al. described in the preceding section above. For each of the eight areas of the SF-36 profile, scores for their sample of 864 disease-free survivors of breast cancer were at or above (indicating similar or more positive outcomes) those from the age-matched population norms for healthy women (Figure 3-2) (Ganz et al., 1998a).

The SF-36 was used in a follow-up study of this cohort of 5- to 10-year survivors of breast cancer (Ganz et al., 2002). Among disease-free survivors, physical well-being and emotional well-being were excellent with minimal changes between the baseline and follow-up assessments reflecting expected age-related changes (Figure 3-3). Energy level and social functioning were unchanged. Past systemic adjuvant treatment was, however, associated with poorer functioning on several dimensions of HRQOL. Among women who had experienced a recurrence of cancer, declines in physical and social functioning were observed from baseline to follow-up, but emotional well-being was stable (Figure 3-4).

The mental health items (referred to as the MHI-5) from the SF-36 might have relevance for screening, since general population and chronic

---

[6]The 36th question (asking respondents to compare present health with that one year before) is not included within the eight scales.

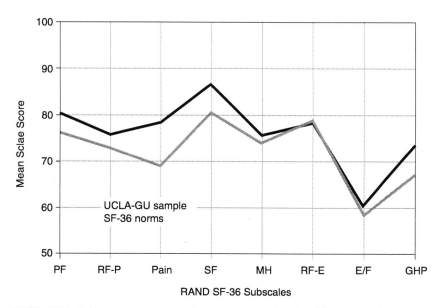

FIGURE 3-2 Breast cancer survivors compared to healthy controls.
SOURCE: Ganz, 1998a.

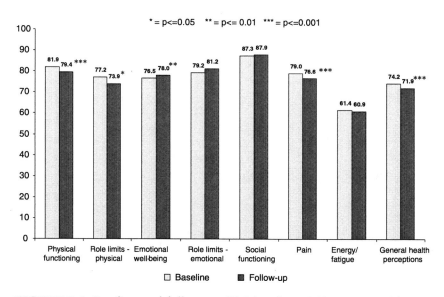

FIGURE 3-3 Baseline and follow-up SF-36 scale or 763 patients without recurrence of cancer.
SOURCE: Ganz et al., 2002.

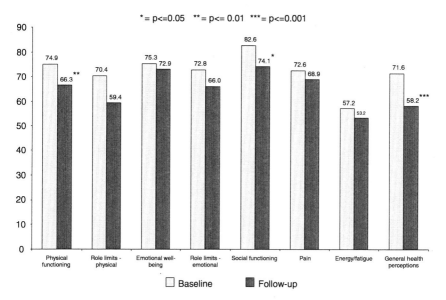

FIGURE 3-4 Baseline and follow-up SF-36 scale scores for 54 patients with recurrence of cancer.
SOURCE: Ganz et al., 2002.

illness norms are available (see Box 3-4) (Ware, 1993). To date the instrument has largely been used for research to characterize groups of patients, including women with breast cancer (Bloom et al., 2000), and not for clinical use for individual patients. Investigators in the United Kingdom tested the use of a computer touchscreen for use in routine oncology practice and found a combination of responses to the MHI-5 and HADS performed best in identifying patients who had been diagnosed through psychiatric interviews as being in need of clinical intervention (Cull et al., 2001; Velikova et al., 1999). This study was conducted among chemotherapy outpatients and was not limited to women with breast cancer.

Brief Symptom Inventory (BSI)

The Brief Symptom Inventory has been used in an early multicenter study of 430 women in the year following initial diagnosis of breast cancer, one cohort of whom was followed longitudinally over 12 months (Bloom et al., 1987). The BSI was able to measure the changes in level of distress over the year as they returned to levels seen in the comparison group of women who had a cholecystectomy, a negative biopsy, or who had no illness in the prior year.

For over a decade the Brief Symptom Inventory (BSI) has been used for psychosocial screening of patients seen at the Johns Hopkins Oncology Cen-

---

BOX 3-4
Mental Health Items from the SF-36

During the past 4 weeks, have you had any of the following problems with your work or other regular daily activities as a result of any emotional problems (such as feeling depressed or anxious)?

a) Cut down the amount of time you spent on work or other activities
b) Accomplished less than you would like
c) Didn't do work or other activities as carefully as usual

These questions are about how you feel and how things have been with you during the past 4 weeks. For each question, please give the one answer that comes closest to the way you have been feeling. How much of the time during the past 4 weeks:

a) Did you feel full of pep?
b) Have you been a very nervous person?
c) Have you felt so down in the dumps that nothing could cheer you up?
d) Have you felt calm and peaceful?
e) Did you have a lot of energy?
f) Have you felt downhearted and blue?
g) Did you feel worn out?
h) Have you been a happy person?
i) Did you feel tired?

NOTE: Items in bold make up the Mental Health Index (MHI-5).
SOURCE: Ware and Sherbourne, 1992.

---

ter (Derogatis et al., 1983; Zabora et al., 2001a, 1990). Using this approach, patients who are identified as showing distress can then be evaluated in greater detail by a trained social worker or mental health professional. The original BSI instrument includes 53 items in nine areas (Zabora et al., 2001a):

1. somatization
2. hostility
3. anxiety
4. depression
5. phobic anxiety
6. interpersonal sensitivity

7. obsessive-compulsive
8. paranoid ideation
9. psychoticism

The BSI is a 53-item measure of psychological distress written at a sixth-grade reading level requiring 5–7 minutes to complete. For each item, the patient responds in terms of "how they have been feeling during the past 7 days" (Zabora et al., 2001a). Using the BSI, psychosocial distress was identified in 35 percent of cancer patients (n = 4,496) seen at the Johns Hopkins Oncology Center with distress more common among patients with cancers associated with higher mortality and morbidity (Zabora et al., 2001a).

A shorter 18-item version of the BSI (BSI-18) has been developed (Zabora et al., 2001b). The BSI-18's sensitivity, specificity, and positive predictive value—important attributes of a screening test—have been examined to evaluate its usefulness as a screening tool, and were found to be adequate (Zabora et al., 2001b). As Zabora suggests, "these findings are an important step in the development of a prospective psychosocial care delivery system for cancer patients" (Zabora et al., 2001b). Indeed, this important work needs replication and specific evaluation in a breast cancer sample, so that it can be considered as a brief clinical screening instrument.

Cancer Rehabilitation Evaluation System (CARES)

The Cancer Rehabilitation Evaluation System (CARES) instrument was one of the first cancer-specific quality of life instruments whose initial development was influenced by the role it would play in identifying the specific rehabilitation needs of cancer patients (Heinrich et al., 1984; Schag et al., 1991, 1990, 1983).[7] Subsequently, Schag and Heinrich (Schag and Heinrich, 1990) developed a computerized report writing program so that the CARES could be used in clinical practice. Two different types of reports are generated: one for health care professionals and the other for the patient/respondent. The CARES has been used by social workers in the Revlon/UCLA Breast Center's follow-up clinic to assist in needs assessment, and it has been used in other clinical centers throughout the United States, includ-

---

[7]The earliest version of the CARES was called the Cancer Inventory of Problem Situations or CIPS. Drs. Coscarelli Schag, Heinrich, and Ganz began a collaboration in 1980—as part of a randomized group intervention trial for patients with cancer—for which the need to develop an instrument to identify cancer specific needs was conceptualized. The instrument evolved over the subsequent decade and was used in research with diverse cancer patient samples and extensively with breast cancer patients. Although used mainly in these research studies, it has also been adopted by clinicians throughout the country in various clinical settings. Unfortunately, there is no widely available database on the clinical experience with the instrument in this setting.

ing a study at UCLA of management of menopausal symptoms in women with a history of breast cancer (Ganz et al., 2000). In this study, a nurse practitioner provided a symptom management intervention and used the CARES as an efficient means to identify psychosocial issues of concern to the patient (Ganz et al., 2000). Use of the CARES in this research study closely simulated the way in which the tool should be used in clinical practice, and efficiently facilitated the assessment of these problems for the nurse's clinical intervention.

Patients complete the CARES by rating problem statements on a 5-point scale ranging from 0 "Not at all" to 4 "Applies very much" during the last month. The instrument contains 139 items, although not all items are rated by every patient (Schag and Heinrich, 1990). Certain subsections apply to some patients and not others. For example, the 9 chemotherapy items are answered only by those patients who have had chemotherapy within the last month. Patients rate a minimum of 93 items and a maximum of 132 items (Box 3-5). It takes approximately 25–30 minutes for patients to complete the full CARES. The CARES is scored into a Global Score, 5 higher order factors referred to as summary scales, or 31 more specific subscales. The 5 higher order summary scales represent the following domains:

1. Physical: the physical changes and disruption of daily activity caused by the disease

2. Psychosocial: psychological issues, communication, relationship (other than partners) problems

---

BOX 3-5
Example of Items from the CARES Assessing
Psychosocial Concerns

How much does it apply to you in the past 4 weeks?

- I frequently feel anxious
- I have difficulty sleeping
- I have difficulty asking friends or relatives to do things for me
- I am uncomfortable with the changes in my body
- I worry about not being able to care for myself

SOURCE: Ganz, workshop presentation, 2002.

3. Medical Interaction: problems interacting and communicating with the medical team

4. Marital: problems associated with any marital or marital-type relationship

5. Sexual: problems related to interest and performance of sexual activity

The Global Score takes into consideration the varying number of possible problems for each patient and in addition has demonstrated its validity as a measure of quality of life (Ganz et al., 1990; Schag et al., 1990). The CARES Global Score and Summary Scales have also been shown to be responsive to change over time in patients with breast cancer (Ganz et al., 1992b, 1992), and in one study the CARES Psychosocial Summary Score administered shortly after diagnosis of breast cancer was helpful in classifying women at subsequent risk for psychosocial distress in the year after breast cancer (Ganz et al., 1993). In another study, women determined to be at risk by a clinical social worker had significantly more problems with greater severity than the low-risk women in all areas measured in CARES (Schag et al., 1993). A short form of CARES was incorporated into the Foundation for Accountability (FACCT) quality measures for breast cancer (Foundation for Accountability, 1997). These measures were developed for health plans and other health-care organizations to assess the quality of several dimensions of care, including the experience of disease (see also Chapter 6).

The CARES has two forms: one for research and one for clinical use. On the clinical form, there is an extra column where the respondent can indicate whether or not she "wants help" with a problem. In addition, the CARES Scoring Manual provides normative data on samples of women with breast cancer so that one can determine where an individual patient scores in comparison to normative values. A short-form of the CARES was developed for use in clinical trial settings (Schag et al., 1991)

In one study, CARES was administered to 235 women with breast cancer representing four treatment phases: new diagnosis, undergoing adjuvant therapy, stable disease, and recurrent cancer (Frost et al., 2000). The overall CARES score and 5 subscores are shown in Figure 3-5. Of note are the relatively stable psychosocial scores by phase. Scores in several areas are high across the phases of care indicating problems, especially in terms of sexual functioning.

Distress Thermometer and Problem List

The National Comprehensive Cancer Network (NCCN), Inc., has published guidelines for distress management in clinical practice (NCCN, 2002)

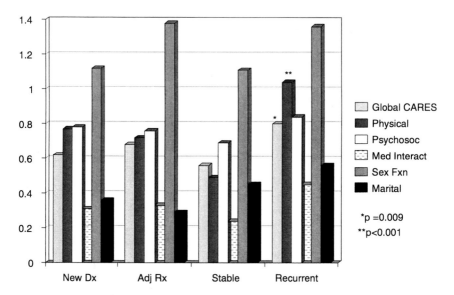

FIGURE 3-5 Influence of disease phase on CARES-SF scores.
SOURCE: Frost et al., 2000.

(see also Chapter 6). They recommend use of the NCCN Distress Thermometer and Problem List that ask patients in the waiting room how distressed they have been during the past week on a scale of 0 to 10 (see Figure 3-6). Accompanying the Distress Thermometer is the Problem List on which patients check the areas of concerns. This can be used by the primary oncology team to determine the particular psychosocial services needed (e.g., mental health, social work, or pastoral counseling). Based on a study in prostate cancer patients (Roth et al., 1998), a score of 5 or greater on the thermometer scale indicated a significant level of distress as assessed by the HADS. The recommendation is that the primary oncology team use 5 or greater as an algorithm to refer a patient for evaluation by a psychosocial professional. This instrument is being further evaluated as part of a 4-center trial to determine appropriate cut-points for screening and to assess levels of functional impairment associated with distress.

This brief screen may be well suited for use in busy oncology clinics because it uses a familiar 0–10 scale that has been successfully used to ask patients about their pain levels. Its administration also provides an opportunity to open a dialogue between patients and their providers about their psychosocial problems.

Needs assessment surveys performed in ambulatory clinics using these screens show that 20–35 percent of patients have significant levels of distress (National Comprehensive Cancer Network, 1999). The sensitivity and specificity have been tested in a three-center study, confirming that a score of 4 to

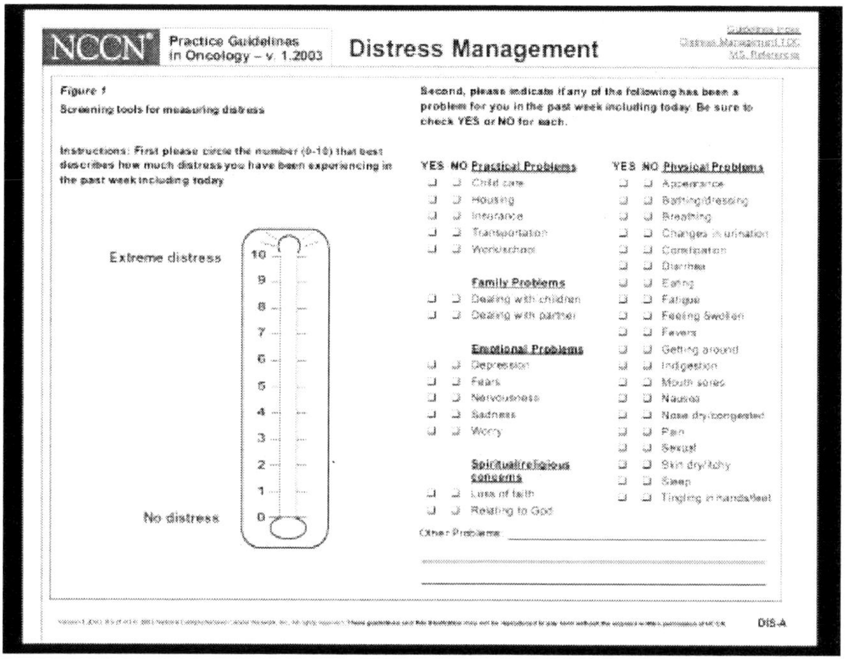

FIGURE 3-6 The NCCN distress thermometer and problem list.
SOURCE: NCCN Guideline, J. NCCN, 2003.

5 offers maximal sensitivity and specificity (P. Jacobsen, personal communication). While this simple screening approach has appeal, it needs further testing in the clinical setting before it can be accepted for widespread use. Specifically, one would need evaluation of its sensitivity and specificity in breast cancer patients at several points along the disease continuum.

Figure 3-7 shows the NCCN recommended use of the brief screening tool (Distress Thermometer and Problem List) and the clinical assessment by the primary oncology team. A score of 4–5 or greater (moderate to severe) serves as the trigger (algorithm) for referral to psychosocial services.

The European Organization for Research and Treatment of Cancer (EORTC) Quality of Life Questionnaire (QLQ-C30)

The European Organization for Research and Treatment of Cancer (EORTC) has developed an integrated, modular approach for evaluating the quality of life of individuals with cancer who participate in international clinical trials. The core instrument, the Quality of Life Questionnaire (QLQ-C30), incorporates nine multi-item scales: five functional scales (physical, role,

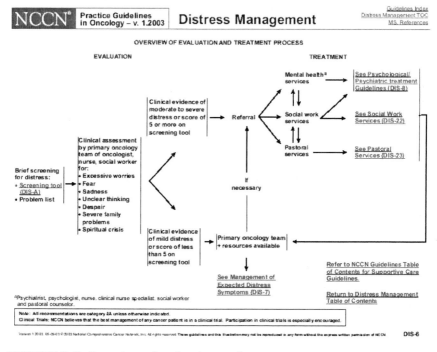

FIGURE 3-7 Overview of evaluation and treatment process.
SOURCE: NCCN Guidelines, 2003.

cognitive, emotional, and social); three symptom scales (fatigue, pain, and nausea and vomiting); and a global health and quality-of-life scale (Aaronson et al., 1993). The QLQ-30 has been used in evaluations of psychosocial interventions for women with breast cancer, and a breast cancer-specific quality-of-life questionnaire module has been developed, the QLQ-BR23, which consists of 23 items covering symptoms and side effects related to different treatment modalities, body image, sexuality, and future perspective (Curran et al., 1998; McLachlan et al., 1998; Sprangers et al., 1996).

The significance of changes in quality-of-life scores was assessed by comparing the extent of change in EORTC scores over time as patients perceived changes in their physical, emotional, and social functioning and overall quality of life. The magnitude of changes in scores was interpreted as small, moderate, and large on the basis of these comparisons (Osoba et al., 1998).

Investigators in the Netherlands conducted a randomized controlled trial (not limited to breast cancer) to test the effect of administering a computerized version of the QLQ-30 as part of routine practice to patients undergoing palliative chemotherapy (Detmar et al., 2002). Incorporating the assessments in daily clinical oncology practice facilitated the discussion of quality-of-life issues and heightened physicians' awareness of their patients' concerns.

Functional Assessment of Cancer Therapy-Breast (FACT-B)

Functional Assessment of Cancer Therapy-Breast (FACT-B) is a 46-item self-report instrument designed to measure multidimensional quality of life (Brady et al., 1997). There are 27 items in five areas of well-being (physical, social/family, emotional, and functional) that are measured on a 5-point rating scale. An additional 19 items are specific to breast cancer, including items assessing breast cancer-related emotional concerns (e.g., worried about risk of cancer in family members, worried about effects of stress on illness), physical concerns (e.g., feeling short of breath, being bothered by swollen/tender arms), body image, and sexual functioning. The FACT instrument is written at a sixth-grade reading level and has been translated into several languages (Bonomi et al., 1996; Cella et al., 1998; Dapueto et al., 2001; Fumimoto et al., 2001; Yu et al., 2000). The authors report that the instrument is easy to administer, brief, reliable, valid, and sensitive to change and recommend its use in oncology clinical trials and clinical practice (Brady et al., 1997). The FACT-G has been administered to patients attending an ambulatory breast cancer clinic at Dana Farber using a hand-held computer. Scores are tabulated and are available to the oncologist prior to the visit thereby facilitating a discussion of psychosocial concerns (Jane Weeks, personal communication to Jimmie Holland, March 2003).

Quality of Life Breast Cancer Instrument

The Quality of Life Breast Cancer Instrument includes 46-items representing four areas of well-being (physical, psychological, social, and spiritual) (Box 3-6). The instrument can be administered in person or by mail and was designed to be used in both clinical practice and research. The instrument has been subjected to assessments and shows reasonably high levels of reliability and validity (Dow et al., 1996; Ferrell et al., 1996, 1997a, 1997b, 1998a, 1998b).

National Population-Based Surveys

According to estimates from the National Health Interview Survey (NHIS), a population-based household survey conducted by the National Center for Health Statistics, adults with a history of cancer (excluding superficial skin cancer) are more likely than others to report psychological problems (Hewitt et al., 2003). To assess psychological problems, inter-

BOX 3-6
Quality of Life Breast Cancer Instrument

We are interested in knowing how your experience of having cancer affects your Quality of Life. Please answer all of the following questions based on your life at this time. Please circle the number from 0 to 10 that best describes your experiences (scale not shown below):

Physical well-being
1. Fatigue
2. Appetite changes
3. Aches or pain
4. Sleep changes
5. Weight gain
6. Vaginal dryness/menopausal symptoms
7. Menstrual changes or fertility
8. Rate your overall physical health

Psychological well-being
9. How difficult is it for you to cope today as a result of your disease?
10. How difficult is it for you to cope today as a result of your treatment?
11. How good is your quality of life?
12. How much happiness do you feel?
13. To what degree do you feel like you are in control of things in your life?
14. How satisfying is your life?
15. How is your present ability to concentrate or to remember things?
16. How useful do you feel?
17. Has you illness or treatment caused changes in your appearance?
18. Has your illness or treatment caused changes in your self concept (the way you see yourself)?

How distressing were the following aspects of your illness and treatment?
19. Initial diagnosis
20. Cancer chemotherapy
21. Cancer radiation
22. Cancer surgery
23. Completion of treatment
24. How much anxiety do you have?
25. How much depression do you have?

To what extent are you fearful of:
26. Future diagnostic tests
27. A second cancer
28. Recurrence of your cancer
29. Spreading (metastasis of your cancer
30. To what degree do you feel your life is back to normal?

Social concerns
31. How distressing has your illness been for your family?
32. Is the amount of support you receive from others sufficient to meet your needs?
33. Is your continuing health care interfering with your personal relationships?
34. Is your sexuality impacted by your illness?
35. To what degree has your illness and treatment interfered with your employment?
36. To what degree has your illness and treatment interfered with your activities at home?
37. How much isolation do you feel is caused by your illness?
38. How much concern to you have for your daughter(s) or other female relatives regarding breast cancer?
39. How much financial burden have you incurred as a result of your illness and treatment?

Spiritual well-being
40. How important to you is your participation in religious activities such as praying, going to church or temple?
41. How important to you are other spiritual activities such as meditation and praying?
42. How much has your spiritual life changed as a result of cancer diagnosis?
43. How much uncertainty do you feel about your future?
44. To what extent has your illness made positive changes in your life?
45. Do you sense a purpose/mission for your life or a reason for being alive?
46. How hopeful do you feel?

SOURCE: Ferrell and Grant, undated memo.

viewers asked about certain feelings (i.e., at least some of the time feeling sad, nervous, restless or fidgety, hopeless, worthless, or that everything was an effort) and whether such feelings had, in the last 30 days, interfered with their life or activities. Cancer survivors were more likely than others to report that these feelings had interfered with their life or activities a lot (5.4 vs. 2.8 percent), but there were no significant differences in prevalence of mental health problems by cancer type (Table 3-3). Cancer survivors without other chronic illness were twice as likely as individuals without cancer or other chronic illnesses to have psychological problems, after controlling for age, history of other chronic illness, age at interview, sex, race/ethnicity, education, health insurance coverage, and marital status. Survivors of cancer with other chronic conditions were 6 times more likely to have psychological problems (Hewitt et al., 2003).

RISK FACTORS ASSOCIATED WITH PSYCHOSOCIAL DISTRESS

A number of risk factors have been identified that are associated with psychosocial distress among women with breast cancer: younger age, a history of pre-existing depression or psychological distress, other serious comorbid conditions, and inadequate social support (Bloom et al., 1987; Ganz et al., 1993, 1992a; Jemal et al., 2002; Leedham and Ganz, 1999; Maunsell et al., 1992, 1995; Schag et al., 1993; Schover, 1994; Shimozuma et al., 1999; Wenzel et al., 1999). In contrast, the specific type of breast cancer surgery does not influence the level of distress (Ganz et al., 1993, 1992a, 1998a, 1998b; Maunsell et al., 1989; Rowland et al., 2000). What makes each of these patient characteristics a risk factor for psychosocial distress after breast cancer?

TABLE 3-3 Prevalence of Psychological Problems Among Adult Survivors of Cancer, by Cancer Type, NHIS, United States, 1998–2000

Characteristic	Psychological Problems Percent (SE)
Total	5.4 (0.4)
Site or Type of Cancer by Sex	
Breast	3.6 (0.6)
Cervix	9.3 (1.3)
Prostate	3.5 (0.8)
Colon, rectum	4.0 (1.0)
Uterus	6.1 (1.2)
Melanoma	5.2 (1.7)
Larynx, lung, pharynx	9.2 (2.6)
Leukemia, lymphoma	6.2 (1.7)
Ovary	9.0 (2.4)
Other	5.4 (0.9)
Male	4.8 (1.0)
Female	6.2 (1.4)

SOURCE: Hewitt et al., 2003.

Younger Age

Most breast cancer occurs in women older than 50 years (about 75 percent of cases), thus for women in their 30s and 40s who are diagnosed with breast cancer, this is a relatively uncommon event, and certainly one that is not expected. In addition, breast cancer in younger women is often temporally related to a recent pregnancy or may occur during pregnancy, and these women often have small children to care for at the same time they must deal with a life-threatening disease. For younger women who have not already had their children, the diagnosis and treatment of breast cancer leads to the specter of death, the likelihood of infertility as a result of treatments, and the symptomatic burden of premature menopause in addition to the acute toxicities of radiation and chemotherapy treatments. All of these medical factors contribute to the risk, and often the reality, of greater psychological distress in these younger women and greater stress for younger husbands (Bloom and Kessler, 1994; Northouse, 1994). In particular, amenorrhea and premature menopause with attendant hormonal changes associated with breast cancer treatment can be linked to mood disorders and complaints of cognitive impairment (Warga, 2000) which may be managed in part by a selective serotonin reuptake inhibitor such as fluoxetine. These kinds of issues which confront younger women were the subject of an NCI conference and monograph in which Bloom and Kessler analyzed the data by decade of age as to distress and dysphoria in a large cohort of women described earlier and reported that they were at greater risk (Bloom and Kessler, 1994). In addition, for those women who do not have a spouse or intimate partner, there may be heightened concerns about femininity, attractiveness, reproduction, and future potential for such a relationship after a breast cancer diagnosis (see following section on sexual problems), for example, the effects of mastectomy, although for those with reconstruction the adjustment problems are no more likely than for those with breast-conserving surgery (Schover et al., 1995). Finally, for younger women this is often their first encounter with the health-care system (other than childbirth or minor health conditions), and this adds considerable anxiety. In contrast, older women may have had other medical conditions or operations, or may have cared for loved ones with cancer, thus blunting some of the initial distress with having to face a new illness. On the other hand, they are more apt to be facing losses of family members or spouse, and reduced economic status.

Sexual Problems

Questions about sexual difficulties and intimacy have been recommended as part of the initial evaluation of patients with cancer. Sexual dysfunction is often not identified by the cancer care team, and most patients receive little or no assistance in dealing with the effects that cancer and cancer treatment have on sexual intimacy (McKee and Schover, 2001). Sexual counseling has been recommended both early and continuing through treatment and recovery for those who need it, but is not routinely provided. Brief counseling can be provided by one of the professionals on the cancer care team. A minority of patient will need more intense interventions, which may be provided in reproductive health clinics in major centers through referral from smaller settings. Brief interventions might include education on the impact of cancer treatment on sexual functioning, suggestions on resuming sex comfortably, advice on mitigating effects of physical handicaps, self help on overcoming specific sexual problems such as painful intercourse or a loss of desire, and treatment for estrogen deficiency (McKee and Schover, 2001; Schover 1999).

Pre-Existing Mental Illness or Psychological Morbidity

Although it appears that cancer, in general, does not heighten the risk for serious depression in women with breast cancer (Lansky et al., 1985; Rowland, 1999), a prior history of depression and the presence of pain and physical limitations are associated with a greater likelihood of depression. An early study (Morris et al., 1977) examined a group of women in the United Kingdom who were attending a clinic because of "breast cancer concerns". They were followed longitudinally and those who had more distress prior to diagnosis tended to be more distressed when studied later after their diagnosis of breast cancer, confirming the importance of psychological and psychiatric comorbidities as a factor in adaptation to breast cancer. In a prospective study of newly diagnosed breast cancer patients, Maunsell and colleagues found that a history of depression and serious life events in the five years preceding the cancer diagnosis were both predictive of higher levels of distress after breast cancer (Maunsell et al., 1992). It is not surprising that the stress associated with a new cancer diagnosis and its treatment would exacerbate preexisting depression or psychological distress. With the prevalence of clinically significant mental disorders among adults estimated at 15 percent (Narrow et al., 2002), it is to be expected that a group of women with breast cancer will be predisposed to more severe cancer-related distress based on psychological morbidity.

Comorbid Physical Conditions

Several studies have indicated that women with comorbid conditions (e.g., cardiac, pulmonary) or impaired performance status report higher levels of psychological distress after a breast cancer diagnosis (Ganz et al., 1993; Lansky et al., 1985). This appears to be independent of age (Ganz et al., 1993), although the likelihood of greater comorbidity at diagnosis is increased with age (Greenfield et al., 1987). Physical recovery after breast cancer surgery may be impaired in women with greater comorbidity (Lash and Silliman, 2000), and this may contribute to greater psychological distress as well.

Social Support

Social support for the woman with breast cancer includes instrumental support, such as transportation to appointments, preparation of meals, help with activities of daily living, and emotional support, meaning the availability of someone to share one's fears, feelings, and concerns. Inadequate levels of either of these two forms of social support increase the likelihood of heightened distress. This may be particularly important in patients with advanced breast cancer (Bloom, 1982; Bloom and Spiegel, 1984; Koopman et al., 1998).

SUMMARY

"Psychosocial distress varies along a continuum from the "normal" reactions to the stress of coping with cancer and its treatment, to symptoms so intense that the person experiencing them meets the criteria for a psychiatric disorder, a severe social or family problem, or significant spiritual distress" (National Comprehensive Cancer Network, 1999: 113). Most of the United States studies upon which available estimates of psychosocial distress are based have been conducted within research-oriented cancer centers and have focused on psychosocial distress or psychiatric illness within the first few years of treatment. It is generally recognized that mental disorders occur relatively frequently among individuals with cancer. Prevalence rates varied from 10 to 25 percent for major depression and depressive symptoms, a rate at least four times higher than in the general population according to one recent review (Agency for Healthcare Research and Quality, 2002). Very little, however, is known from prospective studies of the prevalence of psychosocial distress at the different points along the disease continuum or how levels of distress vary for any particular individual by phase of disease or treatment. Whether women with breast cancer have higher rates of psychosocial distress than others with cancer is also not known, although there is some evidence that distress is greater in cancers with poorer prognoses (e.g., Zabora et al., 2001a). The prevalence of psychosocial distress among women with cancer ranges from roughly 20 to 40 percent, with the variation likely accounted for by differences in study populations and differences in assessment tools as reviewed here (for example, Curran et al., 1998; Ferrell et al., 1996, 1997a, 1997b; Frost et al., 2000;

Fulton, 1998; Ganz et al., 1992, 1996, 1998a, 2000, 2002; Hall et al., 1999; McLachlan et al., 1998; National Comprehensive Cancer Network, 1999; Spranger et al., 1996; Zabora et al., 2001a, 2002b) leading to a probable mid-range estimate in the area of 30 percent. Specific concerns that women with breast cancer have at various points along the care continuum have been well documented, for example, shock and disbelief at diagnosis, anxiety and distress during treatment, fear of recurrence, intrusive thoughts about illness following treatment, and existential concerns following recurrence. Factors that appear to predispose women for psychosocial distress include younger age, a history of pre-existing depression or psychological distress, other serious comorbid conditions, and inadequate social support.

REFERENCES

Aaronson NK, Ahmedzai S, Bergman B, Bullinger M, Cull A, Duez NJ, Filiberti A, Flechtner H, Fleishman SB, de Haes JC, et al. 1993. The European Organization for Research and Treatment of Cancer QLQ-C30: A quality-of-life instrument for use in international clinical trials in oncology. *J Natl Cancer Inst* 85(5):365–376.

Agency for Healthcare Research and Quality. 2002. Management of cancer symptoms: Pain, depression, and fatigue: Summary. *Evidence Report/Technology Assessment* 61:1–9.

Ahles TA, Saykin AJ, Furstenberg CT, Cole B, Mott LA, Skalla K, Whedon MB, Bivens S, Mitchell T, Greenberg ER, Silberfarb PM. 2002. Neuropsychologic impact of standard-dose systemic chemotherapy in long-term survivors of breast cancer and lymphoma. *J Clin Oncol* 20(2):485–493.

American Psychiatric Association. 1994. *Diagnostic and Statistical Manual of Mental Disorders*. Fourth edition. Washington, DC: American Psychiatric Association.

Andersen BL, Anderson B, deProsse C. 1989. Controlled prospective longitudinal study of women with cancer. II. Psychological outcomes. *J Consult Clin Psychol* 57(6):692–697.

Bjelland I, Dahl AA, Haug TT, Neckelmann D. 2002. The validity of the Hospital Anxiety and Depression Scale. An updated literature review. *J Psychosom Res* 52(2):69–77.

Bloom JR. 1982. Social support, accommodation to stress and adjustment to breast cancer. *Soc Sci Med* 16(14):1329–1338.

Bloom JR, Spiegel D. 1984. The relationship of two dimensions of social support to the psychological well-being and social functioning of women with advanced breast cancer. *Soc Sci Med* 19(8):831–837.

Bloom, JR, Cook, M, Flamer, DP, et al. 1987. Psychological response to mastectomy. *Cancer* 59(1):189–196.

Bloom JR, Kessler L. 1994. Risk and timing of counseling and support interventions for younger women with breast cancer. *J Natl Cancer Inst Monogr* 16:199–206

Bloom, JR, Stewart, SL, Banks, PB, et al. 2000.General and specific measures of quality of life in young women with breast cancer. In Baum A, Andersen B, ed. *Psychosocial Interventions for Cancer*. Washington, DC: American Psychological Association. Pp. 37–56,

Bondurant S, Ernster V, Herdman R. 1999. *Safety of Silicone Breast Implants*. Washington, DC: Institute of Medicine, National Academy Press.

Bonomi AE, Cella DF, Hahn EA, Bjordal K, Sperner-Unterweger B, Gangeri L, Bergman B, Willems-Groot J, Hanquet P, Zittoun R. 1996. Multilingual translation of the Functional Assessment of Cancer Therapy (FACT) quality of life measurement system. *Qual Life Res* 5(3):309–320.

Bradley CJ, Bednarek HL, Neumark D. 2002. Breast cancer and women's labor supply. *Health Serv Res* 37(5):1309–1328.

Brady MJ, Cella DF, Mo F, Bonomi AE, Tulsky DS, Lloyd SR, Deasy S, Cobleigh M, Shiomoto G. 1997. Reliability and validity of the Functional Assessment of Cancer Therapy-Breast quality-of-life instrument. *J Clin Oncol* 15(3):974–986.

Breitbart W, Rosenfeld B, Pessin H, et al. 2000. Depression, hopelessness, and desire for hastened death in terminally ill patients with cancer. *JAMA* 284(22) : 2907-2911.

Brennan J. 2001. Adjustment to cancer—coping or personal transition? *Psycho-oncology* 10(1):1–18.

Brezden CB, Phillips KA, Abdolell M, Bunston T, Tannock IF. 2000. Cognitive function in breast cancer patients receiving adjuvant chemotherapy. *J Clin Oncol* 18(14):2695–2701.

Bull AA, Meyerowitz BE, Hart S, Mosconi P, Apolone G, Liberati A. 1999. Quality of life in women with recurrent breast cancer. *Breast Cancer Res Treat* 54(1):47–57.

Butler LD, Koopman C, Cordova MJ, et al. 2003. Psychological distress and pain significantly increase before death in metastatic breast cancer patients. *Psychsom Med* 65(3):416–426

Carroll BT, Kathol RG, Noyes R Jr, Wald TG, Clamon GH. 1993. Screening for depression and anxiety in cancer patients using the Hospital Anxiety and Depression Scale. *Gen Hosp Psychiatry* 15(2):69–74.

Cella D, Hernandez L, Bonomi AE, Corona M, Vaquero M, Shiomoto G, Baez L. 1998. Spanish language translation and initial validation of the functional assessment of cancer therapy quality-of-life instrument. *Med Care* 36(9):1407–1418.

Cella DF. 1995. Methods and problems in measuring quality of life. *Support Care Cancer* 3(1):11–22.

Chou AF. 2002. *Shared Decision Making: The Selection Process of Treatment Options and Resulting Quality of Life Implications for Women with Breast Cancer.* University of California, Berkeley, July 2002.

Chou AF. 2003. *Shared Decision Making: Predictors of Participation in Women with Breast Cancer.* Presented at PAM Conference, Cornell College of Human Ecology. [Online]. Available: http://www.human.cornell.edu/pam/seminars/s03sem/ [accessed September 10, 2003].

Clauson J, Hsieh YC, Acharya S, Redemaker AW, Morrow M. 2002. Results of the Lynn Sage Second-Opinion Program for Local Therapy. Patients with breast carcinoma: Changes in management and determinants of where care is delivered. *Cancer* 94(4):889–894.

Cordova MJ, Cunningham LL, Carlson CR, Andrykowski MA. 2001. Posttraumatic growth following breast cancer: A controlled comparison study. *Health Psychol* 20(3):176–85.

Cull A, Gould A, House A, Smith A, Strong V, Velikova G, Wright P, Selby P. 2001. Validating automated screening for psychological distress by means of computer touchscreens for use in routine oncology practice. *Br J Cancer* 85(12):1842–1849.

Curran D, van Dongen JP, Aaronson NK, Kiebert G, Fentiman IS, Mignolet F, Bartelink H. 1998. Quality of life of early-stage breast cancer patients treated with radical mastectomy or breast-conserving procedures: Results of EORTC Trial 10801. The European Organization for Research and Treatment of Cancer (EORTC), Breast Cancer Co-operative Group (BCCG). *Eur J Cancer* 34(3):307–314.

Dapueto JJ, Francolino C, Gotta I, Levin R, Alonso I, Barrios E, Afonzo Y, Cambiasso S. 2001. Evaluation of the Functional Assessment of Cancer Therapy-General Questionnaire (FACT-G) in a South American Spanish speaking population. *Psycho-oncology* 10(1):88–92.

Day R, Ganz PA, Costantino JP. 2001. Tamoxifen and depression: More evidence from the National Surgical Adjuvant Breast and Bowel Project's Breast Cancer Prevention (P-1) Randomized Study. *J Natl Cancer Inst* 93(21):1615–1623.

Day R, Ganz PA, Costantino JP, Cronin WM, Wickerham DL, Fisher B. 1999. Health-related quality of life and tamoxifen in breast cancer prevention: A report from the National Surgical Adjuvant Breast and Bowel Project P-1 Study. *J Clin Oncol* 17(9):2659–2669.

Derogatis LR. 2000. *BSI-18: Administration, Scoring and Procedures Manual*. Minneapolis: National Computer Systems.

Derogatis LR, Morrow GR, Fetting J, Penman D, Piasetsky S, Schmale AM, Henrichs M, Carnicke CL Jr. 1983. The prevalence of psychiatric disorders among cancer patients. *JAMA* 249(6):751–757.

Detmar SB, Muller MJ, Schornagel JH, Wever LD, Aaronson NK. 2002. Health-related quality-of-life assessments and patient-physician communication: A randomized controlled trial. *JAMA* 288(23):3027–3034.

Dorval M, Maunsell E, Deschenes L, Brisson J. 1998. Type of mastectomy and quality of life for long term breast carcinoma survivors. *Cancer* 83(10):2130–2138.

Dow KH, Ferrell BR, Leigh S, Ly J, Gulasekaram P. 1996. An evaluation of the quality of life among long-term survivors of breast cancer. *Breast Cancer Res Treat* 39(3):261–273.

Evans DL, Staab J, Ward H, Leserman J, Perkins DO, Golden RN, Petitto JM. 1996–1997. Depression in the medically ill: Management considerations. *Depress Anxiety* 4(4):199–208.

Fallowfield L, Fleissig A, Edwards R, West A, Powles TJ, Howell A, Cuzick J. 2001. Tamoxifen for the prevention of breast cancer: Psychosocial impact on women participating in two randomized controlled trials. *J Clin Oncol* 19(7):1885–1892.

Ferrell BR, Grant M, Funk B, Garcia N, Otis-Green S, Schaffner ML. 1996. Quality of life in breast cancer. *Cancer Pract* 4(6):331–340.

Ferrell BR, Grant M, Funk B, Otis-Green S, Garcia N. 1997a. Quality of life in breast cancer. I. Physical and social well-being. *Cancer Nurs* 20(6):398–408.

Ferrell BR, Grant M, Funk B, Otis-Green S, Garcia N. 1998a. Quality of life in breast cancer. II. Psychological and spiritual well-being. *Cancer Nurs* 21(1):1–9.

Ferrell BR, Grant MM, Funk B, Otis-Green S, Garcia N. 1997b. Quality of life in breast cancer survivors as identified by focus groups. *Psycho-oncology* 6(1):13–23.

Ferrell BR, Grant MM, Funk BM, Otis-Green SA, Garcia NJ. 1998b. Quality of life in breast cancer survivors: Implications for developing support services. *Oncol Nurs Forum* 25(5):887–895.

Foley KM. The treatment of cancer pain. 1985. *N Engl J Med* 313(2):84–95.

Foley KM. Controlling cancer pain. 2000, *Hosp Pract* 35(4):101–108.

Foundation for Accountability. 1997. *FACCT Quality Measures: Breast Cancer Measurement Specifications (Version 1.0)*. Portland, OR: Foundation for Accountability.

Frost MH, Suman VJ, Rummans TA, Dose AM, Taylor M, Novotny P, Johnson R, Evans R. 2000. Physical, psychological and social well-being of women with breast cancer: The influence of disease phase. *Psycho-oncology* 9(3):221–231.

Fulton C. 1998. The prevalence and detection of psychiatric morbidity in patients with metastatic breast cancer. *Eur J Cancer Care (Engl)* 7(4):232–239.

Fumimoto H, Kobayashi K, Chang CH, Eremenco S, Fujiki Y, Uemura S, Ohashi Y, Kudoh S. 2001. Cross-cultural validation of an international questionnaire, the General Measure of the Functional Assessment of Cancer Therapy scale (FACT-G), for Japanese. *Qual Life Res* 10(8):701–709.

Ganz PA, Coscarelli A, Fred C, Kahn B, Polinsky ML, Petersen L. 1996. Breast cancer survivors: Psychosocial concerns and quality of life. *Breast Cancer Res Treat* 38(2):183–199.

Ganz PA, Desmond KA, Belin TR, Meyerowitz BE, Rowland JH. 1999. Predictors of sexual health in women after a breast cancer diagnosis. *J Clin Oncol* 17(8):2371–2380.

Ganz PA, Desmond KA, Leedham B, Rowland JH, Meyerowitz BE, Belin TR. 2002. Quality of life in long-term, disease-free survivors of breast cancer: A follow-up study. *J Natl Cancer Inst* 94(1):39–49.

Ganz PA, Greendale GA, Petersen L, Zibecchi L, Kahn B, Belin TR. 2000. Managing menopausal symptoms in breast cancer survivors: Results of a randomized controlled trial. *J Natl Cancer Inst* 92(13):1054–1064.

Ganz PA, Hirji K, Sim MS, Schag CA, Fred C, Polinsky ML. 1993. Predicting psychosocial risk in patients with breast cancer. *Med Care* 31(5):419–431.

Ganz PA, Lee JJ, Sim MS, Polinsky ML, Schag CA. 1992a. Exploring the influence of multiple variables on the relationship of age to quality of life in women with breast cancer. *J Clin Epidemiol* 45(5):473–485.

Ganz PA, Moinpour CM, Cella DF, Fetting JH. 1992b. Quality-of-life assessment in cancer clinical trials: A status report. *J Natl Cancer Inst* 84(13):994–995.

Ganz PA, Rowland JH, Desmond K, Meyerowitz BE, Wyatt GE. 1998a. Life after breast cancer: Understanding women's health-related quality of life and sexual functioning. *J Clin Oncol* 16(2):501–514.

Ganz PA, Rowland JH, Meyerowitz BE, Desmond KA. 1998b. Impact of different adjuvant therapy strategies on quality of life in breast cancer survivors. *Recent Results Cancer Res* 152:396–411.

Ganz PA, Schag CA, Cheng HL. 1990. Assessing the quality of life: A study in newly-diagnosed breast cancer patients. *J Clin Epidemiol* 43(1):75–86.

Ganz PA, Schag CA, Lee JJ, Sim MS. 1992. The CARES: A generic measure of health-related quality of life for patients with cancer. *Qual Life Res* 1(1):19–29.

Gotay CC, Muraoka MY. 1998. Quality of life in long-term survivors of adult-onset cancers. *J Natl Cancer Inst* 90(9):656–667.

Greenfield S, Blanco DM, Elashoff RM, Ganz PA. 1987. Patterns of care related to age of breast cancer patients. *JAMA* 257(20):2766–2770.

Greer S, Morris T. 1975. Psychological attributes of women who develop breast cancer: A controlled study. *J Psychosom Res* 19(2):147–153.

Griff M, Bondurant S, Ernster, V et al. 2000. *Information for Women about the Safety of Silicone Breast Implants.* Washington, DC: Institute of Medicine, National Academy Press.

Groenvold M, Fayers PM, Sprangers MA, Bjorner JB, Klee MC, Aaronson NK, Bech P, Mouridsen HT. 1999. Anxiety and depression in breast cancer patients at low risk of recurrence compared with the general population: a valid comparison? *J Clin Epidemiol* 52(6):523–30.

Hall A, A'Hern R, Fallowfield L. 1999. Are we using appropriate self-report questionnaires for detecting anxiety and depression in women with early breast cancer? *Eur J Cancer* 35(1):79–85.

Hann D, Winter K, Jacobsen P. 1999. Measurement of depressive symptoms in cancer patients: Evaluation of the Center for Epidemiological Studies Depression Scale (CES-D). *J Psychosom Res* 46(5):437–443.

Heinrich RL, Schag CC, Ganz PA. 1984. Living with cancer: The Cancer Inventory of Problem Situations. *J Clin Psychol* 40(4):972–980.

Herrmann C. 1997. International experiences with the Hospital Anxiety and Depression Scale: A review of validation data and clinical results. *J Psychosom Res* 42(1):17–41.

Hewitt M, Rowland JH, Yancik R. 2003. Cancer survivors in the United States: Age, health, and disability. *J Gerontol A Biol Sci Med Sci* 58(1):82–91.

Holland JC, Rowland JH. 1991. Psychological reactions to breast cancer and its treatment. In: Harris JR, Hellman S, Henderson IC, Kinne, DW, eds. *Breast Diseases.* 2nd ed. Philadelphia: Lippincott. Pp 849–866.

Hopwood P, Howell A, Maguire P. 1991a. Psychiatric morbidity in patients with advanced cancer of the breast: Prevalence measured by two self-rating questionnaires. *Br J Cancer* 64(2):349–352.

Hopwood P, Howell A, Maguire P. 1991b. Screening for psychiatric morbidity in patients with advanced breast cancer: Validation of two self-report questionnaires. *Br J Cancer* 64(2):353–356.

Irvine D, Brown B, Crooks D, Roberts J, Browne G. 1991. Psychosocial adjustment in women with breast cancer. *Cancer* 67(4):1097–1117.

Jemal A, Thomas A, Murray T, Thun M. Cancer statistics, 2002. *CA Cancer J Clin* 52(1):23–47.

Justice B. 1999. Why do women treated for breast cancer report good health despite disease or disability? A pilot study. *Psychol Rep* 84(2):392–394.

Katon W, Ciechanowski P. 2002. Impact of major depression on chronic medical illness. *J Psychosom Res* 53(4):859–863.

Katon W, Schulberg H. 1992. Epidemiology of depression in primary care. *Gen Hosp Psychiatry* 14(4):237–247.

Kessler RC, McGonagle KA, Zhao S, Nelson CB, Hughes M, Eshleman S, Wittchen HU, Kendler KS. 1994. Lifetime and 12-month prevalence of DSM-III-R psychiatric disorders in the United States. Results from the National Comorbidity Survey. *Arch Gen Psychiatry* 51(1):8–19.

Koopman C, Hermanson K, Diamond S, Angell K, Spiegel D. 1998. Social support, life stress, pain and emotional adjustment to advanced breast cancer. *Psycho-oncology* 7(2):101–111.

Kornblith AB, Zhang C, Herndon II, JE, Weiss RB, Zuckerman EL, Rosenberg S, Mertz M, Payne D, Massie MJ, Holland JF, Byrd JC, Wingate P, Norton L, Holland JC, for the Cancer and Leukemia Group B (CALGB), Chicago, IL. 2003. Long-term adjustment of survivors of early stage breast cancer 20 years after adjuvant chemotherapy. *Cancer* 98(4):679–689.

Kornblith AB. 1998. Psychosocial adaptation of cancer survivors. In: Holland JC, ed. *Psycho-Oncology*. New York: Oxford University Press.

Krishnan KR, Delong M, Kraemer H, Carney R, Spiegel D, Gordon C, McDonald W, Dew M, Alexopoulos G, Buckwalter K, Cohen PD, Evans D, Kaufmann PG, Olin J, Otey E, Wainscott C. 2002. Comorbidity of depression with other medical diseases in the elderly. *Biol Psychiatry* 52(6):559–588.

Lansky SB, List MA, Herrmann CA, Ets-Hokin EG, DasGupta TK, Wilbanks GD, Hendrickson FR. 1985. Absence of major depressive disorder in female cancer patients. *J Clin Oncol* 3(11):1553–1560.

Lash TL, Silliman RA. 2000. Patient characteristics and treatments associated with a decline in upper-body function following breast cancer therapy. *J Clin Epidemiol* 53(6):615–622.

Leedham B, Ganz PA. 1999. Psychosocial concerns and quality of life in breast cancer survivors. *Cancer Invest* 17(5):342–348.

Love, AW, Kissane DW, Bloch S, Clarke, D. 2002. Diagnostic efficiency of the Hospital Anxiety and Depression Scale in women with early stage breast cancer. *Aust N Z J Psychiatry* 36(2):246–250.

Mandelblatt JS, Eisenberg JM. 1995. Historical and methodological perspectives on cancer outcomes research. *Oncology (Huntingt)* 9(11 Suppl):23–32.

Massie MJ, Holland JC. 1989. *Overview of Normal Reactions and Prevalence of Psychiatric Disorders*. New York: Oxford University Press. Pp. 273–282.

Massie MJ, Holland JC. 1991. Psychological reactions to breast cancer in the pre- and post-surgical period, *Semin Surg Oncol* 7(5):320–325.

Massie MJ, Holland JC. 1992. The cancer patient with pain: Psychiatric complications and their management., *J Pain Symptom Manage* 7(2):99–109.

Maunsell E, Brisson J, Deschenes L. 1989. Psychological distress after initial treatment for breast cancer: A comparison of partial and total mastectomy. *J Clin Epidemiol* 42(8):765–771.

Maunsell E, Brisson J, Deschenes L. 1992. Psychological distress after initial treatment of breast cancer. Assessment of potential risk factors. *Cancer* 70(1):120–125.

Maunsell E, Brisson J, Deschenes L. 1995. Social support and survival among women with breast cancer. *Cancer* 76(4):631–637.

Mausner JS, Kramer S, Bahn AK. 1985. *Epidemiology: An Introductory Text*. 2nd ed. Philadelphia: Saunders.

McEvoy MD, McCorkle R. 1990. Quality of life issues in patients with disseminated breast cancer. *Cancer* 66(6 Suppl):1416–1421.

McGuire WL, Foley KM, Levy MH, et al. 1989. Pain control in breast cancer: A panel discussion. *Breast Canc Res Treat* 13(1):5–15.

McHorney CA, Tarlov AR. 1995. Individual-patient monitoring in clinical practice: Are available health status surveys adequate? *Qual Life Res* 4(4):293–307.

McKee, AL, Schover, LR. 2001. Sexuality rehabilitation. *Cancer* 92(4 Suppl):1008–1012.

McLachlan SA, Devins GM, Goodwin PJ. 1998. Validation of the European Organization for Research and Treatment of Cancer Quality of Life Questionnaire (QLQ-C30) as a measure of psychosocial function in breast cancer patients. *Eur J Cancer* 34(4):510–517.

Meyerowitz BE, Desmond KA, Rowland JH, Wyatt GE, Ganz PA. 1999. Sexuality following breast cancer. *J Sex Marital Ther* 25(3):237–250.

Montazeri A, Gillis CR, McEwen J. 1996. Measuring quality of life in oncology: Is it worthwhile? I. Meaning, purposes and controversies. *Eur J Cancer Care (Engl)* 5(3):159–167.

Montazeri A, Jarvandi S, Haghighat S, Vahdani M, Sajadian A, Ebrahimi M, Haji-Mahmoodi M. 2001. Anxiety and depression in breast cancer patients before and after participation in a cancer support group. *Patient Educ Couns* 45(3):195–198.

Morris T, Greer S, White P. 1977. Psychological and social adjustment to mastectomy. *Cancer* 40:2381–2387.

Musselman DL, Evans DL, Nemeroff CB. 1998. The relationship of depression to cardiovascular disease: Epidemiology, biology, and treatment. *Arch Gen Psychiatry* 55(7):580–592.

Narrow WE, Rae DS, Robins LN, Regier DA. 2002. Revised prevalence estimates of mental disorders in the United States: Using a clinical significance criterion to reconcile 2 surveys' estimates. *Arch Gen Psychiatry* 59(2):115–123.

National Comprehensive Cancer Network. 1999. NCCN practice guidelines for the management of psychosocial distress. *Oncology (Huntingt)* 13(5A):113–147.

NCCN, Practice Guidelines for Breast Cancer, Version 2000. 2000. *NCCN Proceedings, Oncology* 14(11A):33–49

NCCN. 2002. Clinical Practice Guidelines for Management of Distress. *J NCCN* 1(3):344–174

Nemeroff CB, Musselman DL, Evans DL. 1998. Depression and cardiac disease. *Depress Anxiety* 8(Suppl 1):71–79.

Northouse LL. 1994. Breast cancer in younger women: Effects on interpersonal and family relations. *J Natl Cancer Inst Monogr* 16:183–190

Northouse LL, Mood D, Kershaw T, Schafenacker A, Mellon S, Walker J, Galvin E, Decker V. 2002. Quality of life of women with recurrent breast cancer and their family members. *J Clin Oncol* 20(19):4050–4064.

Osoba D, Rodrigues G, Myles J, Zee B, Pater J. 1998. Interpreting the significance of changes in health-related quality-of- life scores. *J Clin Oncol* 16(1):139–144.

Petrie KJ, Buick DL, Weinman J, Booth RJ. 1999. Positive effects of illness reported by myocardial infarction and breast cancer patients. *J Psychosom Res* 47(6):537–543.

Regier DA, Myers JK, Kramer M, Robins LN, Blazer DG, Hough RL, Eaton WW, Locke BZ. 1984. The NIMH Epidemiologic Catchment Area program. Historical context, major objectives, and study population characteristics. *Arch Gen Psychiatry* 41(10):934–941.

Roth AJ, Kornblith AB, Batel-Copel L, Peabody E, Scher HI, Holland JC. 1998. Rapid screening for psychologic distress in men with prostate carcinoma: A pilot study. *Cancer* 82(10):1904–1908.

Rowland JH, Desmond KA, Meyerowitz BE, Belin TR, Wyatt GE, Ganz PA. 2000. Role of breast reconstructive surgery in physical and emotional outcomes among breast cancer survivors. *J Natl Cancer Inst* 92(17):1422–1429.

Rowland, JH, Massie, MJ. 1998. *Breast Cancer in Psycho-oncology*. Holland J, ed. New York: Oxford University Press.

Rowland JH. 1999. Anxiety and the blues after breast cancer: How common are they? *CNS Spectrums* 4(10):40–54.

Santen RJ. 2003. Inhibition of aromatase: Insights from recent studies. *Steroids* 68(7–8):559–567.

Schag CA, Ganz PA, Heinrich RL. 1991. Cancer Rehabilitation Evaluation System—short form (CARES-SF). A cancer specific rehabilitation and quality of life instrument. *Cancer* 68(6):1406–1413.

Schag CA, Ganz PA, Polinsky ML, Fred C, Hirji K, Petersen L. 1993. Characteristics of women at risk for psychosocial distress in the year after breast cancer. *J Clin Oncol* 11(4):783–793.

Schag CA, Heinrich RL. 1990. Development of a comprehensive quality of life measurement tool: CARES. *Oncology (Huntingt)* 4(5):135–138; discussion 147.

Schag CA, Heinrich RL, Aadland RL, Ganz PA. 1990. Assessing problems of cancer patients: Psychometric properties of the cancer inventory of problem situations. Health Psychol 9(1):83–102.

Schag CC, Heinrich RL, Ganz PA. 1983. Cancer Inventory of Problem Situation: An instrument for assessing cancer patients' rehabilitation needs. *Journal of Psychosocial Oncology* 1(4):11–24.

Schagen SB, van Dam FS, Muller MJ, Boogerd W, Lindeboom J, Bruning PF. 1999. Cognitive deficits after postoperative adjuvant chemotherapy for breast carcinoma. *Cancer* 85(3):640–650.

Schover LR. 1994. Sexuality and body image in younger women with breast cancer. *J Natl Cancer Inst Monogr* (16):177–182.

Schover LR, Yetman RJ, Tuason LJ, et al. 1995. Partial mastectomy and breast reconstruction: A comparison of their effects on psychosocial adjustment, body image, and sexuality. *Cancer* 75(1):54–64.

Schover LR, 1999. Couseling cacner patients about changes in sexual function. *Oncology* 13(11):1585–1591.

Shimozuma K, Ganz PA, Petersen L, Hirji K. 1999. Quality of life in the first year after breast cancer surgery: Rehabilitation needs and patterns of recovery. *Breast Cancer Res Treat* 56(1):45–57.

Spiegel D, Bloom JR. 1983. Group therapy and hypnosis reduce metastatic breast carcinoma pain. *Psychosom Med* 45(4):333–339.

Spiegel D, Morrow GR, Classen C, et al. 1999. Group psychotherapy for recently diagnosed breast cancer patients: A multicenter feasibility study. *Psycho-oncology* 8(6):482–493.

Sprangers MA, Groenvold M, Arraras JI, Franklin J, te Velde A, Muller M, Franzini L, Williams A, de Haes HC, Hopwood P, Cull A, Aaronson NK. 1996. The European Organization for Research and Treatment of Cancer breast cancer-specific quality-of-life questionnaire module: First results from a three-country field study. *J Clin Oncol* 14(10):2756–2768.

Stanton AL, Danoff-Burg S, Sworowski LA, et al. 2002. Randomized controlled trial of written emotional expression and benefit finding in breast cancer patients. *J Clin Oncol* 20(20):4160–4168

Stewart AL, Greenfield S, Hays RD, Wells K, Rogers WH, Berry SD, McGlynn EA, Ware JE Jr. 1989. Functional status and well-being of patients with chronic conditions. Results from the Medical Outcomes Study. *JAMA* 262(7):907–913.

Stewart DE, Cheung AM, Duff S, Wong F, McQuestion M, Cheng T, Purdy L, Bunston T. 2001. Attributions of cause and recurrence in long-term breast cancer survivors. *Psycho-oncology* 10(2):179–183.

Syrjala K, Chapko J. 1995. Evidence for a biopsychosocial model of cancer treatment-related pain. *Pain* 61:69–79.

Tchekmedyian NS, Hickman M, Siau J, Greco A, Aisner J. 1990. Treatment of cancer anorexia with megestrol acetate: Impact on quality of life. *Oncology (Huntingt)* 4(5):185–192.

Tomich PL, Helgeson VS. 2002. Five years later: A cross-sectional comparison of breast cancer survivors with healthy women. *Psycho-oncology* 11(2):154–169.

Trimble EL, Rowland J, Varricchio C, Gore-Langton RE. 2001. Clinical trials referral resource. Health related quality of life in cancer clinical trials. *Oncology (Huntingt)* 15(4):456–458, 461–466.

van Dam FS, Schagen SB, Muller MJ, Boogerd W, vd Wall E, Droogleever Fortuyn ME, Rodenhuis S. 1998. Impairment of cognitive function in women receiving adjuvant treatment for high-risk breast cancer: High-dose versus standard-dose chemotherapy. *J Natl Cancer Inst* 90(3):210–218.

van't Spijker A, Trijsburg RW, Duivenvoorden HJ. 1997. Psychological sequelae of cancer diagnosis: A meta-analytical review of 58 studies after 1980. *Psychosom Med* 59(3):280–293.

Velikova G, Wright EP, Smith AB, Cull A, Gould A, Forman D, Perren T, Stead M, Brown J, Selby PJ. 1999. Automated collection of quality-of-life data: A comparison of paper and computer touch-screen questionnaires. *J Clin Oncol* 17(3):998–1007.

Ware JE. 1993. Measuring patients' views: The optimum outcome measure. *BMJ* 306(6890):1429–1430.

Ware JE Jr, Sherbourne CD. 1992. The MOS 36-item short-form health survey (SF-36). I. Conceptual framework and item selection. *Med Care* 30(6):473–183.

Warga CL. 2000. *Menopause and the Mind: The Complete Guide to Coping with the Cognitive Effects of Perimenopause and Menopause, Including Memory Loss, Foggy Thinking, and Verbal Slips.* New York: Simon and Schuster.

Wells KB, Stewart A, Hays RD, Burnam MA, Rogers W, Daniels M, Berry S, Greenfield S, Ware J. 1989. The functioning and well-being of depressed patients. Results from the Medical Outcomes Study. *JAMA* 262(7):914–919.

Wenzel LB, Fairclough DL, Brady MJ, Cella D, Garrett KM, Kluhsman BC, Crane LA, Marcus AC. 1999. Age-related differences in the quality of life of breast carcinoma patients after treatment. *Cancer* 86(9):1768–1774.

Wickman M. 1995. Breast reconstruction: Past achievements, current status, and future goals. *Scand J Reconstr Hand Surg* 29:81–100.

Yu CL, Fielding R, Chan CL, Tse VK, Choi PH, Lau WH, Choy DT, O SK, Lee AW, Sham JS. 2000. Measuring quality of life of Chinese cancer patients: A validation of the Chinese version of the Functional Assessment of Cancer Therapy-General (FACT-G) scale. *Cancer* 88(7):1715–1727.

Zabora J, BrintzenhofeSzoc K, Curbow B, Hooker C, Piantadosi S. 2001a. The prevalence of psychological distress by cancer site. *Psycho-oncology* 10(1):19–28.

Zabora J, BrintzenhofeSzoc K, Jacobsen P, Curbow B, Piantados S, Hooker C, Owens A, Derogatis L. 2001b. A new psychosocial screening instrument for use with cancer patients. *Psychosomatics* 42(3):241–246.

Zabora JR, Smith-Wilson R, Fetting JH, Enterline JP. 1990. An efficient method for psychosocial screening of cancer patients. *Psychosomatics* 31(2):192–196.

Zigmond AS, Snaith RP. 1983. The hospital anxiety and depression scale. *Acta Psychiatr Scand* 67(6):361–370.

4

Psychosocial Services
and Provicers

Psychosocial distress may occur at all points along the cancer continuum: from initial diagnosis through treatment, survivorship, and during advanced illness and end of life. Oncology providers are central to addressing individuals' psychosocial concerns, but primary care providers, who often have longstanding relationships with patients, may provide support to them as they face a diagnosis of cancer and during the post treatment period of care. This section of the report describes the range of psychosocial interventions that are used to alleviate distress and the providers who may deliver them, as well as professional education and training opportunities that are available in the area of psychooncology.

PSYCHOSOCIAL SERVICES

A number of interventions are used to enhance adjustment to cancer by addressing psychosocial concerns and reducing distress. This section presents brief descriptions of the full range of psychosocial services. At the first and essential level is basic social and emotional support provided by health-care providers. More formal interventions, generally provided by professionals with advanced specialized training, include psycho-educational, cognitive, and behavioral approaches, and additionally, psychotherapeutic (group and individual), psychopharmacologic, and complementary therapies.

Basic Social and Emotional Support

Helping individuals cope with illness through personal interaction and empathy is the most basic level of support that all caregivers should provide. Oncologists and other medical professionals responsible for the care of women with breast cancer need to incorporate planning for psychosocial management as an integral part of treatment. Social and emotional support focuses on adjustment to diagnosis, apprehension regarding treatment, and existential concerns. Providing such basic emotional support is the responsibility of those treating women with breast cancer, and it can be enhanced by teams having good communication skills and the ability to recognize significant distress, but it can also be provided individually by peers or clergy, or in group settings such as a support group (Spira, 1998). Providers can take several of the following steps to help individuals cope with "normal" levels of distress (NCCN Distress management Guidelines, 2003):

- clarify diagnosis, treatment options and side effects and ensure that the patient understands the disease and her treatment options,
- acknowledge that distress is normal and expected and inform patients that points of transition can increase distress,
- build trust,
- mobilize resources and direct patient to appropriate educational materials and local resources,
- consider medication to manage symptoms (e.g., analgesics, hypnotics, anxiolytics), and
- ensure continuity of care.

Continued monitoring and re-evaluation are needed to determine if distress symptoms have exceeded "normal" expected levels and if a referral to more specialized psychosocial services is indicated. Signs and symptoms that should signal that a patient needs more help in coping include: excessive worries, excessive fears or sadness, anger or feeling out of control, preoccupation with illness, poor sleep or appetite, unclear thinking, despair, severe family problems, or spiritual crisis (NCCN Distress Management Guidelines, 2003). Figure 4-1 outlines the NCCN symptoms of "expected" distress and the "interventions" that will be helpful and are provided by the primary team.

Psychosocial Interventions

Psycho-Educational Approaches

Psychological and emotional support is often given in conjunction with providing education about breast cancer, its diagnosis and treatment, and

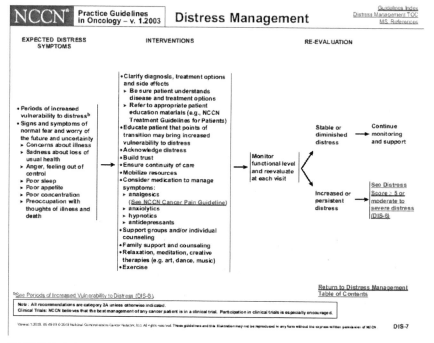

FIGURE 4-1
SOURCE: NCCN Distress Management Guideline [DIS 7].

other pertinent aspects of the cancer experience that affect quality of life. This support provides comfort, instills confidence, and reduces the stress of illness and of having to think through and decide about treatment options (Fawzy and Fawzy, 1998). Given the complexity of breast cancer care, physicians often do not have the time to extensively discuss treatment options and concerns regarding those options. Nurses, psychologists, and social workers are among the providers who augment information from other sources, directly address psychosocial concerns, and aid in the shared decision-making process. Psycho-education is also often a component in cognitive–behavioral interventions (see below).

Cognitive and Behavioral Interventions

Cognitive and behavioral interventions are among the most widely used in cancer centers (Goldman et al., 1998) (see Box 4-1). Based on the theory that physical and mental symptoms are altered by underlying thoughts, feelings and behaviors, several cognitive techniques are employed: distraction,

---

Box 4-1
Cognitive and Behavioral Interventions

Cognitive techniques

Distraction – redirection of attentional processes to reduce awareness of threatening events or aversive sensations.

Cognitive restructuring – critical examination and reevaluation of negative interpretations of events to reduce feelings of distress, helplessness, and hopelessness.

Mental/Guided imagery – use of mental imagery to promote relaxation, enhance perceived control, and improve coping.

Coping self-statements – silent or spoken self-statements used to manage, master, or reinterpret noxious or threatening situations and experiences.

Behavioral techniques

Contingency management – use of positive or negative reinforcement to increase the frequency of desired behaviors or reduce frequency of undesired behaviors.

Systematic desensitization – presenting to a relaxed individual increasingly potent anxiety-arousing stimuli (either in vivo or in imagination) to reduce phobic responses.

Biofeedback – providing relatively immediate information about a normally subliminal aspect of a physiologic function to facilitate learning voluntary control over this function.

Hypnosis – formal induction of a state characterized by sustained attention and concentration, reduced peripheral awareness, and openness to suggestion.

Progressive muscle relaxation – tensing and relaxing specific muscle groups and controlled deep breathing to reduce autonomic activation and induce subjective feelings of relaxation.

Autogenic training – use of suggestion and deep breathing to reduce autonomic arousal and induce a sense of relaxation.

SOURCE: Jacobsen and Hann, 1998.

---

cognitive-restructuring, guided imagery, and coping concepts to foster mastery of threatening situations. These approaches are particularly valuable in three areas: relief of pain, control of anticipatory nausea and vomiting associated with chemotherapy, and in enhancing emotional well-being (Jacobsen and Hann, 1998).

Behavioral interventions are widely used in several ways as outlined in Figure 4-1. Specific techniques for breast cancer patients are hypnosis, progressive muscle relaxation, and autogenic training to induce relaxation. These methods are commonly employed, primarily by psychologists, as adjuncts to pain management and to reduce anxiety, particularly in anticipation of a frightening experience or procedure.

Meditation is another behavioral intervention that has been studied for its effects on physical and emotional symptoms. Kabat-Zinn has popularized mindfulness-based meditation which patients can learn with a therapist and then apply later on their own by use of an audiotape or a self-induced state (Kabat-Zinn et al., 1998). It is often taught in 8–10 group sessions, as well as individual sessions, with exercises to be practiced at home. Frequently, meditation is used in conjunction with other behavioral methods, especially guided imagery and relaxation. Meditation is effective as a means of gaining self-control over distress and anxiety, and helps to control the distress and pain of advanced illness.

Psychotherapeutic Interventions

Psychotherapeutic approaches for women with breast cancer are focused on coping with cancer, but they permit dealing with issues from the past or present that affect the ability to deal with cancer (Sourkes et al., 1998). These approaches involve engaging the patient in a dialogue in which the therapist shows support and empathy, and often uses the range of clinical techniques including some education, cognitive, and psychodynamic components that represent supportive psychotherapy. While theoretical bases may vary by therapist, most experienced clinicians use an "integrative" model of psychotherapy that, at a clinical level, tailors the interventions to the patient's personal needs (Stricker and Gooen-Piels, 2002).

Therapy, psychotherapy, and counseling are terms that are used interchangeably, but the content of these interventions is often not clearly defined, making it difficult to test them in randomized trials. Several types of psychotherapy, however, have been well described so that they can be administered systematically and replicated in research studies (e.g., Expressive–Supportive Psychotherapy [Spiegel et al., 1989], Interpersonal Psychotherapy and Counseling [Weissman, 1997], and Adjuvant Psychotherapy [Moorey et al., 1994]). Outlined below are several psychotherapeutic approaches that can be delivered in individual or group sessions. Chapter 5 describes the most rigorous evidence (randomized trials) on the effectiveness of these interventions, and later chapters, in particular Chapter 6, discuss how women can find out about some of these treatment options and gain access to them.

Crisis counseling The most common form of clinical intervention is brief counseling, which is typically done in relation to coping with a crisis. The crises usually occur around the time of a change in illness status or treatment and result in a transient sense of vulnerability and distress. Counseling at these periods is time-limited and focused on overcoming a present problem or crisis. Underlying personal or psychological problems are not explored (Loscalzo and Brintzenhofeszoc, 1998). The focus is on quickly regaining equilibrium and normal coping ability. Cognitive techniques of problem-solving and restructuring the perception of the crisis may also be employed. The patient may express acute emotional distress, disbelief, anguish, terror, rage, envy, disinterest, or yearning for death. When expressed, these emotions tend to diminish and the illness can be faced more realistically. Although not specific to cancer in general, or breast cancer specifically, Pollin has described medical crisis counseling and funded an institute to advance short-term crisis counseling at Harvard Medical School (Pollin, 1995). This approach has also been reported to have some success in supporting, and enhancing satisfaction among, cancer patients in a small controlled trial (20 experimental, 18 control), and perhaps to decrease the costs of mental health services to this population (Koocher and Pollin, 2001).

Group therapy and counseling The most widely used intervention for psychosocial support is support groups. Groups are available at most cancer centers, at community hospitals, and in voluntary organizations like Gilda's Clubs and The Wellness Community. They can be led by either peers or professionals and usually include 8 to 12 sessions. Groups may be closed with the same individuals or may remain open, permitting patients to enter at any time and continue indefinitely. The latter is more appropriate for more severe stages of illness. For earlier disease, time-limited, focused sessions are held to deal with adjustment or genetic risk, or confronting prophylactic mastectomy. Chapter 5 provides evidence of the effectiveness of group therapy from clinical trials. Clinically, these interventions appear to be helpful to many women because of the social support they provide. Yet there are other women who become more distressed being in a group because of what they hear from patients and because they find it difficult to share their experiences.

Pastoral counseling Some women with breast cancer rely on their spiritual or religious beliefs when dealing with illness. A diagnosis of cancer has been called a "psychospiritual crisis" because it forces the individual not only to cope psychologically, but also to confront the meaning of life and death (Fitchett and Handzo, 1998). Women may choose counseling from a pastoral counselor who can provide spiritual support and help address guilt, loss of faith, fear of punishment, and the need for prayer. Clinical practice guidelines were developed for pastoral counseling by the multidisciplinary panel of the National Comprehensive Cancer Network (NCCN, 2003).

Family therapy and counseling It is well recognized that cancer affects partners and children of women with breast cancer and that psychosocial issues related to breast cancer are often best addressed within the context of the family. Family therapy is frequently the approach of choice when illness forces changes in family roles and contributes to conflict (Lederberg, 1998; Jacobs et al., 1998). At stages of advanced illness when patients are being cared for at home, family issues become more crucial and assistance to the family is a vital aspect of care (Schachter and Coyle, 1998).

Grief therapy Psychological support for surviving family members becomes important when the patient dies. The oncology team that cared for the patient and knows the family is in a good position to monitor the level of grief and determine if a referral is needed for individual or group counseling (see Worden, 2001).

Sexual counseling Women with breast and gynecologic cancers often suffer the most from a sense of loss of femininity and may experience sexual problems secondary to premature menopause and treatment side effects. A skilled sexual therapist can be helpful to a couple in adjusting to such problems (Shell, 2002, and see section on sexual problems in Chapter 3)

Psychopharmacologic Interventions

Subsumed under psychosocial services are those modalities that combine psychosocial support and psychopharmacological intervention. Medication to reduce distress is prescribed to control symptoms in patients with severe symptoms that are not amenable to psychological or behavioral interventions alone. The most common forms of distress that become diagnosable psychiatric disorders (based on the classification system of the Diagnostic and Statistical Manual of Mental Disorders, Fourth Edition [DSM IV]) include dementia, delirium, mood disorder, adjustment disorder, anxiety disorder, substance abuse, and personality disorder. Patients whose psychosocial problems reach this level of severity have often had preexisting psychological or psychiatric problems (e.g., anxiety disorder, early dementia, recurrent depression), and dealing with cancer can easily exacerbate the disorder. Clinical practice guidelines are available to assist providers in the management of these disorders (e.g., NCCN Distress Management Guideline [DIS-8]) (see discussion of clinical practice guidelines in Chapter 6). The guidelines, for example, outline the use of antidepressants in combination with psychotherapy, an effective approach in the management of depression (Costa et al., 1985; Holland et al., 1998). These disorders range from mild to grave, but they clearly have high morbidity, are serious medical conditions that complicate the course of cancer, and often obligate psychopharmacological interventions. They require competent diagnosis and the application of appropriate therapies to properly mange what is medically treatable. An algorithm illustrating the management of mood disorder is shown in Figure 4-2.

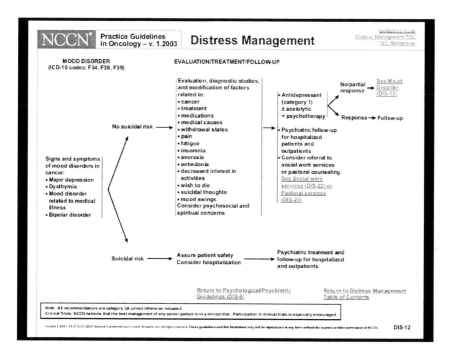

FIGURE 4-2 Clinical management of mood disorder.
SOURCE: NCCN Distress Management Guideline [DIS-12].

Complementary Therapies

Yoga, massage, exercise, acupuncture, and art, music, and dance therapy are examples of complementary therapies used by women with breast cancer to reduce psychosocial distress. Many psychological and behavioral interventions have become identified as complementary therapies. In some schemas, prayer, psychotherapy and nutrition are considered complementary regimens. This variation in defining complementary approaches has made studies of the frequency of their use difficult to interpret. These approaches are available at many clinical centers and in the community from voluntary organizations. Some recent evidence suggests use of alternative or complementary therapies may signal psychosocial distress among women with breast cancer (Burstein et al., 1999; Moschen et al., 2001) and in the general population (Unutzer et al., 2000) In general, there is less stigma attached to using these therapies than there is in seeking psychosocial services. Complementary programs appear to be popular, and randomized trials are underway to evaluate several of these methods.

As with other cancers, complementary or alternative therapies aimed at the physical disease are also often (25–50 percent) used by women with breast cancer. These therapies include nutrition-related measures, mistletoe preparations, trace elements and homeopathy, and others (Burstein et al, 1999, Moschen et al., 2000, U.S. Congress, 1990). Feelings of helplessness, fear, or panic; a desire to gain control, especially of a deteriorating situation; perceived lack of interest on the part of treating physicians; and willingness to try anything that might improve chances of a good outcome are among the reasons that women with breast cancer use complementary or alternative therapies (reviewed in U.S. Congress, 1990).

PROVIDERS OF PSYCHOSOCIAL CARE

Psychosocial services may be provided by the health-care professionals involved in breast cancer care, such as nurses, primary care physicians, surgeons, and oncologists, or by professionals with special training in social work, psychology, psychiatry, or pastoral counseling. Services might be conceptualized as basic, that is, provided as part of routine care by sympathetic and supportive physicians, nurses and clinic and hospital staff who come in contact with the breast cancer patient, supplemented at the next level by others like social workers, support groups, and clergy as needed, and moving in the presence of more serious problems to the highest level of specifically trained mental health professionals such as psychiatrists, psychologists, and clinical social workers (described in Holland, 1990).

Figure 4-3 illustrates the complexity of contemporary breast cancer care, showing the typical progression from screening to therapy and the many providers a woman might encounter as she completes her care. Follow-up care, while not quite the same as the specific disease targeted treatment identified in the figure, is also critical in the management of

Steps in breast cancer treatment				
1. Screening →	2. Diagnosis →	3. Surgery →	4. Adjuvant → therapy	5. Recurrence therapy

• Mammogram
• Ultrasound
	• Fine Needle
	   Aspiration
	• Biopsy
		• Breast
		   conserving
		   surgery
		• Mastectomy
			• Radiation
			• Chemotherapy
			• Hormonal
			   therapy
				• Radiation
				• Chemotherapy
				• Hormonal
				   therapy

Providers of care				

• Primary care
• Radiologist
	• Primary care
	• Radiologist
	• Pathologist
	• Surgeon
		• Surgeon	• Radiation
			   oncology
			• Medical
			   oncology
			• Surgeon
			• Primary care
				• Radiation
				   oncology
				• Medical
				   oncology
				• Surgeon
				• Primary care

FIGURE 4-3 The trajectory of breast cancer care.
SOURCE: Bicknell, IOM Workshop, October 2002.

cancer survivors. The IOM Childhood Cancer Survivorship report (Hewitt et al., 2003) and the forthcoming 2004 IOM Adult Cancer Survivorship report stress the importance of surveillance and interventions to manage late effects and other survivorship concerns by various health professionals

This section of the report describes the education, training, availability, and practice of the professionals involved in providing psychosocial services to women with breast cancer. Chapter 6 discusses the delivery of psychosocial services and points out strengths and weaknesses of various providers and settings. In general, it is clear from that discussion that improvements are needed in both communication by physicians and others and the knowledge base (not to mention the time and resources) to deliver psychosocial services more effectively. This section on professional education and practice provides background and explanation in part for some of the deficiencies identified in Chapter 6.

Nurses

Nursing represents the largest segment of the nation's health care workforce and has a significant role on the "front lines" of cancer care, both in hospitals and ambulatory settings (Ferrell et al., 2003; McCorkle et al., 1998). In 2000, an estimated 2.2 million registered nurses were employed full- or part-time nationwide (HRSA, 2000). Current information on the settings in which nurses practice suggests that the role of nursing in the provision of psychosocial services may have lessened, in the sense that relatively few nurses work in ambulatory and community-based settings, the places where most breast cancer care is delivered. In 2000, only 9 percent of nurses worked in ambulatory settings (HRSA, 2001). In addition, nursing shortages are contributing to short staffing and reducing the time available to assess or respond to other than acute care needs. Nevertheless, some surgeons' offices, most oncologists' offices, and all breast cancer clinics have an oncology nurse, so that for women in these settings, the oncology nurse plays a critical role in being sensitive to and often most aware of her psychosocial needs.

Basic nursing education rarely includes didactic training in oncology (Ferrell and Virani, 2002; McCorkle et al., 1998). Nurses generally receive some exposure to cancer care through coursework related to surgical and medical care of chronic diseases. Nurses may receive general instruction regarding psychology and communications, but their training often inadequately prepares them to work in oncology and gives them a limited understanding of the theoretical content related to psycho-oncology. Burke and Kissane (1998) found this to be the case in Australia and the same is true in the United States (Burke and Kissane, 1998; McCorkle et al., 1998). A cancer nursing curriculum guide for baccalaureate nursing has been developed that addresses psychosocial aspects of cancer care (Sarna and McCorkle, 1995), but the extent of its adoption is not known. Likewise, continuing education opportunities have been described (McCorkle et al., 1998), but the extent of enrollment in such programs is not known. McCorkle is presently developing an online curriculum for oncology nurses in the use of the NCCN Distress Management Guideline to enable them to recognize and assess patients' distress and apply the algorithm for referral to specialized mental health services (McCorkle, personal communication to Jimmie Holland, March 2003). Oncology nurses who are trained in psychiatric nursing are very effective as mental health professionals in cancer care.

Advanced training in oncology nursing is available, but of the 270 nursing graduate programs, only 26 offer a special oncology focus (Ferrell, workshop presentation, October 2002; Brown and Hinds, 1998)). Of these 26 programs, only 18 percent were found in 2000 to cover rehabilitation services, and 68 percent covered pain management. Following initiatives to improve training in end-of-life and palliative care, all programs were found to cover these areas when surveyed again in 2002. This suggests that major changes in curriculum can occur in response to interventions to improve nursing education.

Currently, the Oncology Nursing Society has certified 19,596 nurses as basic level credential adult oncology (OCN®) nurses, 803 basic level credential pediatric oncology (CPON®) nurses, and 1,410 as advanced oncology credential (AOCN®) nurses (Cynthia Miller Murphy, Oncology Nursing Certification Corporation, Executive Director, personal communication to Roger Herdman, September 4, 2003). To be eligible for certification, a nurse must have one-year of nursing experience as an RN, and 1,000 hours of oncology nursing experience. Advanced practice nurses provide models for clinical practice, education, and advocacy. Currently, there are 29,802 members of the Oncology Nursing Society (Cynthia Miller Murphy, Oncology Nursing Certification Corporation, Executive Director, personal communication to Roger Herdman, September 4, 2003).

In the United Kingdom and Australia, a specialty within nursing on breast care has been developed (Liebert et al., 2003; Redman et al., 2003). These breast care nurses provide education, psychosocial interventions, and case management. Nurses with doctoral degrees (including psychology) have made an important contribution to psychosocial oncology clinical research. Several nursing schools have graduate training in psychosocial research, and their faculty provide the field of psycho-oncology with a valuable cohort of senior investigators while also serving as mentors to Ph.D. candidates. Within the Oncology Nursing Society, approximately

150 nurse investigators are identified as a section with specialized interest in this area.

Primary Care Physicians

Primary care physicians, including specialists in internal medicine, family practice, obstetrics and gynecology, and geriatrics, receive little formal training in elements of psychology and essentially none in communication. What training is received is often limited to experience during a residency program when ambulatory management of chronic illnesses is covered. A review of primary care and internal medicine textbooks for content related to cancer survivorship, conducted for the Board, revealed little content on survivorship, and in the area of breast cancer, little mention of psychosocial issues (Winn, 2002). A comprehensive review of primary care for survivors of breast cancer, published in the *New England Journal of Medicine,* addresses all the major domains of breast cancer survivorship, including psychosocial issues (Goldman et al., 1998). There are relatively few continuing medical education (CME) offerings related to cancer survivorship available to primary care providers, according to a review conducted for the Board (Winn, 2002). One important CME resource is a monograph, *Cancer Survivorship*, available through the American Association of Family Practice (AAFP, 2001). The monograph includes information on late effects of treatment, evaluation of common problems in survivors (including depression and anxiety), disability, and discrimination and related issues (Winn, 2002). Annual meetings of professional societies provide other opportunities for education. As part of the Women's Health Session at the 2001 meeting of the American College of Physicians, for example, a module on breast cancer was presented, and it contained a segment on long-term management of breast cancer ,survivors that included psychosocial issues.

Surgeons

A surgeon is often the first physician specialist a woman sees after her diagnosis of breast cancer. The American Board of Surgery had certified 47,000 surgeons as of 2000, and there are about 1,500 members of the American Society of Breast Surgeons (www.breastsurgeons.org, accessed April 2, 2003). Board certification in surgery requires clinical competencies, including interpersonal and communication skills that result in effective information and teaming with patients, their families, and other health professionals.

The American College of Surgeons' Commission on Cancer has a program to approve cancer care facilities that meet certain standards, including standards regarding the provision of psychosocial services (see Chapter 6).

Surgeons' training in communication skills and breaking bad news has been limited. As yet, there has been no national effort to include this in training, though many surgical oncology training programs acknowledge its importance. Trainees learn largely by observing senior members in their interactions with patients.

Radiation Oncologists

Most women with early stage cancer who choose a lumpectomy will be referred to a radiation oncologist after their surgery as part of their primary treatment. Patients with metastatic breast cancer are also often treated by radiation oncologists for control of pain related to bone metastases. The American Board of Radiology had certified 3,540 radiation oncologists as of 2002 (American Board of Medical Specialties, 2002). According to the American Society for Therapeutic Radiology and Oncology, there were 3,174 radiation therapeutic oncologists in 1,400 practices as of 2002. The training of radiotherapists has generally not included communication skills. The daily visits to a radiation oncology unit and daily contact with technicians provide an important setting for positive, sensitive interaction and psychosocial support.

Medical Oncologists

Women with breast cancer usually consult a medical oncologist, especially when contemplating initial treatment for adjuvant chemotherapy in the presence of positive axillary nodes and with recurrence and progressive disease for chemotherapy aimed at palliation with second- and third-line therapy. As of 2003, 8,901 United States medical oncologists had been validly certified by the American Board of Internal Medicine. Roughly 14,000 United States-based physicians belong to the American Society of Clinical Oncology (ASCO), the largest professional society dedicated to clinical oncology issues (www.asco.org, accessed January 21, 2003). The curriculum that is used to train medical oncologists and hematologists is determined by the American Council of Graduate Medical Education. Rehabilitation and psychosocial aspects of clinical management of the cancer patient are core content areas for training. Oncology textbooks contain limited information on psychosocial aspects of care according to a review conducted for the Board (Winn, 2002). The standard general oncology text, *Cancer Principles and Practice of Oncology*, for example, includes a section, Supportive Care and Quality of Life (pp. 2977–3088) with a chapter on psychological issues (Massie et al., 2001) and a chapter on community resources (Indeck and Smith, 2001). *Cancer Medicine* has included a chapter on Principles of Psycho-Oncology in each of its 6 editions (Holland and Gooen-Piels, 2003).

In the text, *Diseases of the Breast* (Harris, 2000), there has been a chapter on psychosocial issues in each edition (Rowland and Massie, 2000). Gynecologic texts also include chapters addressing these issues. Abstracts of new psychosocial and quality-of-life research are presented at the annual meetings of the American Society of Clinical Oncology (ASCO). At the 2002 meeting of ASCO, for example, there were three sessions devoted to issues related to adjustment to cancer (Winn, 2002). ASCO has a communication initiative for oncologists and oncology trainees that offers workshops for interested members. This is being developed into a formal training program that will be conducted annually (Schapira, 2003). There are several formal psycho-oncology training programs that offer fellowships to physicians (e.g., Memorial Sloan-Kettering Cancer Center, Mount Sinai Ruttenberg Cancer Center, Dana-Farber Cancer Institute, University of Pennsylvania). Most oncologists, however, do not have formal training in psycho-oncology and instead may be trained through case management sessions.

Social Workers

Social workers are the primary providers of psychosocial services in hospitals and many cancer centers and are trained to facilitate patient and family adjustment to a cancer diagnosis, its treatment, and rehabilitation (Smith et al., 1998). Social workers may also refer cancer patients and family members who show signs of distress or who have significant family or social problems to psychologists or psychiatrists. In small oncology practices, social workers may be the only professionals available for handling the range of psychological and social problems occurring with cancer. Oncology social workers have a Master of Social Work (M.S.W.) degree and receive training in chronic illness issues in graduate school. Social workers assist cancer patients by addressing the range of psychosocial needs; by providing help with concrete services, such as assisting with insurance and benefits; by serving as case managers to coordinate care and help patients navigate health-care systems; by leading peer support groups; and by referring to community services (Box 4-2). Clinical practice guidelines have been developed by the NCCN to assist social workers in the management of psychosocial distress among patients and families with cancer (NCCN, 2003).

There is no formal accreditation in oncology available for social workers. However, the Association of Oncology Social Work (AOSW) serves as an educational resource. AOSW, with a membership of approximately 1,000 social workers, provides continuing education and online information (www.aosw.org). Psychiatric social workers who have additional training in psycho-oncology are particularly valuable as mental health professionals in oncology. *The Journal of Psychosocial Oncology*, begun in 1983,

---

Box 4-2
Oncology Social Work: Scope of Practice

- Clinical Practice: complete psychosocial assessments; develop multidisciplinary care plans; provide therapeutic interventions and case management; assist with financial, transportation, lodging and other needs; advocate to remove barriers to care and address gaps in service; advance knowledge through research.
- Within Cancer Centers/Institutions: provide education and consultation to professionals and staff regarding psychosocial and other factors affecting cancer care; collaborate in the delivery of psychosocial care, education, and research; develop programs and resources to address the needs of cancer survivors.
- Within the Community: Increase awareness of psychosocial needs of cancer survivors, families, and caregivers; collaborate with community agencies to remove barriers to care; collaborate in the development of special programs and resources to address community-based needs; consult with voluntary agencies to provide community education and develop programs.
- Within the Social Work Profession: teach in the classroom or in clinical settings; supervise and evaluate practitioners; consult with colleagues; participate in research.

SOURCE: http://www.aosw.org/mission/scope.html.

---

reports research findings and clinical observations relevant to the social workers involved in oncology.

A number of structured post-graduate opportunities are available for social workers wishing to specialize in oncology. The American Cancer Society (ACS) offers the following career development grants for social workers (www.cancer.org):

• **Master's Training Grants in Clinical Oncology Social Work:** Awarded to institutions to support training of second-year master's degree students to provide psychosocial services to persons with cancer and their families. One-year awards are made for $12,000 (trainee stipend of $10,000 and $2,000 for faculty/administrative support).

• **Doctoral Training Grants in Clinical Oncology Social Work:** Awarded to doctoral degree candidate to conduct research related to the psychosocial needs of persons with cancer and their families. Awards are made for up to three years with annual funding of $20,000 (trainee stipend of $15,000 and $5,000 for faculty/administrative support).

ACS also offers a number of fellowships that allow social workers to gain experience in palliative and end-of-life care. The International Psycho-Oncology Society provides information about fellowship opportunities to social workers and others (www.ipos-society.org) as well as the American Psychosocial Oncology Society (www.apos-society.org, accessed April 3, 2003).

Psychology

Psychologists are the mental health professionals who, after social workers, are most likely to be available for clinical consultation and management of psychosocial concerns in patients with cancer and their families. They also represent the discipline that contributes predominantly to psycho-oncology and psychosocial oncology research. Psychologists receive a Ph.D. in clinical or health psychology or a Psy.D., Doctorate of Psychology. As of 2003 there were approximately 155,000 members of the American Psychological Association, the professional association that represents psychologists, of which nearly 3,000 belonged to the health division (Mr. Joel Gallardo, Communications Specialist, personal communication to Timothy Brennan, April 3, 2003). Undergraduate programs do not routinely include training in psycho-oncology, except as it might occur in conjunction with clinical rotations. Some health psychology graduate programs have faculty members who do research in psycho-oncology. Graduate students in these programs can elect dissertations dealing with oncology issues. Financial support for pre-doctoral students during their dissertation research has encouraged young investigators to enter the field. (J. Ostroff, personal communication to Jimmie Holland, March 2003).

Psychology internships are not available in the specialized area of oncology. However, many 2-year post-doctoral fellowships exist that permit training in either research or clinical work alone, or a combination of both. A large number of members of The Society of Behavioral Medicine have their career emphasis in some area of psychosocial or behavioral oncology. They have made major contributions in cancer prevention, cancer control, and life-style change, such as smoking cessation.

Counseling

There are many Master's level counselors who are trained in general counseling and who work primarily in family service agencies and corporate Employment Assistance Programs (EAP). A demonstration project, sponsored by Bristol-Myers Squibb Foundation, is underway to train 150 counselors in a "face-to-face" and distance learning program in psychosocial oncology. If successful, the core curriculum, being developed for the program by Cancer Care, Inc., and The American Psychosocial Oncology Society (APOS), can train a new cadre of counselors who will be available in smaller communities and rural areas (J. Holland, personal communication to Maria Hewitt, March 2003).

Psychiatry

Psychiatrists with an interest in diagnosis and treatment of comorbid psychological problems and psychiatric disorders are known as consultation-liaison psychiatrists. The American Psychiatric Association, The American Board of Neurology and Psychiatry, and The American Board of Medical Specialties have given approval for a sub-specialty certification of psychiatry in the care of the medically ill (initial examinations are expected in 2005). Among the 1,000 United States psychiatrists who work primarily with the medically ill, approximately 100 identify oncology as the major focus of their clinical work, and work with cancer patients either on a full-time basis or as a significant part of their clinical care. Control of symptoms that reduce quality of life, such as severe anxiety, depression, and delirium, requires management of psychopharmacologic interventions and awareness of drug–drug interactions in the context of complex oncologic treatment.

Several of the early, major academic departments and divisions of psycho-oncology have been directed by psychiatrists who developed multidisciplinary clinical and research teams. Psychiatric residents must rotate for a period of time, after internship, through the in- and out-patient units, where they learn the common psychiatric disorders of chronically medically ill patients and their psychological and psychopharmacological management. Post-residency clinical fellowships of 1 or 2 years can be taken in psychiatric and psychosocial oncology at a few major academic cancer centers. These few centers have contributed many of the young clinicians and investigators in the field. Psychiatrists, along with psychologists, have contributed to the research portfolio, the development of two textbooks of psycho-oncology (Holland and Rowland, 1989; Holland et al., 1998) and the journal, *Psycho-oncology, Journal of the Psychological, Social and Behavioral Dimensions of Cancer,* begun in 1992. More psychiatrists will have to be encouraged to enter into this area to increase the amount of clinical and research activities in the field.

Pastoral Counseling

Only in recent years have the contributions by pastoral counselors and clergy to psycho-oncology begun to be recognized. A diagnosis of cancer continues to be regarded as a threat to life, bringing the possibility of death into focus. For many patients, confronting issues of life and death constitutes a spiritual or existential crisis. As illness advances, the search for meaning by patients leads many to seek religious or spiritual counselors to assist them in coping. Chaplains, clergy, and pastoral counselors may be preferred to secular counselors. The NCCN *Clinical Practice Guidelines for Management of Distress*, written by a multidisciplinary panel, included pastoral counseling and pastoral counselors as an integral part of psychosocial services and psychosocial professionals involved in supportive services (NCCN, 2003).

Many hospital chaplaincy programs give training in clinical pastoral counseling to young seminarians who spend months to a year gaining experience with hospitalized or ambulatory patients. Certification of these programs is done by a national accrediting body, The National Association of Professional Chaplains, which networks clergy working in medical settings. Several journals cover this overlapping area of medicine and clergy (e.g., *Journal of Psychology and Theology, Journal for the Scientific Study of Religion, Journal of Religion and Health*). Information about spiritual assessment and counseling is now available. An issue of *Psycho-oncology* was devoted to spiritual and religious aspects of psychosocial oncology (Russak et al., 1999).

Specialized Counselors

There are some situations that require counseling services delivered by professionals with specialized skills.

Sexual Counseling.

Women with breast cancer and gynecologic cancer often experience significant problems in sexual self-image and sexual function. Premature menopause and altered breast and/or pelvic organs create significant distress. Counselors knowledgeable about the sexual side effects of cancer treatment (e.g., reduced libido and desire, reduced lubrication, and painful intercourse) can counsel a woman and her partner in both the psychological/psychosexual and practical issues arising from these difficulties. Sexuality counselors, accredited by the American Association of Sex Educators, Counselors, and Therapists, can be located through the Association (www.aasect.org, accessed April 2, 2003).

Grief Counselors

The family caregiver who survives the loss of a loved one to cancer will experience normal symptoms of grief. This grief is sometimes alleviated by group or one-on-one counseling. Grief counselors are skilled at assessment and psychosocial counseling and support. Those who have worked in oncology are particularly helpful in dealing with the family and loss. The Association for Death Education and Counseling provides a registry of accredited grief therapists (www.adec.org, accessed April 2, 2003).

Psychosocial Oncologists

A range of disciplines and specialists provide psychosocial services to women with breast cancer and to patients in general. In addition to the oncologist and oncology nurse, these services may be provided by an oncology social worker, a psychiatric social worker, a psychiatric nurse clinician, psychologist, psychiatrist, pastoral counselor, or veteran patients who become effective volunteer counselors and advocates. This brings a wealth of experience to the field and a diversity of theoretical frameworks and clinical practice. However, it has also served to make it difficult to ensure that there is a core of knowledge about psychosocial oncology that is common to all disciplines and that can serve as a benchmark for expected knowledge/information in the field. The American Psychosocial Oncology Society (APOS) (www.apos-society.org) is developing a core psychosocial oncology curriculum that will be available free online. Lectures will be given by experts in each topic accompanied by slides and a bibliography. The areas to be covered are: Core Courses, Symptom Management, Site-Specific Issues, Psychosocial Interventions, Population-Specific Issues, Research, Medical Ethics. Optional topics will also be available. Those who complete the curriculum and examination will be added to the APOS Referral Directory which, similar to the effort by the American Society of Clinical Oncology, will serve as a national registry of psychosocial oncologists. An example of the curriculum for training in psycho-oncology is shown in Box 4-3 and that for advanced training in Box 4-4.

Continuing education opportunities are provided through several professional organizations: the World Congress of Psycho-Oncology, International Psycho-Oncology Society, Academy of Psychosomatic Medicine, Society of Behavioral Medicine, American Psychological Association, and American Psychiatric Association. Founded in 1986, the American Psychosocial Oncology Society (APOS) has undertaken a new initiative to network all the disciplines mentioned in this chapter that provide psychosocial services to patients with cancer. Its goal is to become a nationally recognized organization that advocates for improvement of psychosocial care for these patients and their families. The consumer advocacy groups (NABCO, NCCS) also voice the importance of these services to their members. Survivors of breast cancer have played a

---

Box 4-3
Objectives of Psycho-oncology Training

- Conduct psychiatric/psychosocial evaluations of cancer patients so as to recognize common psychiatric syndromes, disorders, distress and be aware of cancer-site and treatment-specific psychiatric problems.
- Appropriately apply a range of psychiatric/psychosocial interventions for cancer patients psychotherapy including individual, family, group, supportive, crisis intervention, sexual, bereavement, cognitive-behavioral, psychopharmacology.
- Work effectively in a liaison role, provide support to oncology staff so as to better facilitate understanding of patient and family centered issues.
- Communicate psycho-oncology information to others, oral and written dissemination of clinically based or research-oriented practices/findings, teach medical students, psychiatric interns, residents.
- Be able to critically evaluate and understand and/or conduct research in psycho-oncology.
- Learn organizational and administrative skills needed to administer a psycho-oncology program.

SOURCE: Passik et al., 1998.

Box 4-4.
Curriculum for Advanced Training in Psycho-oncology

I. MEDICAL FACTORS AND THEIR PSYCHOLOGICAL CORRELATES
- Basic concepts in cancer and its treatments
- Cancer development
- Cancer risk factors
- Diagnostic procedures
- Treatment modalities
- Central nervous system complications of cancer
- Cancer pain and its management
- Psychological effects of cancer and its treatment
- Stage-specific issues
- Treatment-specific issues
- Site-specific issues

II. PSYCHOSOCIAL ASPECTS OF CANCER
- Social factors and adaptation to cancer
- Psychological factors
- Coping with a life-threatening illness
- Social support
- Family adaptation to cancer
- Childhood cancer
- The older patient with cancer
- Sexual dysfunctions in cancer patients
- The oncology staff

III. COMMON PSYCHIATRIC DISORDERS AND THEIR MANAGEMENT
- Normal reactions and psychiatric disorders in cancer patients
- Depression
- Suicide
- Anxiety, panic attacks and phobias
- Personality disorders
- Somatoform disorders
- Schizophrenia
- Pharmacological management of psychiatric disorders in cancer patients
- Psychiatric emergencies

iv. ethical issues in cancer care
- Informed consent
- Do Not Resuscitate (DNR) Orders

v. cultural aspects of cancer care
- Varied attitudes towards illness and treatments
- Death and dying
- Mourning rituals and bereavement
- Suicide
- Support systems
- Choice of therapy and treatment compliance

VI. RESEARCH
- Research methods in psycho-oncology

SOURCE: Passik et al., 1998.

strong role in changing national policy regarding health care delivery in Australia (Redman et al, 2003).

SUMMARY

A variety of approaches exist to address psychosocial distress that occurs among individuals with cancer. Some of the more common ones include social and emotional support, psychoeducational approaches, cognitive–behavioral interventions, psychotherapy, crisis counseling, and complementary approaches. Providers of these psychosocial services may include clinicians involved in medical care, such as physicians and nurses, and professionals trained in social work, psychology, and psychiatry. Optimally, these providers work collaboratively to meet the psychosocial needs of women with breast cancer.

Evidence suggests that health-care providers have limited training to provide psychosocial support to individuals with cancer and there are relatively few post graduate or continuing educational opportunities in this area. Given the effectiveness of psychosocial interventions in alleviating psychosocial distress, the Board recommends that:

Sponsors of professional education and training programs (e.g., NCI, ACS, ASCO, ONS, AOSW, ACS-CoC, APOS) should support continuing education programs by designing, recommending, or funding them at a level that recognizes their importance in psycho-oncology for oncologists, those in training programs, and nurses and for further development of programs similar to the ASCO program to improve clinicians' communication skills; and

Graduate education programs for oncology clinicians, primary care practitioners, nurses, social workers, and psychologists should evaluate their capacity to incorporate a core curriculum in psycho-oncology in their overall curriculum. This curriculum should be taught by an adequately trained faculty in psycho-oncology and should include relevant questions in examination requirements.

Education and training opportunities are needed across the cancer care continuum, for providers of primary care and for individuals providing counseling and psychiatric services. While new education and training programs are needed for all cancer care providers, the Board concluded that improvements in access to psychosocial services could most quickly be made with investments in programs for nurses. Nurses play a central role in providing cancer care and currently have very limited oncology training. As a first step, the Board recommends integrating psychosocial content into basic nursing education (baccalaureate and associate degree) programs. Investments in training related to pain management and end-of-life care have led to curricular improvements and new requirements on nursing licensure exams. Continuing education for clinical nurses regarding psychosocial issues is also needed given the limited exposure to this area in undergraduate curriculums. Increased support of oncology specialty education within graduate programs and promotion of certification in oncology nursing through the OCN® and AOCN® examination process could effectively increase the ranks of nurse leaders able to provide supportive care services, train colleagues, and conduct psychosocial research.

REFERENCES

AAFP. 2001. *AAFP Home Study Self-Assessment.* AAFP Monograph 264, Cancer Survivorship. May 2001.

Brown JK, Hinds P. 1998. Assessing master's programs in advanced practice oncology nursing. *Oncol Nurs Forum* 25(8):1433–1434.

Burke S, Kissane DW. 1998. *Psychosocial Support for Breast Cancer Patients: A Review of Interventions by Specialist Providers: A Summary of the Literature 1976–1996.* Sydney: NHMRC National Breast Cancer Centre.

Burstein HJ, Gelber S, Guadagnoli E, Weeks JC. 1999. Use of alternative medicine by women with early-stage breast cancer. *N Engl J Med* 340(22):1733–1739.

Costa D, Mogos I, Toma T. 1985. Efficacy and safety of mianserin in the treatment of depression of women with cancer. *Acta Psychiatr Scand Suppl* 320:85–92.

Fawzy FI, Fawzy NW. 1998. Psychoeducational Interventions. In: Holland JC, ed. *Psycho-Oncology.* New York: Oxford University Press. Pp. 676–693.

Ferrell BR, Virani R, Smith S, Juarez G. 2003. The role of oncology nursing to ensure quality care for cancer survivors: A report commissioned by the national cancer policy board and institute of medicine. *Oncol Nurs Forum* 30(1):E1–E11.

Ferrell BR, Virani R. 2002. *The Role of Oncology Nursing to Insure Quality Care for Cancer Survivors.* Background paper prepared for the National Cancer Policy Board.

Fitchett G, Handzo G. 1998. Spiritual assessment, screening and intervention. In: Holland JC, ed. *Psycho-Oncology.* New York: Oxford University Press. Pp. 790–808.

Goldman W, McCulloch J, Sturm R. 1998. Costs and use of mental health services before and after managed care. *Health Aff (Millwood)* 17(2):40–52.

Harris JR. 2000. *Diseases of the Breast.* 2nd ed. Philadelphia: Lippincott Williams & Wilkins.

Health Resources and Services Administration, Bureau of National Health Professions, U.S. Department of Health and Human Services. March 2000. *The Registered Nurse Population.* Findings from the National Sample of Registered Nurses.

Hewitt, M, Weiner, SL, Simone, JV, eds. 2003. *Childhood Cancer Survivorship: Improving Care and Quality of Life.* Washington, DC: Institute of Medicine, National Academy Press.

Holland JC, Rowland JH. eds. 1989. *Handbook of Psycho-oncology: Psychological Care of the Patient with Cancer.* New York: Oxford University Press.

Holland JC, Romano SJ, Heiligenstein JH, Tepner RG, Wilson MG. 1998. A controlled trial of fluoxetine and desipramine in depressed women with advanced cancer. *Psycho-oncology* 7(4):291–300.

Holland JC, Gooen-Piels J. 2003. Principles of psycho-oncology. In: Holland JF et al., eds. *Cancer Medicine.* 6th ed. Ontario: B.C. Decker.

Holland, JC. 1990. Clinical course of cancer. In: Holland JC, Rowland JH, eds. *Handbook of PsychoOncology: Psychological Care of the Patient with Cancer.* New York: Oxford University Press.

Indeck BA, Smith PM. 2001. Community resources. In: DeVita VT, Hellman S, Rosenberg, SA, eds. *Cancer Principles and Practice of Oncology* 6th ed. Philadelphia: Lippincott. Pp. 3066–3076.

Jacobs J, Ostroff J, Steinglass P. 1998. Family therapy: A systems approach to cancer care. In: Holland JC, ed. *Psycho-Oncology.* New York: Oxford University Press. Pp. 994–1003.

Jacobsen PB, Hann DM. 1998. Cognitive–behavioral interventions. In: Holland JC, ed. *Psycho-Oncology.* New York: Oxford University Press. Pp. 717–729.

Kabat-Zinn J, Ohm Massion A, Rosenbaum E. 1998. Meditation. In: Holland JC, ed. *Psycho-Oncology.* New York: Oxford University Press. Pp. 767–779.

Koocher GP, Pollin I. 2001. Preventive psychosocial intervention in cancer treatment: Implications for managed care. In: Baum A, Anderson BL, eds. *Psychosocial Interventions for Cancer.* Washington, DC: American Psychological Association.

Lederberg MS. 1998. The family of the cancer patient. In: Holland JC, ed. *Psycho-Oncology.* New York: Oxford University Press. Pp. 981–993.

Liebert B, Parle M, Roberts C, Redman S, Carrick S, Gallagher J, Simpson J, Ng K, et al. 2003. An evidence-based specialist breast nurse role in practice: A multicentre implementation study. *Eur J Cancer Care (Engl)* 12(1):91–97.

Loscalzo M, Brintzenhofeszoc K. 1998. Brief Crisis Counseling. In: Holland JC, ed. *Psycho-Oncology.* New York: Oxford University Press. Pp. 662–675.

Massie M, Chertkov L, Roth A. 2001. Psychological issues. In: DeVita VT, Hellman S, Rosenberg SA, eds. *Cancer Principles and Practice of Oncology.* 6th ed. Philadelphia: Lippincott. Pp. 3058–3065.

McCorkle R, Frank-Stromborg M, Pasacreta JV. 1998. Education of nurses in psycho-oncology. In: Holland JC, ed. *Psycho-Oncology.* New York: Oxford University Press. Pp. 1069–1073.

Moorey S, Greer S, Watson M, Baruch JDR, Robertson BM, Mason A, Rowden L, Tunmore R, Law M, Bliss JM. 1994. Adjuvant psychological therapy for patients with cancer: Outcome at one year. *Psycho-Onoclogy* 3(1):1–10.

Moschen R, Kemmler G, Schweigkofler H, Holzner B, Dunser M, Richter R, Fleischhacker WW, Sperner-Unterweger B. 2001. Use of alternative/complementary therapy in breast cancer patients—a psychological perspective. *Support Care Cancer* 9(4):267–274.

NCCN. Clinical Practice Guidelines for Management of Distress. *Journal of the NCCN,* 2003.

Passik SD, Ford CV, Massie MJ. 1998. Training psychiatrists and psychologists in psychooncology. In: Holland JC, ed. *Psycho-Oncology.* New York: Oxford University Press. Pp. 1055–1060.

Pollin I. 1995. *Medical Crisis Counseling: Short Term Therapy for Long Term Illness.* New York: W. W. Norton.

Redman S, Turner J, Davis C. 2003. Improving supportive care for women with breast cancer in Australia: The challenge of modifying health systems. *Psycho-oncology* 12(6): 521–531.

Rowland JR, Massie MJ. 2000. Psychosocial issues and interventions. In: Harris JR et al, eds. *Diseases of the Breast.* 2nd ed. Philadelphia: Lippincott Williams & Wilkins. Pp. 1009–1031.

Russak SM, Lederberg M, Fitchett G, eds. 1999. Spirituality and coping with cancer. Special edition of *Psycho-oncology.* 8(5):375–466.

Sarna L, McCorkle R. 1995. A cancer nursing curriculum guide for baccalaureate nursing education. *Cancer Nurs* 18(6):445–451.

Schachter S, Coyle N. 1998. Palliative home care: Impact on families. In: Holland JC, eds. *Psycho-Oncology.* New York: Oxford University Press. Pp. 1004–1015.

Schapira L. 2003. Communication skills training in clinical oncology: The ASCO position reviewed and an optimistic personal perspective. *Crit Rev Oncol Hematol* 46(1):25–31.

Shell JA. 2002. Evidence-based practice for symptom management in adults with cancer: Sexual dysfunction. *Oncol Nurs Forum* 29(1):53–66.

Smith ED, Walsh-Burke K, Crusan C. 1998. Principles of training social workers. In: Holland JC, ed. *Psycho-Oncology.* New York: Oxford University Press. Pp. 1061–1068.

Sourkes BM, Massie MJ, Holland JC. 1998. Psychotherapeutic issues. In: Holland JC, ed. *Psycho-Oncology.* New York: Oxford University Press. Pp. 694–700.

Spiegel D, Bloom JR, Kraemer HC, Gottheil E. 1989. Effect of psychosocial treatment on survival of patients with metastatic breast cancer. *Lancet* 2(8668):888–891.

Spira JL. 1998. Group therapies. In: Holland JC, ed. *Psycho-Oncology*. New York: Oxford University Press. Pp. 701–716.

Stricker G and Gooen-Piels J. 2002. Research on object relations and an integrative approach to psychotherapy. In: Nolan IS, Nolan P, eds. *Object Relations & Integrative Psychotherapy: Tradition & Innovation in Theory & Practice*. London and Philadelphia: Whurr.

Unutzer J, Klap R, Sturm R, Young AS, Marmon T, Shatkin J, Wells KB. 2000. Mental disorders and the use of alternative medicine: Results from a national survey. *Am J Psychiatry* 157(11):1851–1857.

U. S. Congress, Office of Technology Assessment. 1990. *Unconventional Cancer Treatments*, OTA-H-405. Washington, DC: U.S. Government Printing Office.

Weissman MM. 1997. Interpersonal psychotherapy: Current status. *Keio J Med* 46(3):105–110.

Winn RJ. 2002. *Cancer Survivorship: Professional Education and Training*.

Worden JW. 2001. *Grief Counseling and Grief Therapy: A Handbook for the Mental Health Practitioner*. 3rd ed. New York: Springer Publishing.

5

The Effectiveness of Psychosocial Intervention for Women with Breast Cancer

Health-care providers are offering and women are seeking a range of interventions to manage psychosocial distress following a diagnosis of breast cancer, but there is no strong evidence-based consensus indicating which interventions are effective in reducing distress and improving quality of life. This chapter provides a critical review of the most relevant and highest quality studies of the effectiveness of psychosocial interventions in breast cancer. Included are published randomized trials and selected non-randomized studies that were designed to evaluate the effectiveness of psychosocial interventions for women with breast cancer.[1] Excluded is the psychosocial literature in other cancers or in mixed groups of cancer patients, in which only some patients have breast cancer. Also not covered is the extensive literature relating to psychological issues surrounding breast cancer screening or identification of high-risk individuals. The effectiveness of the treatment of mental disorders such as major depression is not examined, although, according to a recent review, pharmacologic treatment of cancer patients who are clinically depressed is effective if antidepressants are administered appropriately (Agency for Healthcare and Research and Quality, 2002). Underlying psychiatric disorders may worsen or be exacerbated

[1]This chapter is based on a commissioned paper by Pamela J. Goodwin, M.D., M.Sc., FRCPC, Marvelle Koffler Breast Centre, Department of Medicine, Division of Epidemiology, Samuel Lunenfeld Research Institute, Mount Sinai Hospital, University of Toronto and presented at the National Cancer Policy Board workshop *Meeting Psychosocial Needs of Women with Breast Cancer* on October 28–29, 2002 at the Institute of Medicine in Washington, DC.

following a diagnosis of cancer, and psychopharmacologic treatment can reduce distress and improve quality of life.

The chapter begins with a brief history of psychosocial intervention research in breast cancer followed by a discussion of methodological issues that are crucial to assessing the effectiveness of psychosocial interventions. An enumeration of research priorities to address identified knowledge gaps is outlined in Chapter 8.

HISTORY OF PSYCHOSOCIAL INTERVENTION RESEARCH

In the past decade, considerable resources have been allocated to research into the psychosocial aspects of breast cancer. Much of this research has focused on describing the emotional experience of women with breast cancer and developing interventions that reduce the psychosocial distress and improve coping and adjustment. Early intervention studies were done by Ferlic and colleagues (1979) and by Heinrich and Schag (1985), both with positive psychosocial results. A report by David Spiegel et al. that appeared in *The Lancet* in 1989 suggested, for the first time, that a psychological intervention (supportive–expressive group therapy) might prolong survival in women living with metastatic breast cancer (Spiegel et al., 1989). This observation heightened interest in survival effects of psychosocial interventions and led to a series of intervention studies in breast cancer (Classen et al., 2001; Cunningham et al., 1998; Edelman et al., 1999a; Goodwin et al., 2001) and other cancers (Fawzy et al., 1993; Ilnyckyj et al., 1994; Kuchler et al., 1999; Linn et al., 1982), conducted mainly in the 1990s. These studies attempted to confirm a beneficial effect of psychological interventions on survival. None of the subsequent studies in metastatic breast cancer has identified a survival effect of a range of psychological interventions (although one is ongoing) (Cunningham et al., 1998; Edelman et al., 1999a; Edmonds et al., 1999; Goodwin et al., 2001). Three studies in other malignancies (leukemia, melanoma, and mixed GI cancers) have reported survival benefits for brief interventions, delivered around the time of or shortly after diagnosis or during treatment (Fawzy et al., 1993; Kuchler et al., 1999, Richardson et al., 1990). These results have not been replicated. Nonetheless, throughout much of the 1990s, the focus of some members of the psycho-oncology research community shifted from evaluation of psychological effects of interventions to survival and intermediate biomedical effects, including enhancement of immune function. A growing recognition has developed that the survival effect in metastatic breast cancer that was seen by Spiegel et al. (Spiegel et al., 1989) has not been replicated and that little evidence supports the prognostic importance of intermediate outcomes such as cortisol levels that have been linked to psychosocial interventions, although it has been suggested that the Spiegel study at least indicated that these kinds of psychosocial interventions did not damage patients' coping skills in a way that would limit survivals. Spiegel has undertaken a replication study currently in progress.

Research focus is once again returning to the psychological status and quality of life of women with breast cancer, and to the identification of interventions that favorably influence their psychological and social functioning. An example is the report by Kissane and colleagues (2003) of a randomized, controlled trial of cognitive–existential group therapy for women with early breast cancer. It found the women in the intervention group showed significantly lower anxiety, and improved family function. The authors reported self-growth and increased knowledge of cancer and its treatment.

A number of excellent reviews of psychosocial interventions in breast cancer, and cancer in general, have been published recently (Burke and Kissane, 1998; Fawzy et al., 1995; Meyer and Mark, 1995; Newell et al., 2002; Rimer et al., 1985; Wallace, 1997). The majority of these reviews concluded that there are important benefits associated with the use of psychological interventions of various types in various cancer settings, including breast cancer. Fawzy et al. reviewed research into education, behavioral training, individual psychotherapy, and group interventions in cancer patients in general (Fawzy et al., 1995). They concluded that there was evidence of benefit for all of these approaches, reporting that cancer patients may benefit from a range of psychological intervention programs, and suggesting specific interventions at different points along the cancer trajectory. Meyer and Mark conducted a meta-analysis of psychosocial interventions in adult cancer patients (Meyer and Mark, 1995). Effect sizes (treatment mean minus control mean divided by pooled standard deviation) of 0.19–0.28 for emotional adjustment, functional adjustment, and global measures were identified. These effect sizes were in the range considered clinically important, suggesting significant benefit from the interventions. Burke and Kissane prepared a review of psychosocial interventions provided to breast cancer patients by specialist providers (including both published and unpublished data), drawing fairly extensively from the general cancer literature (Burke and Kissane, 1998). They concluded that the benefits of psychosocial interventions in breast cancer were clearly established and recommended that such interventions be an "integral part of comprehensive medical care." They presented a series of recommendations for future research and made more specific recommendations regarding integration of psychosocial interventions into the treatment setting. These were published in an overview paper outlining the need to challenge the health delivery system to improve and implement psychosocial and supportive care (Redman et al, 2003). Two targeted reviews concluded beneficial effects were present for relaxation and imagery interventions (Wallace, 1997) and for educational interventions in patients with cancer (Rimer et al., 1985). All of these reviews identified important areas for additional research.

One recent review reached somewhat different conclusions (Newell et al., 2002). The authors of this review undertook an extensive review of psychological therapies in all types of cancer—they applied a series of rigorous methodological standards and retained only those reports that scored one-third or more of the total possible points. This resulted in exclusion of the majority of published studies. They also took a very conservative approach to evaluation of benefits, requiring that at least half of the outcome measures for a specific attribute (e.g., mood) yield significant results for the effect to be classified as significant. This assumes that all of the questionnaires were equally responsive to change, a situation that is not likely. They examined the short, medium, and long-term impact of interventions on a large number of outcomes including anxiety, depression, hostility, general or overall affect, stress or distress, general or overall functional ability or quality of life, coping or coping skills, vocational or domestic adjustment, interpersonal or social relationships, sexual or marital relationships, nausea, vomiting, pain, fatigue, overall physical symptoms, conditioned nausea, conditioned vomiting, survival, and immune outcomes. They did not distinguish the effects of interventions among different types of cancers. These authors concluded that "only tentative recommendations about the effectiveness of psychosocial therapies for improving cancer patients' outcomes" were possible and recommended that future trials adhere to minimum methodological standards. Examples of their tentative recommendations included the use of music therapy to reduce anxiety and enhance overall affect, group therapy to enhance coping skills, counseling to enhance social or interpersonal relationships, and hypnosis to reduce conditioned nausea and vomiting. Further research was recommended into the benefits of these and other forms of therapy, including cognitive behavioral therapy, education, individual therapy, and interventions involving significant others. This review was thorough, but it did not focus on a specific type of cancer or a specific type of treatment, and its strict application of exacting methodologic criteria (some of which may not have been well suited to psychosocial research) places it at the conservative end of the spectrum of analyses and may have resulted in important effects of psychosocial interventions being missed or undervalued. Nevertheless, the Board realizes that attention needs to be paid to stronger research designs in future studies. Relatively few studies among those reviewed in this chapter may relate to a specific intervention, so that expanded research will be needed to strengthen evidence for a particular treatment.

METHODOLOGICAL ISSUES

There are a number of key methodological characteristics that are critical to the success of studies assessing the effectiveness of psychosocial interventions. Many of these methodological characteristics are similar in studies evaluating biomedical or psychosocial interventions. Others, notably those related to measurement and to standardization of the intervention, are unique challenges for researchers conducting psychosocial intervention trials.

Study Design

The gold standard design for studies that evaluate effectiveness of various interventions is the randomized controlled trial. The purpose of randomized allocation of patients is to avoid bias or confounding in the assignment of study treatments, thereby insuring that patients in each arm of the study are as comparable as possible with respect to all characteristics except for the specific intervention(s) being studied. When baseline patient characteristics are potentially associated with effects of the intervention being studied (e.g., severity of anxiety or depression), methodological approaches to ensure balance between study arms (e.g., stratification) are recommended as part of the randomization process. This is particularly important in studies with a small sample size.

Although randomized trials have been recognized as the gold standard since the mid-twentieth century, concerns have been raised that they may not be the most appropriate study design for evaluation of psychosocial interventions in cancer patients, in part because patient commitment to the intervention is deemed an important predictor of benefit from the intervention (Cunningham et al., 1998). It has been argued that if patients are willing to be randomized to a control arm, they are not as strongly committed to the intervention, and this will lead to an underestimation of the benefits of the intervention. Although this is possible, it is difficult to overcome self-selection biases (which may be powerful predictors of psychosocial outcomes) without using a randomized study design.

It has also been argued that cancer patients may not be willing to accept randomization. This might occur not only in psychosocial trials but also in biomedical intervention trials. However, the success of the many randomized trials reviewed below argues against this as a major obstacle to successful conduct of randomized psychosocial intervention trials in breast cancer.

When a randomized design is selected, it is important that the randomization not be compromised for logistical, or other, reasons. In the studies reviewed here, an example of compromised randomization occurred in an otherwise well conducted trial of the contribution of coaches to support groups for women with breast cancer when re-randomization was permitted in the two intervention arms (but not the control arm) if logistics of group meetings for the original randomized allocation were not convenient (Samarel et al., 1997). Another potential example occurred when assignment to a specialist nursing intervention versus control was according to the week women were admitted for surgery (weeks, not patients, were randomized) (Maguire et al., 1980). Theoretically, advance knowledge of whether the intervention was being administered in a given week could have influenced admission dates for individual women, leading to non-comparable study groups.

The issue of selection of an appropriate control or comparison arm is also challenging in randomized psychosocial intervention trials. Although many researchers select a "no treatment" or "standard treatment" control group, others argue that the control group should receive a similar amount of attention to that received by the intervention group, so that beneficial effects of attention (as opposed to the "active" components of the intervention) are not falsely labeled as benefits of the intervention. Selection of a no-treatment (or standard treatment) control arm versus attention control arm should probably reflect the specific study question. If the purpose of the study is to evaluate the overall benefits of adding the psychosocial intervention being studied to routine clinical care, then a no-treatment (or standard treatment) control group would be most appropriate. If, however, researchers are attempting to delineate which aspects of the intervention (e.g., attention versus teaching of coping skills or a specific cognitive–behavioral therapeutic approach) are important determinants of benefit, then selection of an attention control group may be more appropriate. The selection of control conditions will become an even more challenging issue as the benefits of psychosocial interventions are increasingly accepted by the medical community and these interventions become standard care; these interventions will then become the control or comparison arm in future studies. To facilitate this selection of comparison arms, agreement will be necessary regarding which interventions are considered standard care.

Some studies reviewed used "wait-list" controls. These controls were offered the study intervention after all study measurements were completed. Other studies passively offered educational materials to control subjects. Although these approaches may enhance acceptability of the study design to investigators, potential participants, and ethics committees alike, they are not truly no-treatment approaches and their use may tend to diminish treatment effects or, in the case of "wait-list" controls, make it difficult to examine long-term effects of interventions. These issues should be considered in both design and interpretation of trials.

Finally, there are situations when non-randomized designs may be desirable. These include studies whose purpose is to develop and standardize an intervention, studies whose purpose is to demonstrate that an intervention is feasible and can be delivered in a standard fashion by more than one investigator, and pilot studies looking for early evidence of treatment effectiveness, before full commitment is made to an expensive, long-term randomized trial. Non-randomized designs may also be important for studies seeking to obtain descriptive information about patient experiences or information about change over time, as well as for studies examining prognostic effects of psychosocial status. Such non-randomized designs may also be used when randomization is difficult, such as in the evaluation of peer support, novel and/or alternative therapies (e.g., reiki, yoga or t'ai chi), or participation in Internet chat support rooms where access to the intervention may be available to controls outside of the study. However, when assessment of treatment effectiveness is the primary purpose of a study, a randomized design is optimal. Use of alternative designs may lead to biased or inaccurate results.

Study Population

Many published psychosocial intervention studies involve patients with more than one type of cancer or patients with the same type of cancer in various stages of their illness (for example, early stage curable and late stage metastatic). Although, in the long term, intervention studies may demonstrate that the effectiveness of psychosocial interventions does not vary across cancer type or cancer stage, this is not known a priori. More sharply focused trials include patients with one type of cancer, and, in most circumstances, one stage of cancer. In the reports reviewed here, only randomized trials that restricted study entry to breast cancer patients are included. Once the population of interest is identified (e.g., women with recently diagnosed breast cancer), the study population should be as representative of that population as possible. The characteristics of the women in the trials reported here are listed (Phase/Stage of Disease) in Appendix B. Although the review of Newell and colleagues (Newell et al., 2002) was critical of low reporting of randomization (about 25 percent) in the trials they reviewed, in the present case with the exceptions noted earlier, randomization appears acceptable. Furthermore, the populations offered the trials were drawn consecutively from, responded to advertisements or other solicitations to, or were identified through records of, patient groups similar to those that might be offered the intervention in routine practice, although this was not specifically stated in those words, with the caveat that many of the studied populations were in academic health centers. It would be interesting to study patients in a larger cross-section of settings.

It is possible that attributes of the study population, such as age, medical treatment received, or baseline psychological characteristics will be predictors of effectiveness of psychosocial interventions. This was the case in a recent study in which the psychological benefits of supportive–expressive group therapy on mood were present in women who were distressed at study entry, but not in non-distressed women (Goodwin et al., 2001). Patient attributes that are potential predictors of benefit from the study intervention should be identified and their contribution to study outcomes carefully examined. Ideally, randomization should be stratified for these key baseline characteristics, as was discussed above.

Finally, attempts are warranted to design research on larger sample sizes. About half the 31 trials reviewed in this chapter involved fewer than 100 subjects, in many cases 50 or fewer, weakening their power to provide strong evidence. The largest trial involved 312 women randomized to four arms and did not demonstrate lasting effects (Helgeson et al., 1999, 2000, 2001). The recent study from Australia by Kissane and colleagues randomized 303 women to group and relaxation versus relaxation alone. Positive findings of reduced anxiety and better function were found in this large cohort.

Study Intervention

Standardization of the study intervention is a particular challenge when the intervention is psychosocial in nature. As much as possible, investigators should use a well described, standardized therapy that has the potential to be delivered in routine practice by other trained and qualified practitioners who will be the end-users of the study results. When describing the intervention, the skills and the qualifications of the therapists must be included along with details of the intervention. Furthermore, it should be demonstrated that the therapy is delivered in a standardized fashion throughout the study. Ideally, investigators should provide evidence of compliance with the intervention as well as evidence of the competence of therapists delivering it. They should also report the dose/duration of exposure to the study intervention, and designs of longer duration should be considered for future studies. These issues are more straightforward when interventions are biomedical because investigators can simply describe the number of doses and number of milligrams of a drug that are administered. The challenge is much greater when the intervention is psychosocial.

The interventions that were investigated in the reports reviewed here often involved more than one potentially active component. For example, group therapy, relaxation/self-hypnosis, and teaching of coping skills were included in a single intervention (Cunningham et al., 1998). When interventions have multiple components, it may be difficult for investigators to determine whether one, or all, of the components is responsible for the outcome. This is not a problem if it is the overall effectiveness of the intervention that is being investigated. However, if evidence of effectiveness of individual components is sought, it may be necessary to study each component separately.

Study Measures

Measurement of psychological outcomes is as exact a science as measuring biomedical outcomes, and requires the same attention to accuracy. There are many well validated, standardized instruments available that measure quality of life and psychosocial status. However, not all of these instruments measure attributes that are likely to be altered by specific study interventions (see Chapter 3 for a description of selected instruments). For example, an intervention targeting anxiety would not necessarily be expected to enhance role functioning. Furthermore, not all of the available instruments are sufficiently sensitive to detect clinically important change resulting from an intervention that is, in fact, efficacious. This was demonstrated in a recent randomized trial of supportive–expressive group therapy in metastatic breast cancer (Goodwin et al., 2001). Beneficial effects of the intervention on mood were readily detected using the Profile of Mood States. Similar benefits were not detected using the Emotional Functioning Subscale of the European Organization for Treatment and Research of Cancer (EORTC) QLQ-C30 (see Chapter 3). The selection of quality of life and psychosocial outcome measures in randomized trials in breast cancer patients, and the ability of these instruments to identify changes when various interventions are delivered, has recently been reviewed by Ganz and Goodwin (Ganz and Goodwin, 2003).

It is recommended that investigators select, whenever possible, standardized, well validated, and well accepted outcome measures that are sensitive to clinically important change and that target attributes that are likely to be influenced by the intervention. For example, if the intervention is designed to reduce anxiety, then an instrument that specifically measures anxiety and is responsive to changes in anxiety should be used. As noted above, a general health-related quality of life (HRQOL) instrument that measures emotional functioning in a general way with a small number of items and limited response categories may miss important changes in mood that can be detected with other instruments. Thus, use of these general HRQOL instruments as sole outcome measures in psychosocial intervention studies is not recommended. At times, it will be necessary for investigators to develop new instruments or new modules of existing instruments in order to ensure they are targeting key attributes. When this is the case, care should be taken to validate these new measures before they are used as study outcomes. However, wholesale development of new instruments when acceptable instruments already exist is not recommended because it reduces the ability to compare results across studies.

An additional challenge in psychosocial intervention research relates to compliance with study measurements. A balance must be reached between patient burden and comprehensiveness. Every effort should be made to encourage patients to comply with study measurements. The problem of missing data points has been a troublesome issue in psychosocial research. This is particularly challenging when patients are seriously ill, or undergoing complex medical treatments, or when multiple outcome measures are being used.

Blinding should be used in outcome assessments to the extent possible, given the study design. When outcomes are self-reported, patients should be unaware of the specific study hypothesis (if possible), and research staff who score the questionnaires should be unaware of subjects' randomization allocation. When outcomes are interview-based, interviewers should be blinded to randomization allocation.

Finally, cost and feasibility assessments to allow the possible balancing of benefits against costs of psychosocial interventions or programs should be included insofar as is possible and consistent with the abilities of the investigators, time and money resources available, and capacities of the settings. It is recognized that this is easier said than done, and that with the exception of an occasional study or mention in reports is rarely accomplished (Koocher and Pollin, 2001; Simpson et al., 2001)

Outcome/Analysis

Each randomized trial should have a clearly stated hypothesis and a clearly stated primary outcome; sample size calculations and statistical analyses should reflect this primary study question. The description of the primary outcome should include a description of the specific questionnaire and/or questionnaire item/scale as well as the specific time-point(s) in the study that will be used to define this outcome. If more than one primary study outcome (or time-point) is selected, allowances must be made for multiple testing in statistical analysis and sample size calculations. At times, the issue of multiple time-points can be overcome using statistical methods, such as repeated measures analysis of variance or slopes analysis, that incorporate measurements performed at multiple times into a single statistical analysis. Thus, although studies may use multiple instruments administered at multiple time-points with a plan for multiple approaches to analysis, the primary endpoint, time-point, and analytic approach must be stated a priori, and the sample size and significance cut-points must reflect these decisions. Other endpoints and/or analyses should then be viewed as secondary or hypothesis-generating. This will overcome the common criticism of psychosocial intervention studies that use of multiple outcomes, all of which are treated equally in the analysis, leads to multiple, and at times conflicting, study results with a high experiment-wide type-1 error (the probability of incorrectly accepting a study hypothesis that is not true) (Newell et al., 2002).

In evaluating outcomes, it might also be useful to consider whether the length of follow-up should be related to the length of time that the treatment's effect is expected to be needed. For example, if the intervention being tested is intended to deal with a current problem, like getting through physical treatments like surgery, radiation, of chemotherapy, a long follow-up may not be required and could lead to an erroneous conclusion that the treatment was not effective because its effects did not last until the final follow-up. Also, since trials of psychosocial interventions evaluated here are often applied to the whole population of women with breast cancer, they may include some women who would not have, or would not develop, psychosocial problems. This might dilute results and explain lack of effect in some trials.

The majority of the published psychosocial intervention studies in breast cancer reviewed here have selected psychosocial outcomes as their primary outcome measure, but some have also included biomedical outcomes, notably survival, treatment response, and immune factors. As with psychosocial outcomes, when biomedical outcomes are being studied, the primary outcome must be identified a priori. The only exceptions to this rigorous approach occur in hypotheses generating studies such as pilot studies, or in studies designed to standardize interventions. Descriptive qualitative–analytic studies of cancer patients' narratives, or correlative studies examining inter-relationships of psychosocial variables that are designed to generate, rather than confirm, hypotheses are also excluded. Nonetheless, such studies provide important hypotheses that are generated and subjected to confirmation in future trials.

REVIEW OF THE LITERATURE

Methods

Literature searches were conducted using computerized databases (MedLine, Cancer Lit) between March 2002 and August 2002 using the following headings:

1. breast cancer and psychological intervention
2. breast cancer and psychosocial intervention
3. breast cancer and relaxation intervention
4. breast cancer and hypnosis intervention
5. breast cancer and group therapy intervention
6. breast cancer and individual therapy intervention
7. breast cancer and psychotherapy intervention

Searches were also made for reviews in each of these areas. The articles were obtained, and their reference lists were reviewed to identify additional reports. This process continued in an iterative fashion until no new reports were identified. Studies reported in abstract form only were not included as they provided insufficient information on methodology for adequate critical review.

The reports thus identified were included in this review if they described randomized trials of psychosocial interventions in breast cancer patients, and they provided information on psychosocial and/or biomedical outcomes. Pilot studies were included if they met these criteria, but not if they did not compare study arms (i.e., presentation of before/after data within study arms as the only outcome was not adequate). Studies in mixed cancer patients were not included (though some of these studies are briefly cited if they provide key data not otherwise available).

In total, 31 randomized trials of psychosocial interventions meeting these criteria were identified, some of which were reported in a series of publications (Cunningham et al., 1998; Edelman et al., 1999b; Goodwin et al., 2001; Maguire et al., 1983, 1980; Samarel et al., 1997; Spiegel et al., 1989). Potentially important problems with randomization in two of these trials were noted above (Maguire et al., 1980; Samarel et al., 1997). These trials are summarized in Table 5-1 according to year of publication and phase of breast cancer (early, metastatic, healthy survivor). The majority of the published studies (24 of 31) have focused on early phases of breast cancer, that is, initial diagnosis and treatment, including surgery, chemotherapy, and radiation therapy. The pace of publication is increasing, with about 80 percent (25 of 31) of the studies appearing since 1995. This un-

TABLE 5-1 Randomized Trials of Psychosocial Interventions in Breast Cancer

	Year of Publication					
Phase of Illness	1980 to 1984	1985 to 1989	1990 to 1994	1995 to 1999	2000 to mid-2002	Total
"Early"*	2	1	1	9	11**	24
"Metastatic"	1	0	1	2	2	6
"Healthy Survivors"	0	0	0	1	0	1
Total	3	1	2	12	13	31

*Includes all reports that enrolled patients at diagnosis during initial treatment (surgery, chemotherapy, radiation therapy.
**One trial included a small number of women with metastatic breast cancer (Targ and Levine, 2002).

doubtedly reflects a growing interest in psychosocial intervention in breast cancer patients in the scientific, medical, and lay communities.

The studies are further subdivided in Table 5-2 according to the type of intervention studied and the country in which the research was conducted. The majority of this psychosocial intervention research in breast cancer has been conducted in the United States (16 of 31 studies, 52 percent), and 13 of the studies examined group interventions (Antoni et al., 2001; Bultz et al., 2000; Classen et al., 2001; Cunningham et al., 1998; Edelman et al., 1999a, 1999b; Edmonds et al., 1999; Fukui et al., 2000; Goodwin et al., 2001; Helgeson et al., 1999, 2000, 2001; Richardson et al., 1997; Samarel and Fawcett, 1992; Samarel et al., 1993, 1997; Spiegel and Bloom, 1983; Spiegel et al., 1989). These group interventions varied in nature; some were supportive only, some involved manual-based supportive–expressive therapy, some examined cognitive–behavioral interventions or a combination of cognitive–behavioral and supportive interventions, while one examined psycho-education and peer discussion and one investigated a mind-body–spirit complementary medicine intervention. The next largest group of studies evaluated individual therapies (Allen et al., 2002; Burton et al., 1995; Cimprich, 1993; Lev et al., 2001; Maguire et al., 1983, 1980; Marchioro et al., 1996; Maunsell et al., 1996; Richardson et al., 1997; Ritz et al., 2000; Sandgren et al., 2000; Walker et al., 1999; Wengstrom et al., 2001, 1999; McArdle et al., 1996). The interventions used in these studies were diverse and included telephone support and screening, a series of nursing interventions, couples therapy, cognitive–behavioral interventions, and others. Relaxation/hypnosis with or without imagery was also a major focus of several reports; in total six studies examined interventions of this type as their primary focus (several others included relaxation/hypnosis as part of multifaceted intervention) (Bridge et al., 1988; Arathuzik, 1994; Kolcaba and Fox, 1999; Molassiotis et al., 2002; Richardson et al., 1997; Walker et al., 1999). Although only one study formally evaluated the use of education as a form of psychosocial support, a number of other studies provided educational materials in a passive fashion to women randomized to control groups (Fukui et al., 2000; Helgeson et al., 2000, 2001). The study that formally evaluated education was also the only randomized trial to evaluate facilitated peer discussion; one other study (McArdle et al., 1996) evaluated support from a lay breast cancer organization.

Given the characteristics of these studies, their results should be highly relevant to women with breast cancer receiving care in the United States today. The focus of many studies on the early phases of breast cancer reflects the fact that this is often a stressful time for women diagnosed with breast cancer. It is a phase of breast cancer that affects all women, and it is a phase of the illness in which intervention is facilitated by the fact that women attend for treatment on a regular basis. The paucity of studies in

TABLE 5-2 Randomized Trials of Psychosocial Interventions in Breast Cancer

Phase of Illness	Country		Type(s) of Intervention Investigated (some studies investigated more than one intervention)				
			Education*	Group Therapy†	Individual Therapy**	Relaxation Imagery	Other***
"Early" (n=24)	United States	12	1	8	10	5	11
	Canada	4					
	UK/Europe	6					
	Asia	2					
"Metastatic" (n=6)	United States	3	0	5	1	1	0
	Canada	2					
	Australia	1					
"Healthy Survivors" (n=1)	United States	1	0	0	0	0	1
Total			1	13	11	6	2

*** Educational materials provided passively to control groups not included.
** Includes telephone support, nursing intervention, cognitive-behavioral interventions, other.
* Includes telephone screening in early breast cancer, videotapes in healthy survivors.
† Includes supportive or supportive-expressive group therapy, cognitive-behavioral interventions, peer discussion.

healthy survivors is a potential concern; the one study that has been reported used this group as a convenience sample to evaluate the psychosocial benefit derived from viewing a videotape that projected an empathic interaction (enhanced compassion) (Fogarty et al., 1999). This study did not specifically address psychosocial issues of healthy survivors. One additional study evaluated the benefits of managing menopausal symptoms in breast cancer survivors using a comprehensive menopausal assessment with subsequent recommendations for management (Ganz et al., 2000). Because the main focus of this trial was on medical symptom management, it was not included as a psychosocial intervention trial, even though a portion of the intervention was psychosocial in nature (pharmacologic interventions were also used). Survivors are a relatively understudied group in general (although research on survivorship is growing), and descriptive studies that focus on identifying psychosocial problems in this group and that determine the prevalence of these problems, as well as those at risk, are probably needed to guide development of interventions that can be tested in full-fledged randomized trials.

Review of Clinical Trials

This section of the chapter reviews each of the 31 randomized trials of psychosocial interventions in women with breast cancer identified in the literature search. Trials are first grouped into those taking place in the early phases of breast cancer, metastatic breast cancer, and during survivorship. Key characteristics, methodologic limitations and findings of each trial are presented (a detailed summary of each trial is included in Appendix B). Trials are then regrouped according to the intervention approach used (e.g., group, individual, relaxation/hypnosis). Table 5-3 provides definitions of the most common types of interventions used in these trials.

Early Breast Cancer

The first, and largest, group of trials involves those conducted in early breast cancer (see Table B-1). These 24 trials include patients enrolled at cancer diagnosis and those enrolled during initial treatment, including surgery, chemotherapy, and radiation therapy. One of these studies (Targ and Levine, 2002) included a small number of patients with metastatic breast cancer. In general, patients on these trials were within 1 to 2 years of breast cancer diagnosis and, in most trials, they were within a few weeks or months of diagnosis. These trials are listed chronologically in Table B-1 along with information on the number of women studied, the type of intervention evaluated, and the duration of the intervention, as well as study outcomes and the length of follow-up.

TABLE 5-3 Definitions of Psychosocial Interventions

Supportive-expressive psychotherapy	A group therapy developed by Spiegel and colleagues in which social support is given in the context of encouraging expression of feeling, following a manualized format.
Supportive-existential psychotherapy	A group therapy developed by Kissane and colleagues which provides both social support and encouragement to explore existential fears, e.g., recurrence, and the need for meaning in the face of serious illness.
Psychoeducational interventions	Providing information to individuals and groups about illness in a social, supportive interaction.
Interpersonal psychotherapy/counseling	An intervention that uses a manual approach to focus on role changes and problems caused by illness, exploring constructive efforts to accommodate.
Cognitive-behavioral interventions	(See Chapter 4, Box 4-1). Use of cognitive restructuring, distraction, mental guided imagery, coping-enhancing interpretations along with common behavioral interventions of relaxation, hypnosis, desensitization.
Mind-body-spiritual interventions	This approach by Targ and Levine combines psychosocial and complementary medicine interventions (dance, meditation, imaging).
Restorative interventions	A structured nursing intervention to help women give attention to and participate in activities while reducing attention to negative aspects of illness and treatment resulting in attentional fatigue.
Supportive group with coaching	A group intervention in which women were "coached" to improve self-concept, physical function, roles, and relationships.

SOURCE: Jimmie Holland, personal communication.

Maguire et al. reported the first randomized psychosocial intervention trial in breast cancer (Maguire et al., 1980, 1983), but randomization was not performed on individual patients. Instead, weeks during a 24 month period were randomized. Thus, it is possible surgeons or patients may have been aware of randomization allocation for a given week and that knowledge may have influenced admission dates. This might have led to bias in treatment allocation and non-comparability of study arms. The intervention involved individual counseling by a nurse before and after mastectomy, with subsequent home visits every 2 months until the woman had "adapted well." The focus of the intervention was on adaptation to the scar, arm morbidity, and breast prosthesis as well as encouraging women to be open regarding the effect of the surgery on themselves and their emotional status. The comparison patients received usual treatment. Outcomes were evaluated using an interviewer administered Present State Exam and Life Events Scale, as well as a linear analog scale of mood. Patients were followed for up to 12 to 18 months. Counseling failed to prevent morbidity; however, the nurses' regular monitoring of the women led to more appropriate psychiatric referral, and subsequent psychiatric intervention reduced psychiatric morbidity as well as anxiety and depression. This early trial provides the first evidence of benefit of a psychosocial intervention in women with breast cancer.

Christensen randomized 20 husband and wife pairs after mastectomy to receive four weekly counseling sessions or to a control condition (Christensen, 1983). The intervention focused on the impact of mastectomy on the couple's relationship, and it was tailored to each couple's needs. No overall treatment effects were identified, although the small sample size may have precluded identification of clinically important effects. Despite the absence of overall effects, adjusted analyses suggested that there might be some benefits in terms of enhanced sexual satisfaction and psychological status in both husbands and wives and reduced depression in wives. Follow-up was short—only 1 week post intervention. Effects of this short intervention on longer-term outcomes cannot be assessed.

Cimprich studied an individualized, but structured nursing intervention designed to enhance attentional capacity in women with recently diagnosed breast cancer (Cimprich, 1993). The restorative intervention was designed to "minimize or prevent attentional fatigue through regular participation in activities that engage fascination or have other restorative properties." The intervention resulted in significantly improved attentional capacity and total attentional score over a 90-day period. There were no effects on mood.

Bridge et al. randomized 154 women undergoing local radiotherapy for early stage breast cancer to one of three arms: (1) structured teaching of relaxation techniques including diaphragmatic breathing, supplemented by audiotapes; (2) the above plus imagery of a peaceful scene; or (3) a control arm in which individuals were seen individually and encouraged to talk about themselves (Bridge et al., 1988). The interventions took place weekly for 30 minutes for a total of 6 weeks. They were delivered by the researchers, one of whom was a psychiatrist. Immediately post intervention, the relaxation with imagery intervention resulted in lower total mood disturbance on the Profile of Mood States than relaxation alone, and both interventions resulted in enhanced mood compared to the attention control arm.

Similar findings were found for the individual item "relaxed." This study provides evidence of short-term benefits of relaxation, and it suggests that the addition of imagery to muscular relaxation further enhances psychological benefits.

Burton et al. randomized 200 women who were about to undergo mastectomy to an interview with a psychologist (a Present State Examination that focused on worries, concerns, or beliefs), or to the interview plus a half-hour individual psychotherapy session provided by a surgeon that dealt with the effects of breast cancer on the woman's life situations and her feelings, or to the interview with a 30-minute chat with the surgeon that focused on patients' holidays and the like, or to a control arm (Burton et al., 1995). Psychological outcomes were obtained up to 1 year after the intervention. The preoperative interviews with the psychologist resulted in a lasting reduction in body image distress, reduced overall distress, anxiety, and depression, reduced upset regarding the loss of the breast as well as enhanced use of fighting spirit coping style. The psychotherapy versus the chat was superior among patients who had experienced stressful life events, but not in the overall study group. The control subjects in this study were not informed that they were participating in a study until the final 1-year measurement. Therefore, no baseline data were available on controls. Thus, results should be interpreted with caution, as the comparability of intervention and control groups at baseline was not demonstrated. It is notable that 80 women randomized to the intervention declined. There were no such decliners in the control group because the control subjects did not know that they were part of a study. This further increases the possibility that study groups were not comparable at baseline.

Maunsell et al. randomized 259 women with newly diagnosed, local, or regional breast cancer to receive telephone screening every 28 days or to routine care (Maunsell et al., 1996). Telephone screening, performed by a research assistant, involved administration of the General Health Questionnaire. If a score >5 was obtained, patients were referred to a social worker who then intervened by telephone to confirm distress, identified the cause for the distress, and offered support. Screening continued for 1 year. No significant effects of this brief screening intervention performed by a non-mental health professional were identified, despite the use of a fairly large number of outcome measures.

Marchioro et al. randomized 36 women with newly diagnosed non-metastatic breast cancer to weekly, psychologist led individual cognitive psychotherapy combined with bi-monthly family counseling, or to standard care (Marchioro et al., 1996). The duration of the intervention was not described. Follow-up continued to 9 months. The intervention was reported to reduce depression and enhance quality of life. Changes in some aspects of personality were also identified. This study provides evidence of psychological benefit for an individual intervention; information on duration of the intervention would have been helpful.

McArdle et al. randomized 272 women at the time of breast cancer diagnosis to receive either (1) support from a breast cancer nurse, (2) support from a voluntary organization (Tak Tent) that provided individual counseling and support groups, (3) support from both the nurse and the voluntary organization, or (4) usual care (McArdle et al., 1996). Outcomes (general health, social function, and depression) were best in those randomized to receive support from the nurse, providing clear evidence of benefit for support provided by a breast cancer nurse specialist; no benefit was seen in those randomized to the voluntary organization, and dropout rates were also higher among this latter group.

In a small pilot study, Richardson et al. randomized 47 subjects to a non-structured support group that focused on stress reduction, reducing feelings of isolation, and enhancing self-esteem or to an imagery relaxation group that received instruction on relaxation, imagery, and basic breathing with supplemental discussion of stress and coping. In the latter arm, group meetings were supplemented by one individual relaxation/imagery session (Richardson et al., 1997). A third arm received standard care. The support group and relaxation imagery group sessions occurred weekly for 6 weeks, each lasting 1 hour. They were led by Master's level social workers; a hypnotist participated in the relaxation imagery group. Although this was a small pilot study, there was evidence of enhanced coping skills in both the support and the relaxation/imagery groups (more significant in the former), and there was evidence that women in both intervention arms sought more support from others than women in the control arm. There was also a greater acceptance of death in women participating in the support groups. There was no evidence of an effect of either intervention on quality of life, mood, or immune parameters and no evidence of a differential effect of the support group versus the imagery relaxation group. Psychological outcomes were measured in the short-term only, the final evaluation was conducted immediately after the intervention was completed. No information was available on long-term effects.

Samarel et al. randomized 228 women with recently treated stage I or II breast cancer to a support group, a support group with coaching (each woman was invited to bring a significant other—a spouse, friend, or family member), or to a control arm (Samarel and Fawcett, 1992; Samarel et al., 1993, 1997). The support groups were led by a nurse and social worker and were structured and designed to assist women to adapt in physiological, self-concept, role function, and interdependent response modes. The intervention took place weekly for 8 weeks. Psychological outcomes were measured up to 8 weeks after the end of the intervention. It was reported that the addition of coaching to the support groups resulted in higher quality relationships at the end of the intervention compared to the other arms of the study, but this effect did not persist 8 weeks later. The interventions had no effect on symptom distress, mood, or functional status, although an effect on symptom distress and mood might have been expected in view of the large size of the study and the use of psychological measures shown to be responsive to change in other studies (Profile of Mood States, Symptom Distress Scale). In this study, randomization was not straightforward since women randomized to one of the two intervention arms could be re-randomized to one of the two remaining arms if they were unable to attend the assigned group for any reason, but re-randomization was not possible for women allocated to the control arm. This may have led to non-comparability of the study groups and interference with detection of potential psychological benefits.

Kolcaba and Fox randomized 53 women to use a guided imagery audiotape daily during radiation therapy and for three weeks later or to a no treatment control arm (Kolcaba and Fox, 1999). The audiotape included 20 minutes of verbal guided imagery focusing on comfort, as well as 20 minutes of soft jazz. Psychosocial follow-up continued until 3 weeks after radiation was completed. The intervention significantly improved comfort (psycho-spiritual, environmental, social) throughout the duration of the study.

Walker et al. randomized 96 women with newly diagnosed locally advanced breast cancer to relaxation training with guided imagery or to standard care (Walker et al., 1999). The relaxation training included the use of audiocassettes and cartoon images of host defenses destroying cancer cells. The relaxation component focused on progressive muscular relaxation and cue controlled relaxation. The first 20 women in the study received "live" training, and the remaining women used the audiocassettes and cartoon images alone. Women were encouraged to use these materials daily during six chemotherapy cycles. Follow-up was to the end of the sixth chemotherapy cycle. The intervention reduced overall emotional repression as well as unhappiness, and it enhanced global quality of life. It had no effect on mood. There was no effect of the intervention on tumor size or response to chemotherapy. This relatively simple intervention had a beneficial psychological effect in women with locally advanced breast cancer, but no biomedical effect was observed.

Wengström et al. randomized 134 women to a nursing intervention based on Orem's model for self-care versus standard care (Wengstrom et al., 1999, 2001). The intervention, based on individual patient contact, included education; support and guidance regarding self-care, psychological support, coping strategies, body image; and treatment. Patients received a total of five 30-minute sessions weekly for 5 weeks. They were followed throughout radiation and for 3 months post radiation. The intervention group had fewer distress reactions as measured using the Impact of Events Scale, but there were no overall effects on quality of life or toxicity. In women over 59 years of age, the intervention was reported to result in "stronger motivation to be emotionally involved."

Sandgren et al. randomized 62 women to telephone-based individual cognitive–behavioral therapy or to assessment only (Sandgren et al., 2000). The telephone based cognitive–behavioral therapy, delivered by Master's level clinical psychology students, provided support, addressed coping skills and strategies to manage anxiety and stress, and helped patients solve problems. Cognitive restructuring and emotional expression were encouraged. Women randomized to the intervention received weekly interventions for 4 weeks, then every 2 weeks for 6 weeks. Each intervention averaged 20 to 25 minutes. Women were followed for a total of 10 months. There were no consistent effects of the intervention over time. Some borderline and transient effects were seen; for example, there was an early reduction in stress followed by a late increase in stress, and early benefits for mental health but early deterioration in physical functioning. These inconsistent and borderline results may reflect the small sample size of this study or the lack of experience of the therapists. Further investigation in a larger group of patients, or with more experienced therapists, might yield more stable results.

Bultz et al., in a unique study, randomized 36 partners of breast cancer patients to a psycho-educational group led by two psychologists that took place weekly for 6weeks or to a control arm (Bultz et al., 2000). Both patients and their partners were followed until 3 months after the completion of the intervention. There were no statistically significant effects.

Ritz et al. randomized 210 women who had been diagnosed with either invasive or non-invasive breast cancer within the preceding 2 weeks to receive advanced practice nursing interventions or to standard care (Ritz et al., 2000). The advanced practice nursing interventions included written and verbal information about breast cancer. They addressed what to expect in consultation with physicians; they assisted with decision-making, provided support, answered questions, and enhanced continuity of care. The intervention was provided in person, by telephone, and during home visits. The number of contacts per patient and the duration of these contacts were not specified. Patients were followed for a total of 24 months. The intervention was reported to reduce uncertainty at 1, 3, and 6 months with the effect being greatest in unmarried women. There were benefits in a number of uncertainty subscales including complexity, inconsistency, and unpredictability. There was no overall effect on mood, although a beneficial effect on mood was seen at 1 and 3 months in women without a family history of breast cancer. There were no effects on quality of life or on overall health-care costs. This nursing intervention, which in some centers may be considered the standard of care, reduced uncertainty, at least in the short term.

Fukui et al. randomized 50 Japanese women to cognitive–behavioral group therapy or to a wait-list control arm (Fukui et al., 2000). Women had been diagnosed with high-risk invasive breast cancer 4 to 18 months earlier, and none had received chemotherapy. The cognitive–behavioral group therapy was led by a psychiatrist and a psychologist; it included education, coping skills training, stress management (including muscle relaxation and guided imagery), and psychosocial support. Sessions lasted 90 minutes and were held weekly for 6 weeks. The intervention significantly improved vigor and overall mood, and it significantly enhanced fighting spirit coping at the end of 6 weeks, but effects were marginal 6 months later. Additionally, there were no significant effects on depression or anxiety. This brief intervention appeared to have short-term, but not long-term, beneficial psychological effects.

Helgeson et al. randomized 312 women to four arms using a factorial design. The three treatment arms consisted of (1) education, (2) facilitated peer discussion, and (3) education and facilitated peer discussion. There was also a non-treatment control arm (Helgeson et al., 1999, 2000, 2001). The education intervention was group-based and involved a lecture as well as a question and answer session with an expert presenter and an oncology nurse or social worker. Interaction between group members was not encouraged. The peer discussion was also in a group format with a nurse or social work facilitator who did not direct the conversation but encouraged women to focus on expression of feelings and self-disclosure. Both interventions lasted 60 minutes weekly for 8 weeks. Follow-up continued for 48 months. The education intervention resulted in a number of psychological benefits over both facilitated peer discussion and control. These benefits included enhanced vitality, social functioning, and mental health as well as reduced bodily pain. There were no early or late benefits for the facilitated peer discussion group, and the beneficial effects of the educational intervention dissipated over time. This study demonstrated early benefits for an educational intervention but provided no evidence of benefit for a facilitated peer discussion group. This is the only randomized trial that included a peer discussion group (although professional facilitators were present). The findings at 48 months are harder to interpret because of attrition in the groups over time.

Simpson et al. randomized 89 women with early stage breast cancer who had completed their treatment up to 2 years earlier to either a group intervention or to a control arm that received a book *Helping Yourself—A Workbook for People Living with Cancer* (Simpson et al., 2001). The intervention arm participated in structured group psychotherapy, 90 minutes weekly for 6 weeks, with weekly themes. A psychiatrist and two survivors led the groups, which included up to 10 subjects. Follow-up continued for 2 years. This brief intervention reduced depression, enhanced mood and quality of life, and diminished psychiatric symptoms at 2 years but not at 1 year. Furthermore, health care billing was reduced by $147 (Canadian dollars) in each intervention subject (a 23.5 percent reduction). These results suggest that a brief intervention may result in psychological benefits and reduction of health-care costs.

Lev et al. randomized 53 women with stage I or II breast cancer who were receiving their first cycle of chemotherapy to an "efficacy enhancing intervention" or to receive an educational booklet on cancer chemotherapy (Lev et al., 2001). The efficacy enhancing intervention included a 5-minute videotape, a self-care educational booklet, and five monthly efficacy enhancing counseling interventions over 8 months. Patients were followed for a total of 8 months. No formal tests of statistical significance were performed. The authors reported effect sizes only: small to large effect sizes for functional or social concerns on the Functional Assessment of Cancer Therapy–B, as well as small to large effect sizes on the Symptom Distress Scale and a scale called "Strategies Used by Patients to Promote Health." The lack of statistical significance testing and a dropout rate over 50 percent make interpretation of these results highly problematic.

Antoni et al. randomized 136 women with stage 0 to II breast cancer who were within 8 weeks of surgery to a structured group intervention that included cognitive–behavioral and stress management therapy that met weekly for 2 hours for a total of 10 weeks or to a control arm (Antoni et al., 2001). The intervention also included didactic/experiential exercises as well as homework. Women randomized to the control arm participated in a 1-day seminar during which they received information relating to stress reactions and successful adjustment. The interventions and seminars were led by psychology fellows and doctoral students. Only the 100 women who completed all psychological assessments were included in the analysis. Thus, the larger group of women who were randomized was not fully described. The authors reported that there were no overall effects of the intervention, although they noted that it reduced the prevalence of moderate depression (but not mean depression scores) and that it increased benefit finding and optimism, the latter effect being maximal in women who had low baseline optimism scores. A large number of secondary analyses were presented. The selection of only the 100 women who completed all psychological assessments may have led to non-comparable study groups, and may have made it difficult to identify overall effects of the intervention similar to those found by other investigators.

Molassiotis et al. randomized 71 women receiving their first cycle of chemotherapy for stage I to III breast cancer to a relaxation/imagery intervention or to a control arm (Molassiotis et al., 2002). The intervention involved progressive muscle relaxation training and guided imagery that was provided in six standardized sessions with a therapist (1 hour before chemotherapy and days 1 to 5 post chemotherapy). This intervention was supplemented with individual audiocassettes as well as a 30-minute video teaching program. Psychological assessments were obtained up to 14 days post chemotherapy. The intervention resulted in a significant decrease in total mood disturbance, as well as a significant decrease in the duration of nausea and vomiting and a trend towards lower frequency of nausea and vomiting; however, it had no effect on the intensity of nausea and vomiting. These findings suggest that this brief, simple intervention had important effects on symptom control and the psychological well being of women receiving adjuvant chemotherapy.

Allen et al. randomized 164 women under the age of 50 who were receiving adjuvant chemotherapy for stage I to III breast cancer to a brief intervention with an oncology nurse or to a control arm (Allen et al., 2002). The intervention consisted of two in-person and four telephone sessions over a 12-week period. The nurse provided problem-solving skills training as well as informational materials. Women were followed up to 8 months. There were no overall effects of the intervention in either univariate or multivariate analyses. Some subgroup effects were seen; in particular, women who had good baseline, inate problem-solving ability had a significant decrease in the number and severity of difficulties they experienced. A similar effect was not seen in women with poor baseline, inate problem-solving abilities. This suggests that a more focused and/or more intensive intervention may be necessary in women with poor baseline problem-solving abilities, and it highlights the importance of targeting interventions to the needs and characteristics of specific populations.

Finally, Targ and Levine (2002) recently reported an important study comparing a standard psychoeducational group to a mind–body–spirit group that included a number of complementary and alternative medicine (CAM) interventions, including dance, meditation, imagery, and ritual (Targ and Levine, 2002). The standard group with two leaders, one of whom was a psychologist, met for 90 minutes weekly for 12 weeks. The CAM group, led by nurses and social workers, met twice weekly for 150 minutes each time for 12 weeks. The CAM sessions included health discussions, meditation and guided imagery, experiential work, group discussion, and a movement/dance program. Despite that greater time commitment, dropouts were fewer and satisfaction was greater among women randomized to the CAM group. Psychosocial status including mood, coping, and HRQOL improved in both groups. The only significant between-group difference was in a novel measurement, spiritual integration, or the degree to which a person makes spirituality an integral part of their coping. Because the standard group had more dropouts than the CAM group even before that intervention began, it was suggested that the study may have attracted participants who were particularly interested in CAM interventions. Although the authors concluded there was "equivalence on most psychosocial outcomes," this study does describe the acceptability of complementary and alternative medicine interventions to women with breast cancer.

Metastatic Breast Cancer

There have been six randomized trials of psychosocial interventions in metastatic breast cancer (Arathuzik, 1994; Classen et al., 2001; Cunningham et al., 1998; Edelman et al., 1999a, 1999b; Edmonds et al., 1999; Goodwin et al., 2001; Spiegel et al., 1989, 1981; Spiegel and Bloom, 1983). Many of these trials have included both survival outcomes and psychosocial outcomes. As noted earlier, this interest in effects of psychosocial outcomes on survival reflects the publication by Spiegel et al. of an unexpected survival benefit for a group psychosocial intervention in metastatic breast cancer (Spiegel et al., 1989).

Spiegel et al. reported the first randomized trial of a psychosocial intervention in metastatic breast cancer (Spiegel et al., 1989, 1981; Spiegel and Bloom, 1983). He randomized 86 women to participate in weekly expressive–supportive group therapy that included hypnosis for pain control or to a control arm. There was a high dropout rate pre-intervention (28 of 86 women dropped out before the intervention began, largely because of illness). The group therapy sessions lasted for 90 minutes and were led by a psychiatrist and social worker. Women were asked to participate for 1 year, longer if possible. The intervention was reported to improve mood, to reduce maladaptive coping responses, and to reduce phobias. Furthermore, in an unplanned survival analysis conducted after prolonged follow-up, the intervention was reported to significantly increase survival—the mean survival being 36.6 months in the intervention arm and 18.9 months in the control arm. Although these results were exciting and provided the first evidence of psychological benefit for a psychological intervention in metastatic breast cancer, while also showing the feasibility of a psychological intervention in this seriously ill population of patients, the study was not designed to examine survival effects. Fox pointed out in a critique of the study that using SEER data for survival of women from metastatic breast cancer in that geographic area at that time resulted in the same survival curve for both the women in the intervention group and the women in the SEER database. In fact, for unknown reasons, the control group had a poorer survival. The apparent survival advantage appeared to be attributable to this fact (Fox, 1998). Replication of these results, particularly the results of the unplanned survival analysis, was recommended and is underway by Spiegel and the subject of the Goodwin study described below.

Arathuzik reported a very small randomized trial, essentially a pilot study, involving 24 women who were randomized to relaxation/visualization, relaxation/visualization plus cognitive–behavioral therapy, or to a control arm (Arathuzik, 1994). The relaxation and visualization was a structured intervention that involved individual sessions during which women were taught progressive relaxation and encouraged to perform visualization exercises. The cognitive–behavioral component was also delivered individually, and it included discussion and a written handout describing 23 methods of pain distraction. Each intervention was administered once by the nurse investigator. There were no between-group differences in pain or mood. However, both treatment groups reported an interesting finding, an enhanced perceived ability to decrease pain. The lack of significant between-group effects on pain or mood might reflect the extremely small sample size in this study.

Edelman et al. randomized 121 women with metastatic breast cancer to a group cognitive–behavioral therapy program or to a control arm (Edelman et al., 1999a, 1999b). The cognitive–behavioral intervention included a support group that met weekly for 8 weeks, then monthly for 3 weeks, and involved one family session. There was a focus on cognitive restructuring, relaxation, communication and coping strategies, group interaction and support, relationships, and self-image. The group meetings were delivered by two therapists, one of whom was a psychologist, and were supplemented by a structured, manual-based set of homework exercises. Survival and psychosocial effects were examined. Patients were followed for at least 12 months post intervention; there was evidence of improved mood (depression, total mood disturbance) and enhanced self-esteem at the end of therapy, but no benefits were present at 3 and 6 months. There was no evidence of survival benefits.

Edmonds et al. and Cunningham et al. randomized 66 women to a group intervention that involved discussion, supportive strategies, and cognitive–behavioral therapy (Cunningham et al., 1998; Edmonds et al., 1999). The latter included 20 cognitive–behavioral assignments. In addition, participants were asked to attend a coping skills weekend and to practice relaxation exercises. The group intervention lasted 35 weeks for 2 hours each week and was led by a psychologist and either a social worker or psychology doctoral student. The control arm received a home cognitive–behavioral therapy package which included a coping skills workbook, relaxation tapes as well as supportive phone calls at 2, 4, 5, 10, and 12 months. Patients were followed for 12 months. This intervention resulted in "little" psychometric benefit compared to the control arm. Intervention subjects experienced increased anxious preoccupation coping and reduced helplessness coping. The control arm involved an important degree of intervention. This makes interpretation of the absence of a psychological benefit from the group intervention difficult. No survival effects were seen in this study.

Classen et al. have reported psychological outcomes of a randomized trial attempting to replicate Spiegel's earlier report of a survival benefit of supportive–expressive therapy in metastatic breast cancer (Classen et al., 2001). One hundred and twenty-five women with metastatic breast cancer were randomized to the same weekly supportive–expressive group therapy used in Spiegel's original study, each session lasting 90 minutes. Women were encouraged to participate to the end of life. Sessions were led by psychiatrists, psychologists, and social workers. The control arm was offered educational materials. Psychological outcomes were reported; the intervention significantly reduced traumatic stress symptoms but had no significant effects on overall mood. However, if the final assessment performed during the last year of life was excluded, a significant improvement in mood was seen. Survival data have not yet been reported.

Goodwin et al. reported the results of a multicenter randomized trial of group supportive–expressive therapy in 235 women with metastatic breast cancer (Goodwin et al., 2001). Women randomized to the intervention arm received supportive–expressive therapy following Spiegel's manual-based description. The therapy fostered support and encouraged emotional expressiveness and confronting effects of illness and change in self-image. Women were encouraged to examine roles, relationships, and the life altering nature of their illness, and to enhance communication and coping. Women attended weekly 90-minute sessions led by psychiatrists, psychologists, social workers, and nurse clinicians until death. The intervention was reported to enhance mood (total mood, anger, anxiety, depression, confusion) and to reduce pain. No survival effects were seen despite greater than 90 percent power to identify the survival effects that had been reported in 1989 by Spiegel et al. This study represents the largest attempt to replicate Spiegel's survival results—the successful delivery of the intervention is evidenced by the psychological benefits that were seen—however, an important effect of the intervention on survival was ruled out.

Healthy Survivors

Only one trial has been reported in healthy breast cancer survivors (not included in Tables B-1 or B-2). In this trial, Fogarty et al. randomized 123 subjects to view a dramatized videotape of a treatment consultation that enhanced compassion, or a dramatized videotape of a treatment consultation that did not enhance compassion; women who viewed the enhanced compassion videotapes reported reduced anxiety but also reduced information recall (Fogarty et al., 1999). There were also differences in perception of compassion and physician attributes in the expected direction. Women with no history of breast cancer participated as a second comparison group; results from these women were similar to those in breast cancer survivors.

Summary of Effectiveness of Psychosocial Interventions According to Type of Intervention

As was discussed in the preceding section, many of the published reports have identified psychological benefits of a variety of psychosocial interventions. These studies are reorganized in Appendix B, Table B-3 into three groups. The first group involves studies that primarily evaluated relaxation and/or imagery, whether the approach was individual or group based. The second category of interventions involved therapy delivered in a group setting; the specific type of therapy varied across studies. It included cognitive–behavioral therapy, structured group therapy, supportive–expressive group therapy, education with or without peer discussion, and mind-body–spirit groups. In the final section of Table B-3, studies of interventions in individuals are listed. These individual interventions were delivered in person or by telephone. Interventions included psychological assessment, telephone screening, cognitive–behavioral counseling, and several of these studies evaluated a variety of nursing interventions, focusing mainly on women with early stage breast cancer. Consideration was given to grouping studies by type of therapy evaluated (e.g., supportive, cognitive–behavioral). However, many of the interventions included components of more than one type of therapy (e.g., Cunningham), and some could not be easily classified into a specific therapeutic approach (e.g., telephone screening). Furthermore, the classification of interventions into group or individual approaches reflects current interest in group approaches for women with breast cancer. Studies involving couples counseling or partners of breast cancer patients are not included in these tables (Bultz et al., 2000; Christensen, 1983).

Studies evaluating relaxation with or without imagery appear in the first section of Table B-3.. Studies in early breast cancer are listed first (Arathuzik, 1994; Bridge et al., 1988; Kolcaba and Fox, 1999; Molassiotis et al., 2002; Richardson et al., 1997; Walker et al., 1999). With a single exception (Arathuzik, 1994), all of these studies provided evidence of effectiveness of the intervention, including improvements in mood, relaxation, comfort, overall quality of life, acceptance of death, enhanced coping, as well as reduced nausea and vomiting. The effective studies were all conducted in early phase breast cancer, the majority during initial treatment. Most of these interventions were short-term (6 days to 6 months), and the majority involved the use of relaxation audiotapes. One study utilized a group intervention (that study is also listed in the group intervention section of Table B-3) (Richardson et al., 1997). Taken together, these studies provide evidence of the effectiveness of relaxation with or without imagery in relieving psychologic distress or side effects of treatment (including nausea) in the early phases of breast cancer, effects that were present during active treatment with radiation and/or chemotherapy. The failure of

Arathuzik to identify significant effects may reflect the fact that the intervention was delivered in one session, that the study involved only 24 women (the power may have been inadequate to identify significant effects), or that the study was conducted in the setting of metastatic breast cancer, a setting in which a longer intervention may be needed (Arathuzik, 1994). Because of these limitations, further research would be needed to clarify the effectiveness of relaxation as a sole modality or combined with brief (single session) cognitive–behavioral therapy in metastatic breast cancer.

The second section of Table B-3 lists studies that evaluated a variety of group interventions. Studies of supportive therapy (including a study that compared supportive therapy to mind–body–spirit group therapy) are listed first, followed by those of supportive–expressive therapy, and then those that evaluated interventions having cognitive–behavioral therapy as a component (studies in early breast cancer are listed first in each grouping). These studies are roughly evenly split between early stage (seven studies) and metastatic (five studies) breast cancer. Four of these studies included cognitive-behavioral therapy either as the sole treatment modality, or as a major treatment modality. Three utilized a manual-based form of therapy: supportive–expressive therapy, combined with relaxation. One evaluated the benefits of therapist facilitated peer discussion groups, comparing them to education alone or to education combined with therapist-facilitated peer discussion, and one investigated a mind–body–spirit (CAM) group intervention. The interventions in early stage breast cancer tended to be shorter (6 to 12 weeks) than those conducted in metastatic breast cancer (5 months to end of life).

Despite the differences among these studies, the majority demonstrated important psychosocial benefits, although some of the studies conducted in early stage disease evaluated psychological outcomes for only a brief period of time (6 weeks) (Richardson et al., 1997). The benefits reported in these studies included improved mood, enhanced coping, reduced phobias, reduced traumatic stress symptoms, enhanced vitality, social and role functioning, reduced severity of psychiatric symptoms, enhanced quality of life, and enhanced spiritual integration. One study reported prolongation of survival (this is discussed in greater detail in the next section) (Spiegel et al., 1989). In at least one study beneficial effects of the intervention (an educational intervention) dissipated over time (Helgeson et al., 2001). In contrast to these largely positive findings, there were some studies that did not identify significant overall effects. For example, Edmonds et al., studying 66 patients evaluating supportive plus cognitive–behavioral group therapy versus home cognitive–behavioral study, reported "little psychometric effects" although there were some minor changes in coping style (Edmonds et al., 1999). The fact that the control group in this study also received interventions such as a home cognitive–behavioral study package and supportive telephone calls may have contributed to these negative results. Antoni et al. also failed to identify overall effects for a structured cognitive–behavioral group intervention, although they did find some beneficial effects in subgroups (Antoni et al., 2001). In evaluating Antoni's results, it must be noted that only the 73 percent of randomized women that completed all study assessments were included in the analysis; this could have introduced bias and made it difficult to identify important effects of the intervention.

Two studies evaluated the benefits of facilitated peer discussion or the use of coaches in support groups. Samarel, evaluating the addition of coaches to a structured support group, found higher quality relationships in the short-term when coaches were incorporated into the groups; however, these effects did not last beyond 8 weeks (Samarel and Fawcett, 1992; Samarel et al., 1993, 1997). In this study, some patients were re-randomized if their initial randomization resulted in an allocation that posed logistical difficulties. Because of this, these results must be interpreted with caution. Helgeson is the only investigator to have evaluated a facilitated peer discussion group in women with breast cancer (Helgeson et al., 1999, 2000, 2001). No benefits of facilitated peer discussion were identified in this large study in which women were followed for up to 4 years after randomization. Firm conclusions about facilitated peer discussion groups will require more than a single study.

Targ and Levine demonstrate comparability of psychoeducational group support to a complex CAM group support that addressed the mind–body–spirit continuum for most key psychosocial and HRQOL outcomes (Targ and Levine, 2002). Enhanced satisfaction and spiritual integration were reported in those who participated in the CAM group.

Overall, there was little evidence that the type of group therapy used led to different therapeutic effects; psychological benefits of various types were reported in cognitive–behavioral group interventions, supportive–expressive group interventions, and other interventions. There have been no head-to-head comparisons of the two most commonly utilized types of support groups: cognitive–behavioral and supportive–expressive. Such a comparison might lead to an enhanced understanding of the relative benefits of each type of intervention. On the basis of evidence currently available, selection of one type of intervention could probably be based on therapist and/or patient preference.

Finally, individual interventions have been listed in the third section of Table B-3. All of these were conducted in early breast cancer. The interventions evaluated in these studies were quite variable, including psychological interviews, telephone screening, individual cognitive–behavioral therapy, and problem skills training as well as a variety of nursing interventions. These nursing interventions yielded somewhat mixed results. In a very early study, Maguire et al. showed that nurse specialist counseling increased recognition of the need for psychiatric referral and that subsequent psychiatric intervention reduced psychiatric morbidity (Maguire et al., 1980, 1983). McArdle et al. identified important psychosocial and quality of life benefits for support from a breast cancer nurse compared to support from a voluntary organization of usual care (McArdle et al., 1996). Similarly, Wengström et al. reported fewer distress reactions and a stronger motivation to be emotionally involved in women who received a nursing intervention based on Orem's model for self-care (Walker et al., 1999; Wengstrom et al., 2001; Wengstrom et al., 1999). Ritz et al., evaluating advanced practice nursing interventions, identified reduced uncertainty, as well as beneficial subgroup effects on mood in those without a family history of breast cancer (Ritz et al., 2000). Cimprich reported beneficial effects of an unusual intervention designed to restore attentional capacity (Cimprich, 1993). In contrast, Sandgren et al. reported no overall beneficial effects of telephone-based cognitive–behavioral therapy (Sandgren et al., 2000). Similarly, Allen et al., evaluating problem-solving skills training (two sessions in person, four by telephone), identified no overall effects, although subgroup analysis suggested that there may be some benefit in women with good problem-solving skills at baseline (Allen et al., 2002). Finally, Lev et al., evaluating nurse counseling supplemented with videotape and a self-care booklet, reported "small to large effect sizes" for quality of life outcomes and psychiatric symptoms but did not perform any significance testing in their small study (Lev et al., 2001).

A single study of individual cognitive–behavioral counseling identified improved depression and quality of life in women receiving the intervention, similar to the findings reported for group cognitive–behavioral therapy (Marchioro et al., 1996). Similar effects were noted for a brief (one session) psychological interview, with or without a subsequent brief psychotherapy session (Burton et al., 1995). Maunsell's study of telephone screening for psychologic distress with referral of distressed patients to a social worker did not lead to any identifiable psychological benefits (Maunsell et al., 1996). Use of a health-care professional to provide screening (as opposed to a research assistant) and closer coordination of referrals to a therapist (rather than forwarding the patient's name to a social worker who attempted to contact the patient by telephone) may have led to better screening and counseling and different results. Further research in this area is needed. Taken together, these studies of individual interventions have identified some important psychological benefits; however, their results are not as consistent as those of relaxation/imagery interventions or group interventions.

It is probably too early to make comparisons across types of interventions, particularly since there have been no head-to-head comparisons of individual versus group interventions. It is notable that trials of individual interventions have been conducted in early stage breast cancer only, that some of the interventions have been extremely brief, and that the variety of the interventions studied has been much broader than the variety of interventions used in the group setting. Furthermore, although many reports in the metastatic setting in particular have examined long-term benefits, some, especially those in early stage breast cancer, have examined extremely short-term benefits (Arathuzik, 1994; Goodwin et al., 2001; Molassiotis et al., 2002; Richardson et al., 1997; Spiegel et al., 1989; Walker et al., 1999). In general, there is fairly good support for a short to intermediate term benefit for many group and individual interventions in early breast cancer (up to six months). However, the long-term benefits of interventions (apart from group interventions in the metastatic setting) have not been adequately evaluated.

Review of Selected Studies Using Non-randomized Designs

There is an extensive literature describing a variety of psychosocial interventions in cancer using non-randomized designs. Some of these studies focus on breast cancer patients. Others, including some that used randomized designs, involve patients with many different types of cancer. These studies are too numerous to review in detail; a small selection that highlights key points will be reviewed here.

Devine and Westlake have published an excellent meta-analysis[2] of over 100 studies of psycho-educational care in cancer patients (Devine and Westlake, 1995). These studies were conducted in a variety of settings, in patients with a variety of cancers, and they evaluated a range of interventions. The majority of the studies reviewed were conducted in the United States, and the most common setting for the intervention was the outpatient treatment department. Some of the interventions involved education only; others included muscle relaxation, guided imagery, and other behavioral interventions. Statistically significant benefits were found for anxiety, depression, overall mood, nausea, vomiting, pain, and knowledge in the meta-analysis. It was concluded that psycho-educational care was of benefit to adults with cancer, but that it was difficult to differentiate the effectiveness of various types of psycho-educational care.

The results of this meta-analysis are consistent with the findings of Helgeson et al. reported above in which a psycho-educational group intervention administered to women with breast cancer was found to be effective for a variety of psychosocial outcomes (Helgeson et al., 2001, 1999, 2000). They are also consistent with a recent non-randomized study by

---

[2]The term "meta-analysis" refers to the statistical analysis of the results from many individual studies for the purpose of integrating the findings.

Sepucha et al. in which breast cancer patients were assigned either to a control intervention (productive listening) in which a researcher listened to and prompted patients to reflect on their experiences communicating with physicians or to an experimental intervention (consultation planning) in which a researcher actively assisted patients in preparing for an upcoming consultation, generating a printed agenda, and developing techniques to improve communication with their physicians (Sepucha et al., 2002). Patients who received the experimental intervention reported significantly higher satisfaction, a sentiment that was echoed by the patients' physicians, suggesting that psycho-educational interventions and/or interventions that prepare patients for consultations with their physicians in a structured fashion may result in psychological benefit.

A series of studies conducted by Hosaka et al. in Japan evaluated a structured intervention that included psycho-education, problem-solving, psychological support, relaxation training, and guided imagery (Hosaka et al., 2001a, 2001b, 2000a, 2000b, 2000c). Using non-randomized before-after designs, these investigators first demonstrated psychological benefits of a 5 week intervention in women with node-negative breast cancer who did not have adjustment disorders but not in those with positive nodes or adjustment disorders. They later added three sessions at two monthly intervals and were able to show persistent benefit in all women regardless of nodal status or presence of an adjustment disorder. Additionally, they identified a series of psychological attributes predictive of improvement (good relationship with doctors, family support/ understanding, no co-morbid adjustment disorders). Although these results should be confirmed in a randomized trial, this pilot work suggested characteristics of women who needed a longer intervention and the efficacy of a longer intervention.

There are a number of interventions of potential psychosocial value that have not undergone adequate scrutiny in a randomized trial. Some patients are interested in these interventions, and some are used with increasingly frequency; for example, Internet chat groups, art therapy, music therapy, yoga, reflexology, and t'ai chi. Evidence supporting the benefits of these interventions is lacking. Targ and Levine (2002) evaluated a multi-factorial mind–body–spirit group intervention and suggested that these alternative therapy interventions will be well received by women with breast cancer and they may provide psychosocial benefit similar to more traditional psychosocial interventions. Haun and colleagues reported results of a non-randomized comparison of women awaiting breast biopsy who were exposed to either a 20 minute music-based intervention or to usual care (Haun et al., 2001). The music intervention involved a selection of "new age music" from which participants chose a 20-minute segment which they listened to via headphones. Women who received the intervention had a lower level of anxiety (measured using the State Trait Anxiety Inventory) and a lower respiratory rate. Similar information regarding other complementary interventions is likely to be forthcoming. Formal evaluation of the benefit, both in the long-term and short-term, of some of these interventions will be of interest.

Ashbury et al. evaluated a Canadian Cancer Society post-mastectomy peer visitor program, Reach to Recovery (Ashbury et al., 1998). They reported that patients were generally satisfied with the program and presented evidence of enhanced quality of life for participants. This non-randomized study suggests a beneficial effect of peer support shortly after breast cancer diagnosis.

Finally, there is a growing number of reports of benefit from a range of psychological interventions in breast cancer. In this literature, either the intervention or the subject population is novel. For example, Spiegel et al. have evaluated supportive–expressive group therapy in early stage breast cancer using a pre-, post-test design; they indicate that mood is enhanced, anxiety and depression are reduced, and traumatic stress symptoms reduced over a 6 month period (Spiegel et al., 1999). Because the study design was pre- and post-test and not randomized, it cannot be concluded that these benefits arose from the supportive–expressive group therapy intervention and not from spontaneous improvement as women adapted to their diagnosis. Similar benefits were seen in the metastatic setting, suggesting that at least some of these benefits might have arisen from the group intervention. Donnelly et al. carried out a pilot study of interpersonal psychotherapy administered by telephone to cancer patients receiving high dose chemotherapy and their partners (Donnelly et al., 2000). They reported the feasibility of the intervention and that participants were satisfied with the intervention. Further exploration of this approach could be useful for a number of reasons. It uses a therapeutic approach that has not been evaluated in a randomized trial in breast cancer patients (interpersonal psychotherapy), the intervention is telephone-based (some of the randomized trials of telephone-based interventions have not been successful in breast cancer patients), and it intervenes not only with breast cancer patients but also with partners—a group that has not received as much attention in the randomized trials setting.

This brief, and selective, presentation of findings outside of the clinical trials setting is not intended to be comprehensive. Instead, it is intended to demonstrate that there is currently a broad spectrum of interesting and potentially useful research that is looking at a spectrum of novel interventions. Additional research is recommended to address research gaps, to evaluate the generalizability of research findings across gender and cancer type, and to examine the translation of research findings into community practice. The Board's priorities for future research are described in Chapter 8.

SUMMARY

The results of 31 randomized trials in women with breast cancer and two meta-analyses, supported by observations in non-randomized studies, provide evidence of beneficial effects of a range of psychosocial interventions in both early and metastatic breast cancer. Notably, there is evidence for the benefit of relaxation/hypnosis/imagery interventions in early stage breast cancer, for group interventions in both early and metastatic breast cancer, and for individual interventions, primarily in the early setting. Although it needs strengthening, this evidence supports the conclusion that psychosocial interventions can be expected to reduce psychiatric symptoms and improve quality of life in routine clinical care of breast cancer.

REFERENCES

Agency for Healthcare Research and Quality. 2002. Management of cancer symptoms: Pain, depression, and fatigue: Summary. *Evidence Report/Technology Assessment* (61):1–9.

Allen SM, Shah AC, Nezu AM, et al. 2002. A problem-solving approach to stress reduction among younger women with breast carcinoma: A randomized controlled trial. *Cancer* 94(12):3089–3100.

Antoni MH, Lehman JM, Kilbourn KM, et al. 2001. Cognitive–behavioral stress management intervention decreases the prevalence of depression and enhances benefit finding among women under treatment for early-stage breast cancer. *Health Psychol* 20(1):20–32.

Arathuzik D. 1994. Effects of cognitive–behavioral strategies on pain in cancer patients. *Cancer Nurs* 17(3):207–214.

Ashbury FD, Cameron C, Mercer SL, Fitch M, Nielsen E. 1998. One-on-one peer support and quality of life for breast cancer patients. *Patient Educ Couns* 35(2):89–100.

Bridge LR, Benson P, Pietroni PC, Priest RG. 1988. Relaxation and imagery in the treatment of breast cancer. *Br Med J* 297(6657):1169–1172.

Bultz BD, Speca M, Brasher PM, Geggie PH, Page SA. 2000. A randomized controlled trial of a brief psychoeducational support group for partners of early stage breast cancer patients. *Psycho-oncology* 9(4):303–313.

Burke S, Kissane DW. 1998. Psychosocial impact of breast cancer: A review of interventions by specialist providers: A summary of the literature 1976–1996. NHMRC National Breast Cancer Center, NSW, Australia. [Online]. Available http://www.nbcc.org.au/pages/info/resource/nbccpubs/psych/interv/contents.htm [accessed October 23, 2003].

Burton MV, Parker RW, Farrell A, Bailey D, Conneely J, Booth S, Elcombe S. 1995. A randomized controlled trial of preoperative psychological preparation for mastectomy. *Psycho-oncology* 14:1–19.

Christensen DL. 1983. Postmastectomy couple counseling: An outcome study of a structured treatment protocol. *Journal of Sex and Marital Therapy* 9:266–275.

Cimprich B. 1993. Development of an intervention to restore attention in cancer patients. *Cancer Nurs* 16(2):83–92.

Classen C, Butler LD, Koopman C, et al. 2001. Supportive–expressive group therapy and distress in patients with metastatic breast cancer: A randomized clinical intervention trial. *Arch Gen Psychiatry* 58(5):494–501.

Cunningham AJ, Edmonds CV, Jenkins GP, Pollack H, Lockwood GA, Warr D. 1998. A randomized controlled trial of the effects of group psychological therapy on survival in women with metastatic breast cancer. *Psycho-oncology* 7(6):508–517.

Devine EC, Westlake SK. 1995. The effects of psychoeducational care provided to adults with cancer: Meta-analysis of 116 studies. *Oncol Nurs Forum* 22(9):1369–1381.

Donnelly JM, Kornblith AB, Fleishman S, et al. 2000. A pilot study of interpersonal psychotherapy by telephone with cancer patients and their partners. *Psycho-oncology* 9(1):44–56.

Edelman S, Bell DR, Kidman AD. 1999a. A group cognitive behaviour therapy programme with metastatic breast cancer patients. *Psycho-oncology* 8(4):295–305.

Edelman S, Lemon J, Bell DR, Kidman AD. 1999b. Effects of group CBT on the survival time of patients with metastatic breast cancer. *Psycho-oncology* 8(6):474–481.

Edmonds CV, Lockwood GA, Cunningham AJ. 1999. Psychological response to long-term group therapy: A randomized trial with metastatic breast cancer patients. *Psycho-oncology* 8(1):74–91.

Fawzy FI, Fawzy NW, Arndt LA, Pasnau RO. 1995. Critical review of psychosocial interventions in cancer care. *Arch Gen Psychiatry* 52(2):100–113.

Fawzy FI, Fawzy NW, Hyun CS, et al. 1993. Malignant melanoma. Effects of an early structured psychiatric intervention, coping, and affective state on recurrence and survival 6 years later. *Arch Gen Psychiatry* 50(9):681–689.

Ferlic M, Goldman A, Kennedy JJ. 1979. Group counseling in adult patients. *Cancer* 43:760–766.

Fogarty LA, Curbow BA, Wingard JR, McDonnell K, Somerfield MR. 1999. Can 40 seconds of compassion reduce patient anxiety? *J Clin Oncol* 17(1):371–379.

Fox BH. 1998. A hypothesis about Spiegel et al.'s 1989 paper on psychosocial intervention and breast cancer survival. *Psycho-oncology* 7(5):361–370.

Fukui S, Kugaya A, Okamura H, et al. 2000. A psychosocial group intervention for Japanese women with primary breast carcinoma. *Cancer* 89(5):1026–1036.

Ganz PA, Goodwin PJ. 2003. Quality of life in breast cancer. What have we learned and where do we go from here? In: Lipscomb J, Gotay C, Snyder C, eds. *Outcome Assessments in Cancer*. Cambridge: Cambridge University Press 2003.

Ganz PA, Greendale GA, Petersen L, Zibecchi L, Kahn B, Belin TR. 2000. Managing menopausal symptoms in breast cancer survivors: Results of a randomized controlled trial. *J Natl Cancer Inst* 92(13):1054–1064.

Goodwin PJ, Leszcz M, Ennis M, et al. 2001. The effect of group psychosocial support on survival in metastatic breast cancer. *N Engl J Med* 345(24):1719–1726.

Haun M, Mainous RO, Looney SW. 2001. Effect of music on anxiety of women awaiting breast biopsy. *Behav Med* 27(3):127–132.

Heinrich RL, Schag CC. 1985. Stress and activity management: Group treatment for cancer patients and spouses. *J Counsel Clin Psychol* 53;439–446.

Helgeson VS, Cohen S, Schulz R, Yasko J. 1999. Education and peer discussion group interventions and adjustment to breast cancer. *Arch Gen Psychiatry* 56(4):340–347.

Helgeson VS, Cohen S, Schulz R, Yasko J. 2000. Group support interventions for women with breast cancer: Who benefits from what? *Health Psychol* 19(2):107–114.

Helgeson VS, Cohen S, Schulz R, Yasko J. 2001. Long-term effects of educational and peer discussion group interventions on adjustment to breast cancer. *Health Psychol* 20(5):387–392.

Hosaka T, Sugiyama Y, Hirai K, Okuyama T, Sugawara Y, Nakamura Y. 2001a. Effects of a modified group intervention with early-stage breast cancer patients. *Gen Hosp Psychiatry* 23(3):145–151.

Hosaka T, Sugiyama Y, Hirai K, Sugawara Y. 2001b. Factors associated with the effects of a structured psychiatric intervention on breast cancer patients. *Tokai J Exp Clin Med* 26(2):33–38.

Hosaka T, Sugiyama Y, Tokuda Y, Okuyama T. 2000a. Persistent effects of a structured psychiatric intervention on breast cancer patients' emotions. *Psychiatry Clin Neurosci* 54(5):559–563.

Hosaka T, Sugiyama Y, Tokuda Y, Okuyama T, Sugawara Y, Nakamura Y. 2000b. Persistence of the benefits of a structured psychiatric intervention for breast cancer patients with lymph node metastases. *Tokai J Exp Clin Med* 25(2):45–49.

Hosaka T, Tokuda Y, Sugiyama Y, Hirai K, Okuyama T. 2000c. Effects of a structured psychiatric intervention on immune function of cancer patients. *Tokai J Clin Med* 25(4–6):183–188.

Ilnyckyj A, Farber J, Cheang MC WBH. 1994. A randomized controlled trial of psychotherapeutic intervention in cancer patients. *Ann CRMCC* 27:2:93–96.

Kissane D, Bloch S, Smith GC, et al. 2003. Cognitive–existential group psychotherapy for women with primary breast cancer: A randomized controlled trial. *Psycho-oncology* 12(6):532–546.

Kolcaba K, Fox C. 1999. The effects of guided imagery on comfort of women with early stage breast cancer undergoing radiation therapy. *Oncol Nurs Forum* 26(1):67–72.

Koocher, GP, Pollin, I. 2001. Preventive Psychosocial Intervention in Cancer Treatment: Implications for Managed Care, in *Psychosocial Interventions for Cancer*, Baum, A and Anderson, BL. eds. American Psychological Association: Washington DC.

Kuchler T, Henne-Bruns D, Rappat S, et al. 1999. Impact of psychotherapeutic support on gastrointestinal cancer patients undergoing surgery: Survival results of a trial. *Hepatogastroenterology* 46(25):322–335.

Lev EL, Daley KM, Conner NE, Reith M, Fernandez C, Owen SV. 2001. An intervention to increase quality of life and self-care self-efficacy and decrease symptoms in breast cancer patients. *Sch Inq Nurs Pract* 15(3):277–294.

Linn MW, Linn BS, Harris R. 1982. Effects of counseling for late stage cancer patients. *Cancer* 49(5):1048–1055.

Maguire P, Brooke M, Tait A, Thomas C, Sellwood R. 1983. The effect of counselling on physical disability and social recovery after mastectomy. *Clin Oncol* 9(4):319–324.

Maguire P, Tait A, Brooke M, Thomas C, Sellwood R. 1980. Effect of counselling on the psychiatric morbidity associated with mastectomy. *Br Med J* 281(6253):1454–1456.

Marchioro G, Azzarello G, Checchin F, Perale M, Segati R, Sampognaro E, Rosetti F, Franchin A, Pappagallo GL, Vinante O. 1996. The impact of a psychological intervention on quality of life in non-metastatic breast cancer. *Eur J Cancer* 32A(9):1612–1615.

Maunsell E, Brisson J, Deschenes L, Frasure-Smith N. 1996. Randomized trial of a psychologic distress screening program after breast cancer: Effects on quality of life. *J Clin Oncol* 14(10):2747–2755.

McArdle JM, George WD, McArdle CS, Smith DC, Moodie AR, Hughson AV, Murray GD. 1996. Psychological support for patients undergoing breast cancer surgery: A randomised study. *Br Med J* 312(7034):813–816.

Meyer TJ, Mark MM. 1995. Effects of psychosocial interventions with adult cancer patients: A meta-analysis of randomized experiments. *Health Psychol* 14(2):101–108.

Molassiotis A, Yung HP, Yam BM, Chan FY, Mok TS. 2002. The effectiveness of progressive muscle relaxation training in managing chemotherapy-induced nausea and vomiting in Chinese breast cancer patients: A randomised controlled trial. *Support Care Cancer* 10(3):237–246.

Newell SA, Sanson-Fisher RW, Savolainen NJ. 2002. Systematic review of psychological therapies for cancer patients: Overview and recommendations for future research. *J Natl Cancer Inst* 94(8):558–584.

Redman S, Turner J, Davis C. 2003. Improving supportive care for women with breast cancer in Australia: The challenge of modifying health systems. *Psycho-oncology* 12(56):521–531..

Richardson MA, Post-White J, Grimm EA, Moye LA, Singletary SE, Justice B. 1997. Coping, life attitudes, and immune responses to imagery and group support after breast cancer treatment. *Altern Ther Health Med* 3(5):62–70.

Richardson JL Shelton DR, Krailo M, et al. 1990. The effect of compliance with treatment on survival among patients with hematologic malignancies. *J Clin Oncol* 8(2):356–364.

Rimer B, Keintz MK, Glassman B. 1985. Cancer patient education: Reality and potential. *Prev Med* 14(6):801–818.

Ritz LJ, Nissen MJ, Swenson KK, et al. 2000. Effects of advanced nursing care on quality of life and cost outcomes of women diagnosed with breast cancer. *Oncol Nurs Forum* 27(6):923–932.

Samarel N, Fawcett J. 1992. Enhancing adaptation to breast cancer: The addition of coaching to support groups. *Oncol Nurs Forum* 19(4):591–596.

Samarel N, Fawcett J, Tulman L. 1993. The effects of coaching in breast cancer support groups: A pilot study. *Oncol Nurs Forum* 20(5):795–798.

Samarel N, Fawcett J, Tulman L. 1997. Effect of support groups with coaching on adaptation to early stage breast cancer. *Res Nurs Health* 20(1):15–26.

Sandgren AK, McCaul KD, King B, O'Donnell S, Foreman G. 2000. Telephone therapy for patients with breast cancer. *Oncol Nurs Forum* 27(4):683–688.

Sepucha KR, Belkora JK, Mutchnick S, Esserman LJ. 2002. Consultation planning to help breast cancer patients prepare for medical consultations: Effect on communication and satisfaction for patients and physicians. *J Clin Oncol* 20(11):2695–2700.

Simpson JS, Carlson LE, Trew ME. 2001. Effect of group therapy for breast cancer on healthcare utilization. *Cancer Pract* 9(1):19–26.

Spiegel D, Bloom JR. 1983. Group therapy and hypnosis reduce metastatic breast carcinoma pain. *Psychosom Med* 45(4):333–339.

Spiegel D, Bloom JR, Kraemer HC, Gottheil E. 1989. Effect of psychosocial treatment on survival of patients with metastatic breast cancer. *Lancet* 2(8668):888–891.

Spiegel D, Bloom JR, Yalom I. 1981. Group support for patients with metastatic cancer. A randomized outcome study. *Arch Gen Psychiatry* 38(5):527–533.

Spiegel D, Morrow GR, Classen C, et al. 1999. Group psychotherapy for recently diagnosed breast cancer patients: A multicenter feasibility study. *Psycho-oncology* 8(6):482–493.

Targ EF, Levine EG. 2002. The efficacy of a mind–body–spirit group for women with breast cancer: A randomized controlled trial. *Gen Hosp Psychiatry* 24(4):238–48.

Walker LG, Walker MB, Ogston K, et al. 1999. Psychological, clinical and pathological effects of relaxation training and guided imagery during primary chemotherapy. *Br J Cancer* 80(1–2):262–268.

Wallace KG. 1997. Analysis of recent literature concerning relaxation and imagery interventions for cancer pain. *Cancer Nurs* 20(2):79–87.

Wengstrom Y, Haggmark C, Forsberg C. 2001. Coping with radiation therapy: Effects of a nursing intervention on coping ability for women with breast cancer. *Int J Nurs Pract* 7(1):8–15.

Wengstrom Y, Haggmark C, Strander H, Forsberg C. 1999. Effects of a nursing intervention on subjective distress, side effects and quality of life of breast cancer patients receiving curative radiation therapy—a randomized study. *Acta Oncol* 38(6):763–770.

6

Delivering Psychosocial Services

Important advances in the diagnosis and treatment of breast cancer over the last quarter century have changed the makeup of the population of women surviving with breast cancer and dramatically altered how care is delivered, moving it from largely in-hospital to primarily ambulatory care. This chapter reviews the implications of these advances with respect to the prevalence and management of psychosocial distress. This chapter describes the structure and delivery of psychosocial services to women with breast cancer, including information on how services are delivered and the extent to which clinical and psychosocial services are integrated. Lastly, evidence is presented on how frequently women with breast cancer use psychosocial services.

THE EVOLUTION OF BREAST CANCER CARE AND ITS IMPLICATIONS FOR THE PROVISION OF PSYCHOSOCIAL SERVICES

Quality of life following a diagnosis of breast cancer is influenced by how and when the disease is diagnosed, the treatment, and the manner in which care is delivered. Breast cancer diagnosis, treatment, and care delivery have evolved greatly in the past 25 years, altering the composition of the population of women living with breast cancer, the health status of survivors of the disease, and how care is delivered. In the area of diagnostics, the widespread use of mammographic screening has resulted in women being diagnosed at younger ages and with smaller tumors. The 20 to 30 percent decrease in mortality associated with mammographic screening has contributed to a growing population of breast cancer survivors, estimated at 2.1 million women as of 1997. High screening rates have also resulted in more women being diagnosed with ductal carcinoma in situ (DCIS), a type of non-invasive breast cancer (see Chapters 2 and 3). In 2002, there were an estimated 47,700 women diagnosed with DCIS (54,300 with in situ cancer: lobular and ductal) (American Cancer Society, 2001, 2002). These women were not counted as among the 203,500 cases of invasive breast cancer, but because women with DCIS usually receive the same treatment as women with invasive early breast cancer, the rise in DCIS detection has increased the use of breast-cancer-related services and created a new cohort of women worried about their future risk of invasive disease.

Research conducted in the 1980s and early 1990s demonstrating that breast-conserving therapy followed by radiation is an efficacious alternative to mastectomy in most women has contributed to less disfigurement and reduced morbidity among women. This evolution in treatment has also reduced hospital stays and shifted care to outpatient settings. This trend has been accelerated with the dominance of managed care since the 1980s and efforts to reduce health-care costs. Mastectomy and other breast surgical procedures have been increasingly performed in outpatient day-hospital settings. According to one study, cancer-related complete mastectomies were rarely outpatient procedures in 1990, but by 1996, 8 percent of these procedures were outpatient in Connecticut, 13 percent were outpatient in Maryland, and 22 percent were outpatient in Colorado. By 1996, 43 to 72 percent of cancer-related subtotal mastectomies were outpatient procedures in these states, and 78 to 88 percent of lumpectomies were performed on an outpatient basis (Case et al., 2001). The implication of this shift in site of care is that women cared for in outpatient settings no longer have access to the many supportive care personnel that are hospital-based, such as social workers, nurse educators, psychologists, and clergy. The move to outpatient care and shorter hospital stays also has implications for caregivers and families. Much of the assistance with post-surgery recovery and rehabilitation is now assumed by families rather than by nursing personnel.

A greater reliance on pharmacological interventions for women with breast cancer follows findings that adjuvant systemic therapy reduces the risk of distant recurrence by about 40 percent and reduces mortality by 10 to 20 percent. New chemotherapeutic and hormonal agents have been introduced that are active in both early and metastatic breast cancer. These developments, while beneficial, have contributed to increased complexity of breast cancer care. Women treated for breast cancer in the 1960s would have typically been treated surgically with mastectomy in the hospital, with cancer care managed by a surgeon. In contrast, a woman with breast cancer today is likely to encounter a surgeon, radiation oncologist, and medical oncologist during her initial breast cancer treatment. With a number of treatment options to consider, women have increasingly become active participants in their care and often seek second opinions regarding treatment options. The breast cancer advocacy movement has encouraged informed decision-making among women facing alternative treatment choices (Lerner, 2001; National Breast Cancer Coalition, 2002).

The many steps along the trajectory of contemporary breast cancer (see Figure 4-1 in Chapter 4) and the multiple providers a woman encounters as she completes her care add to the complexity of cancer and highlight the need for care coordination. The complexity of care and the absence of coordination are often in themselves a source of psychosocial distress. The question of "Who is my doctor?" arises often and adds to the sense of vulnerability and uncertainty.

The evolving nature of breast cancer treatment has resulted in a heterogeneous group of breast cancer survivors. Elderly survivors treated 20 to 30 years ago, for example, had fewer treatment options and likely experienced radical mastectomy. The issues of concern to those women were often linked to late effects of surgery such as lymphedema and body image. Younger cohorts of women, in contrast, have benefited from a wider range of options, but may be concerned about a broader set of late effects related to their treatment. Among the late effects of contemporary breast cancer treatments are cognitive deficits, early menopause, heart conditions, and sexual dysfunction. During the late 1990s, many women with metastatic breast cancer underwent bone marrow transplantation, which was later shown not to be more effective than chemotherapy alone for advanced disease. Women who survived this treatment experienced not only the late effects but also the financial costs of this expensive procedure.

Evidence emerged in the mid 1990s that there was no medical benefit of frequent specialized follow-up of women after initial breast cancer in terms of time to diagnosis of recurrence and quality of life (Rosselli Del Turco et al., 1994; The GIVIO Investigators, 1994). Prior to that time, women with breast cancer visited their surgeon or oncologist for as many as 10 years after diagnosis for history taking, physical examination, blood tests, imaging, and mammography. It was thought that women preferred specialized care and intensive follow-up after primary treatment, but according to a randomized controlled trial conducted in England in 1996, routine, less intensive follow-up care could be provided by primary care practitioners without compromising patient satisfaction (Grunfeld et al., 1999, 1996). Professional guidelines now recommend against extensive blood tests and imaging and encourage periodic physical examinations, mammography, and pelvic exams (www.PeopleLivingWithCancer.org). This plan for follow-up implies that primary care physicians and not oncology providers will be responsible for addressing long-term issues related to late effects and psychosocial distress. In the United States, however, follow-up by oncologists continues as common clinical practice, driven perhaps by their availability and patient preferences, among other things. Women are still fearful about reduced frequency of visits and continue to believe that earlier diagnosis of recurrence is clinically important for a better outcome.

THE STRUCTURE AND DELIVERY OF PSYCHOSOCIAL SERVICES TO WOMEN WITH BREAST CANCER

Patterns of Breast Cancer Care

Assessing how well psychosocial services are being delivered depends on knowing where women with breast cancer seek care and who provides that care. There are very few descriptions of cancer-related health care delivery, but according to national population-based surveys, each year an estimated 4.8 million ambulatory care visits are made and 150,000 hospitalizations occur for breast cancer care (Table 6-1). These sources do not provide a great deal of clinical data, making it difficult to distinguish primary treatment from longer-term survivorship care. These data do provide rough estimates of who is getting care, where it is delivered, and some characteristics of care, for example, the source of payment for care.

Information on ambulatory care comes from two large population-based surveys conducted by the National Centers for Health Statistics, the National Ambulatory Medical Care Survey and the National Hospital Ambulatory Care Survey (NCPB special tabulations of NAMCS and NHAMCS, 1995–2000). Each year, data are collected on a sample of 20,000 to 40,000 visits to physicians' offices and a sample of 25,000 to 30,000 visits to hospital outpatient departments. Data are provided by physicians in their offices or by their office staff. Estimates of ambulatory care use are somewhat hampered by the exclusion of radiologists from the sampling frame of providers (some cancer-related radiology care is identified from data from hospital outpatient departments). According to these two surveys, the vast majority of ambulatory care occurs in private practice settings, with 90 percent of visits made to physician's offices and 10 percent to hospital outpatient departments. Of the visits to physicians' offices, 52 percent are made to oncologists, 19 percent to general surgeons, 5 percent to specialty surgeons, and 23 percent to specialists in medicine and primary care. Visits to hospital outpatient departments are most often to general medicine and surgery clinics. These findings suggest that efforts to improve the provision of psychosocial care should target oncology and surgery providers in private practice settings.

Although 45 percent of new cases of cancer occur among women age 65 and older, more than half of cancer-related outpatient visits are made by women under age 65 (Table 6-2). This likely reflects the use of ambulatory

TABLE 6-1 Characteristics of Breast Cancer-Related Ambulatory Care Visits, by Site of Care, United States, 1995-2000 [preliminary data][a]

Characteristic	Annual number of visits (in 1,000s)	Percent distribution
Site of visit		
All visits	4,836	100.0
Physician office-based visits	4,353	90.0
Hospital outpatient department visits	483	10.0
Physician office-based visits		
All physicians	4,353	100.0
Oncology/hematology	2,252	51.7
General surgery	811	18.6
Specialty surgery	228	5.2
Medical specialty	327	7.5
Primary care	726	16.7
Hospital outpatient department visits		
All clinic visits	483	100.0
General medicine	396	81.9
Surgery	68	14.2
Other	19	3.9

[a]Analyses of the National Ambulatory Medical Care Survey (NAMCS) and National Hospital Ambulatory Medical Care Survey (NHAMCS), 1995-2000. Breast cancer-related visits are those for which breast cancer (ICD-9-CM = 174) was recorded as the first, second, or third diagnosis associated with the visit. The sample size for breast cancer-related visits to physician offices was 904 and the sample size for visits to hospital outpatient departments was 1,169.
SOURCE: NCPB staff analyses of NAMCS and NHAMCS. Physician office-based visits are visits made to non-federally-employed physicians (excluding those in the specialties of anesthesiology, radiology, and pathology) in private offices, non-hospital-based clinics, and HMOs.
SOURCE: Special tabulations of NAMCS NHAMCS, NCPB staff.

care services by cancer survivors, who as a group are younger than women who are newly diagnosed (incident cases). The age and racial/ethnic distribution of patients seen in physician offices and hospital outpatient departments differs. Younger women and members of minority racial/ethnic groups are more likely to frequent hospital outpatient departments. Patients seen in outpatient departments are also more likely to be uninsured or insured through the Medicaid program. Any effort to improve services to members of minority racial/ethnic groups could focus on these sites of care.

Reasons for visits (as stated by patients) were similar by site. Generally, they were to monitor progress, to obtain breast cancer care and examinations, and to receive post-operative care. Patients visiting hospital outpatient departments are more likely to spend more time with the physicians—

TABLE 6-2 Characteristics of Breast Cancer-Related Ambulatory Care Visits, by Site of Care, United States, 1995-2000[a]

Characteristic	Physician Office-Based Visits (percent)	Hospital Outpatient Department Visits (percent)
Total number of visits	4,353,000	483,000
Percent	100.0	100.0
Age		
Less than 45	13.0	20.2
45 to 64	45.5	50.4
65 to 74	25.0	17.6
75 and older	16.5	11.8
Race/ethnicity		
White, non-Hispanic	86.3	76.5
White, Hispanic	4.7	7.3
Black	6.3	13.5
Other	2.6	2.7
Main source of payment		
Private insurance	59.8	57.6
Medicare	25.0	14.5
Medicaid	2.5	6.9
Other, unknown source	8.8	10.5
Uninsured (self pay/no charge)	3.9	10.6
Reason for visit (as reported by patient)		
Progress visit	14.3	19.5
Breast cancer care	13.2	18.1
General medical exam/breast exam	8.8	9.2
Post-operative visit	8.2	4.4
Chemotherapy	7.3	10.6
Medical counseling	—	3.7
Radiation therapy	—	2.5
Other	48.1	32.0
Time spent with doctor[b]		
Less than 15 minutes	20. 3	27.0
15 to 29 minutes	54.9	17.9
30 minutes and longer	24.7	55.1
Saw RN, PA, NP during visit		
Yes	37.7	59.6
No	62.3	40.4
Services provided during visit		
Mental health and psychotherapy[c]	4.8	5.3
Breast self exam instruction	50.0	34.5
Diet counseling/education	15.7	7.6
Exercise counseling/education	13.3	4.7

[a]Analyses of the National Ambulatory Medical Care Survey (NAMCS) and National Hospital Ambulatory Medical Care Survey (NHAMCS), 1995–2000. Breast cancer-related visits are those for which breast cancer (ICID-9-CW=174) was recorded as the first, second, or third diagnosis associated with the visit.
[b]Time spent with physician is not available in hospital outpatient clinics in 1995.

for more than half (55 percent) of visits, patients were seen for half an hour or longer as compared to 25 percent in physicians' offices. This may reflect the complexity of cases seen in outpatient departments, the provision of more extensive counseling, or the fact that many outpatient departments have teaching functions. Visits to outpatient departments are more likely than those made to physicians' offices to bring patients into contact with registered nurses, nurse practitioners, or physician assistants (60 vs. 38 percent of visits). According to these ambulatory care surveys, mental health-related services are rarely provided in the context of cancer-related care (in 5 percent or less of visits), and generally are less likely to be provided than counseling regarding breast self-exam, diet, and exercise. These estimates, may, of course, be artificially low if providers failed to document the provision of counseling on the survey.

In the past decade, comprehensive breast centers and breast care programs have been developed to put under one roof the many providers and services that a woman with breast cancer might need to make breast care simpler and to provide "one stop" care. Typically, these programs employ social workers, clinical nurse specialists, or psychologists affiliated with them, who provide some form of systematic psychosocial intake or assessment, education, and counseling. Because the physical and the psychological impacts of the disease and treatment are often inter-related, having psychosocial services available within the breast care setting allows for the flow of patient-centered information to be shared among the center practitioners. For example, if a woman suddenly develops lymphedema of her arm, she will need a variety of physical interventions to address the problem, and she will need someone to assist her with the psychological distress that often accompanies this experience. Women understandably like the comprehensive breast care approach, and it appears to be gaining in popularity. However, it is not known what proportion of women receive care in these settings, but it is surely a small minority given that most visits are to a physician's office and the small number of comprehensive cancer centers and their uneven geographic distribution (Frost et al., 1999; Rabinowitz, 2002). Furthermore, while multidisciplinary care in breast clinics has gained wide acceptance in theory, in practice it can be a complicated situation. There can be economic constraints as well as turf issues among surgery, medical oncology, and radiology, requiring that some sacrifices be made by at least one or two of these major players so that the patient may be best served. Specifically, this means that one or more of the three players may have to give up their turf and perhaps efficiency in working in the clinic. For example, a member of the treatment team may have to wait while patients move through a surgery clinic, some of whom are not diagnosed with breast cancer and therefore may not be in need of multidisciplinary collaboration. Collaboration can be limited if salaries are at stake and one member of the team stands to gain or lose money depending on how the clinic is managed.

Information on breast cancer-related hospital care is available from the National Hospital Discharge Survey (NHDS), a population-based survey conducted by the Centers for Disease Control and Prevention. Presented here are results of analyses of a sample of 1,850 discharges for which breast cancer was the primary diagnosis associated with the hospitalization (a total of 613,719 hospital discharges [all causes] were in the combined sample from the 1999 and 2000 surveys). According to the NHDS, there were an estimated 106,600 United States hospitalizations annually with the associated principle diagnosis of female breast cancer (Table 6-3). Half (50.1 percent) of the breast cancer-related hospital care was for women age 65 and older. Nearly two-thirds of breast-cancer-related hospitalizations were for mastectomy (65.2 percent), 7.2 percent for subtotal mastectomy, 10.1 percent for lumpectomy, and 17.5 percent are for other indications. Breast cancer-related stays in the hospital were relatively short, with 39.2 percent of women discharged within a day. As many as 7,500 women with breast cancer who were over the age of 75 were discharged from the hospital to their home within one day. The implications of this are that post-surgical care for elderly women, who are often frail and have other chronic illnesses, has to be managed at home, usually by family members and caregivers. Medicare is the predominant payer for hospital care, responsible for 45.0 percent of breast cancer-related discharges. One-in-five (22 percent) of discharges related to breast cancer care were from hospitals with fewer than 100 beds. This has implications for psychosocial care insofar as smaller hospitals are less likely to have extensive support service personnel immediately available.

This descriptive information on ambulatory and hospital care does not fully capture breast-cancer related care. Increasingly breast cancer surgical care is being delivered in free-standing ambulatory surgery centers. There are few sources of national data on care provided in these facilities. A national survey of ambulatory surgery centers was conducted by NCHS in 1995, but it has not been repeated. As mentioned earlier, by 1996, roughly 10 to 20 percent of cancer-related complete mastectomies were outpatient procedures, 40 to 70 percent of subtotal mastectomies were outpatient procedures, and 80 to 90 percent of lumpectomies were performed on an outpatient basis (Case et al., 2001). While much of the surgical care provided to women may be absent in the estimates above, it is likely that pre- and post-surgical consultations take place in ambulatory settings for which data are available and where psychosocial issues would most likely be addressed.

PSYCHOSOCIAL SERVICE USE

While evidence suggests that roughly 20 to 40 percent of women with breast cancer will exhibit psychosocial distress (see Chapter 3), it is not well

TABLE 6-3 Characteristics of Breast Cancer-Related Hospitalizations, United States, 1999–2000

Characteristic	Annual Number	Percent Distribution
Total	106,600	100.0
Age		
Under 45	12,200	11.5
45–64	41,000	38.5
65–74	27,200	25.6
75 and older	26,100	24.5
Principle procedure'		
Mastectomy	69,500	65.2
Subtotal mastectomy	7,700	7.2
Lumpectomy	10,700	10.1
Other	18,700	17.5
Discharge status		
Routine/discharged home	93,500	87.8
Long-term care institution	3,900	3.7
Dead	2,000	1.9
Other	7,200	6.7
Length of stay		
1 day	41,800	39.2
2 days	31,200	29.2
3 days	16,500	15.4
4 or more days	17,100	16.1
Main source of payment		
Medicare	47,900	45.0
Medicaid	6,000	5.6
Private	29,000	27.2
HMO/PPO	15,400	14.5
Uninsured	3,000	2.8
Other	5,300	5.0
Size of hospital (number of beds)		
6–99	23,400	22.0
100–199	28,700	26.9
200–299	14,900	14.0
300–499	25,600	24.0
500 and over	14,000	13.1
Hospital ownership		
Proprietary	8,100	7.6
Government	11,200	10.5
Nonprofit	87,200	81.9

[a]ICD-9-CM codes for procedures: mastectomy (85.4), subtotal mastectomy (85.23), lumpectomy (85.21).
NOTE: 1,850 of 613,719 sample hospital discharges were for women whose primary diagnosis was breast cancer (International Classification of Diseases, 9th Revision, Clinical Modification [ICD-9-CM] code 174).

understood how often women with breast cancer are referred for services, how accessible services are to women, and how often services are actually sought. Evidence from the field of mental health suggests that a majority of individuals with mental disorders do not receive mental health services (U.S. Department of Health and Human Services, 2000). According to one of the largest studies of mental health needs and service use, 28 percent of individuals can be expected to have mental or addictive disorders in the course of a year, but only 15 percent of the population obtains services to address these disorders (U.S. Department of Health and Human Services, 2000). When mental health services are obtained, they are largely obtained in the health sector (either mental health specialty or general health sector). Other sectors such as human services or voluntary support networks are also important providers of services.

The National Coalition for Cancer Survivorship (NCCS), an advocacy organization, as a part of its published "Imperatives for Quality Cancer Care" stressed the importance of meeting the psychosocial needs of cancer survivors. The NCCS recommends that psychosocial services be provided for every person with cancer including (http://www.canceradvocacy.org):

• Availability of a psychosocial program and case manager who provides assessment, education, support, and referral for services;
• Screening for psychosocial risk and in-depth individual and family assessments conducted on a regular and continuous basis across the disease spectrum by qualified psychosocial specialists and, in conjunction with the medical plan, the development of a psychosocial treatment plan;
• A choice of intervention modalities including individual, family, marital, peer, and pastoral counseling and access to complementary therapies;
• Training in cancer-related self-advocacy including information seeking, negotiation, communication, and problem-solving skills.

The NCCN further recommends that the patient and the family be seen as the unit of care and receive:

• Culturally appropriate education about cancer, its treatment and side effects, and the necessary physical care responsibilities that need to be assumed by the patient and family; and
• Information about local, state, and national organizations that provide support, education, and concrete services including how to access legal information and services for workplace, insurance and other cancer-related discrimination.

Judging how close the cancer care community is in meeting these goals is difficult because of a relative lack of information on the content of cancer care. The extent of psychosocial service use among women with breast cancer is hard to gauge because of limited data from large representative samples and because survey and regional study data vary in different reports and time periods. The National Cancer Institute added a special supplement to the National Health Interview Survey (NHIS) in 1992 to assess issues related to cancer survivorship. The NHIS is a population-based survey of 49,401 households conducted by the National Center for Health Statistics, Centers for Disease Control and Prevention. According to this supplement, which sampled 24,040 households, only 14 percent of 656 individuals who had had any cancer (excluding non-melanoma skin cancer) within the past 10 years reported that they had received counseling or participated in a support group following their diagnosis (Hewitt et al., 1999). Among those who did not receive counseling, most (64 percent) felt that they did not need it, 12 percent did not want it, and 9 percent did not know that it was available. Another 15 percent said that they did not get counseling for some other reason. Controlling for sociodemographic characteristics, women with breast cancer (and individuals with any cancer diagnosed more recently) were found to be twice as likely as those with other cancers to have received counseling or to have participated in a support group. More than a quarter (27 percent) of women with a history of breast cancer had received psychosocial services following their diagnosis (Hewitt et al., 1999).

In a more recent analysis of data from the NHIS, cancer survivors (4,878) were more likely than individuals without a history of cancer to report using a mental health service within the past year (7.2 versus 5.7 percent) (Hewitt and Rowland, 2002). A mental health service was defined as contact with a mental health professional such as a psychiatrist, psychologist, psychiatric nurse, or clinical social worker. Participation in support groups was not ascertained, and the reason for the mental health visit was not asked. Controlling for socio-demographic characteristics, cancer survivors without other chronic illness were 1.6 times more likely to use a mental health service, and cancer survivors with other chronic illness were 3.0 times more likely to use a mental health service as compared to those without cancer or other chronic disease. According to these results, based on 3 years of NHIS data (1998 to 2000), survivors of breast cancer were not more likely (6.3 percent) than survivors of other cancers to have used a mental health service (Hewitt and Rowland, 2002). This latter might seem at variance with the increased likelihood found in earlier surveys, but the intervention, mental health services for any reason, differed from cancer related counseling and support group participation as did the time period.

Information from regional studies confirms findings of relatively low mental health service use among women with breast cancer. According to a survey of 233 women (151 completed responses, 65 percent response rate) conducted at a regional breast care center in upstate New York and contacted within 3 years of their breast cancer diagnosis, relatively few had used formal psychosocial services. Only 15 percent of women had talked to a professional counselor (e.g., psychologist), 25 percent had participated in a support group, and the majority (60 percent) of women had talked to a friend who had breast cancer (Table 6-4), although there is overlap in these percentages. Of those who did not seek services, the majority did not feel it

TABLE 6-4 Survey of Breast Cancer Patients Regarding Use of Psychosocial Services

Question	Sample size	Percent
Since your diagnosis, have you talked to:		
A professional counselor (e.g., psychologist)?		
• Yes	22	15.2
• No, not necessary	95	65.5
• No, but helpful	28	19.3
A volunteer counselor?		
• Yes	42	29.4
• No, not necessary	81	56.6
• No, but helpful	20	14.0
A friend who had breast cancer?		
• Yes	89	59.7
• No, not necessary	42	28.2
• No, but helpful	18	12.1
A "support group"?		
• Yes	36	24.5
• No, not necessary	78	53.1
• No, but helpful	33	22.4
When was counseling most needed for you?		
• Didn't need counseling	49	23.7
• At time of diagnosis	85	41.1
• During treatment	44	21.2
• After treatment	29	14.0
Counseling services you would have been interested in the past:		
• Talking to a professional counselor	55	23.7
• Talking to a volunteer counselor (another woman with breast cancer)	84	36.2
• Attending a monthly support group as necessary	45	19.4
• Attending a professionally led group therapy program	48	20.7

NOTE: Cases do not always total 151 because of omitted responses and multiple responses.
SOURCE: Trief and Donohue-Smith, 1996.

was necessary (Trief and Donohue-Smith, 1996). Women were more likely to report needing counseling at the time of diagnosis (41 percent), but a substantial proportion of women felt that counseling was needed during treatment (21 percent) and after treatment (14 percent) (Table 6-4). Among this sample, 28 percent reported a great deal of anxiety, and 14 percent reported a great deal of depression as they had coped with their illness. The percentage that experienced both a high degree of anxiety and depression was not reported, so it is not clear that the percentages can be summed to a level of distress of 42 percent. The authors concluded that although a sizable minority of women need formal psychosocial services, many women work their way through the stressful periods using available support and their own coping skills.

This conclusion is consistent with work of Worden and Weisman, investigators who developed a screening survey to identify cancer survivors at risk for poor coping and distress. Of 372 patients screened, 124 (33 percent) were found to be at risk and about half (60) accepted counseling. There did not appear to be any clear way to differentiate among those who did or did not accept counseling (Worden and Weisman, 1980). A German study conducted among 132 oncology outpatients (72 percent of whom had breast cancer) found that 28 percent participated in psychosocial support, with younger patients more likely to participate (Plass and Koch, 2001). The main reason for not participating was sufficient support from family, friends, or doctors. In an Australian study involving 202 individuals (115 males) with cancer seen in an outpatient setting (all cancer sites), counseling was offered to 48 percent of patients but was only accepted by 28 percent of patients to whom it was offered. A frequently reported reason for refusal of services was "not now" indicating that the offer of psychosocial services needs to be repeated (Curry et al., 2002).

Relatively few long-term survivors of breast cancer continue to receive psychosocial support, according to a large cohort study of women conducted in Los Angeles and Washington DC. In this study of 5- to 10-year survivors, fewer than 13 percent of women reported that they were currently using psychosocial or counseling therapies, while many more said that they had used them in the past. Only 6 percent of the women were currently in individual therapy. Only 5 percent were currently active in cancer support groups, although 30 percent said that they had used them in the past (Ganz et al., 2002).

Other research points to an unmet need for psychosocial services. Ferrell and colleagues asked nearly 300 women, "What resources do you feel you did not receive and are most needed to improve QoL?" (Ferrell et al., 1998; Simmons, 1998). Respondents identified 9 resources related to psychosocial support that were lacking in their care:

1. Support groups (peer-led, newly diagnosed, single women, long-term survivors)
2. Individual counseling
3. Family support
4. Education on delayed side effects
5. Management of menopause/hormone changes
6. Spiritual support
7. Support from/for spouse
8. Sexuality counseling
9. Support for fear of recurrence

In summary, it is difficult to judge the extent of use of psychosocial services among women with breast cancer, but available evidence from national surveys and regional studies of cancer patients' use and acceptance of psychosocial services suggests that: use is relatively low (perhaps 10 percent and at the most 30 percent, and often of relatively informal nature) (Hewitt et al., 1999; Ganz et al., 2002: Plass and Koch, 2001; Trief and Donohue-Smith, 1996; Worden and Weisman, 1980); it seems to diminish with time; and most individuals who refuse services want to cope using their own resources, or to receive help at another time.

The Delivery of Psychosocial Services

Psychosocial services can be delivered by primary care and cancer care providers, specialty providers such as mental health professionals (psychologists and psychiatrists), advanced practice nurses, social workers, community-based programs, and increasingly by telephone or online computer services (see Chapter 4 for a description of psychosocial providers). Psychosocial services may or may not be integrated with breast cancer clinical care. Some settings such as comprehensive breast care centers have psychosocial providers on staff (Sorensen and Liu, 1995), while in other settings there are parallel systems for clinical and psychosocial care. This section describes examples of the delivery of psychosocial services in private practice, a managed care setting, through community-based programs, and via computer. The examples are drawn from presentations of program providers at the Board's October 2002 workshop (see agenda in Appendix A).

Private Practice

Most women receive their breast cancer care in community-based private practice settings. Psychosocial services may be provided by primary care physicians or oncology providers in the context of clinical care, but relatively few clinicians have psychologists or social workers available on site, unless they work in a large group practice or have a hospital-based practice. Physicians may refer individuals experiencing psychosocial distress to a local psychologist or psychiatrist or to community-based support programs available through a local hospital or breast cancer group. A model that is infrequently used, but which holds promise for making psychosocial services more accessible to patients seen in private physicians' offices is "collaborative practice," which involves a psychologist in private practice regularly rotating to private oncology, primary care, and other practices (e.g., obstetrics/gynecology) to work in partnership with referring physicians.

At the NCPB October 2002 workshop, the Board heard from Dr. Helen Coons, a psychologist in private practice who works collaboratively with a number of oncology care clinicians to provide psychosocial support services. Among the services that psychologists working in this fashion may provide are counseling related to treatment, depression, body image concerns, symptoms (e.g., hot flashes), sexual, reproductive and parenting issues, and substance abuse problems. Dr. Coons reported that commonly addressed issues in her practice include fears of recurrence, concerns about symptoms, anxiety, and adjustments at the end of life.

Managed Care

The majority of Americans receive their care within a managed care plan. Managed care can be defined as an entity that assumes both the clinical and the financial responsibility for the provision of health care for a defined population (Donaldson, 1998). With an increasingly complex health care system, a number of types of managed care have emerged, and it is difficult to distinguish one type of managed care organization from another (Landon et al., 1998). There is no information regarding how psychosocial care is delivered within managed care plans across the country, but there are a few programs that have been described as improving the quality of breast cancer care, including patient satisfaction with care. The American Association of Health Plans recognized one supportive care program as exemplary; it is offered by one of its members, a large group-model HMO in Southern California (Geiger et al., 2000)

The Southern California Kaiser Permanente Medical Group in collaboration with Women's Information Network Against Breast Cancer (WIN-ABC) improved patient satisfaction with care following the introduction of a breast cancer patient information and support program (Geiger et al., 2000). The program, called Breast Buddy Care Program, featured a coordinator, information resources, and mentoring from a breast cancer survivor. Following implementation of the program, participants were more likely than non-program respondents to be very satisfied with their care (71 percent versus 56 percent). Use of the program resources was relatively high, with 75 percent of

women using materials from the clinic-based library and 60 percent request-
ing a patient mentor. Investigators estimate that the annual cost of a fully
functioning program at a single hospital with several hundred new breast
cancer cases annually would probably range from $25,000 to $75,000.

Cancer Center-Based Programs

Many women with breast cancer will receive at least some of their care
within a hospital, either as an inpatient or when visiting an outpatient hospital-based practice or clinic. There are two sets of standards that address
cancer-related quality of care, those of the American College of Surgeons'
(ACoS) Commission on Cancer (CoC), and those of the Association of Community Cancer Centers (ACCC). Of the two, the standards of the CoC
affect more individuals with cancer because an estimated 82 percent of new
cases of cancer are seen in the 1,428 hospitals approved by the CoC. Relatively few individuals with cancer are seen within the 47 NCI-designated
comprehensive cancer centers, but these institutions are where many of the
research, education, and training programs are located, making them important models of care. This section of the report describes the availability
of psychosocial services within hospitals that provide cancer care.

The American College of Surgeons' Commission on Cancer The CoC sets standards for quality multidisciplinary cancer care delivered primarily in hospitals,
surveys hospitals to assess compliance with those standards, collects standardized and quality data from approved hospitals to measure treatment patterns
and outcomes, and uses the data to evaluate hospital provider performance and
develop effective educational interventions to improve cancer care outcomes at
the national and local level (http://www.facs.org/dept/cancer/coc/cocar.html,
accessed January 24, 2003). Selected standards of the Commission related to
the provision of psychosocial care are shown in Box 6-1).

The CoC had, by 2003, approved 1,428 cancer programs which, as
mentioned earlier, are estimated to provide care for 82 percent of the
nation's newly diagnosed patients (http://www.facs.org/dept/cancer/coc/
whatis.html, accessed May 1, 2003). The Commission conducts extensive
reviews of cancer programs through onsite visits at least every 3 years. Findings of the CoC survey are used as part of the Joint Commission for the
Accreditation of Healthcare Organizations (JCAHO) accreditation process
for JCAHO-accredited organizations that house a cancer center. The collaboration between the American College of Surgeons' CoC and JCAHO is
an attempt to increase the visibility of approved cancer programs, share
information on standards and survey process, and increase consumer access
to performance information about health care organizations. CoC staff provided information on supportive care services from institutions surveyed by

BOX 6-1
Selected Standards of the American College of Surgeons' Commission on Cancer Related to Psychosocial Services

Cancer patients have access to rehabilitative, supportive, and continuing care services. (standard 5.1.0)
- Education is provided for patients and their families through structured programs.
- Referral to support services is available to patients and their families.
- A home care agency(ies) exists to provide professional services to patients and their families in the home.
- A clinical nutritionist works with patients and their families.
- Pastoral care services are available to meet the needs of patients and their families.
- A hospice program exists to provide professional and volunteer services to terminally ill patients and their families.
- Information and programs specific to survivorship issues are available to patients with cancer and their families.

Site-specific services are based on the needs of the patients (standard 5.2.0).

There is a multidisciplinary team approach to planning and implementing supportive and continuing care services (standard 5.3.0).
- A multidisciplinary recovery/rehabilitation team is in place.
- The team meets regularly.
- The team is an essential part of patient care.
- The team actively participates with families.

Oncology services provide multidisciplinary care (standard 4.1.0).
- A multidisciplinary team approach is available (including a multimodality assessment of medical treatment, nursing interactions, nutritional, and psychosocial needs).
- Patients have access to the following care providers or services, either in-house or by referral: counseling, discharge planning, hospice care, nutritional care, oncology nursing, pain control, pastoral care, patient education, pharmacy, rehabilitation/support, social work, specialty physicians).
- The patient and families are assessed to determine physical, psychosocial, and spiritual needs; appropriate interventions and referrals are in evidence.
- Patient education and supportive care activities, comprehensive multidisciplinary discharge planning, and referral to community agencies and services are available.

Nursing care is provided by nurses with specialized knowledge and skills in oncology (standard 4.8.0).

SOURCE: American College of Surgeons' Commission on Cancer, 1997.

TABLE 6-5 Support Services Offered by Cancer Programs Approved and Surveyed by the American College of Surgeons' Commission on Cancer, 1999–2001

Service[a]	Programs Offering Service (N = 1170)[b]	
Support services:	Number	Percent
Home care	1081	92
Hospice	1037	87
Nutrition[c]	869	74
Pain management	1081	92
Lymphedema rehabilitation	396*	85
Providers:		
ONS certified nurses on staff	994	85
Physical/occupational therapist	455*	98
Pastoral care	1152	98
Psychiatrist	1114	95
Psychologist	1062	91
Social worker	1155	99
Rehab therapist	1101	94
Stomal therapist	1082	92
Support activities:		
Breast cancer specific:		
Reach to Recovery[d]	1048	90
Prostate cancer specific:		
Man to Man[e]	489	42
US Too[f]	304	26
Any cancer type:		
CanSurmount[g]	194	17
I Can Cope[h]	651	56
Other Support Groups	359	77

[a]Services may be available directly from the institution or by referral to appropriate resource.
[b]Combinedsample results from CoC approved programs surveyed in 1999 (N = 325), 2000 (N = 380), and 2001 (N = 465).
[c]In 1999 13% of surveyed programs reported nutrition services as compared to 98 percent in both 2000 and 2001. This significant change could not be explained by CoC staff.
[d]A support group sponsored by ACS for women with breast cancer.
[e]A support group sponsored by ACS for men who are prostate cancer survivors.
[f]US TOO provides information, local support groups, counseling and educational meetings to assist people with prostate cancer as they make decisions about their treatment and continued quality of life.
[g]A program that puts a patient in touch with a person who has experienced the same kind of cancer.
[h]A 7-week educational series for cancer patients and their families sponsored by ACS.

CoC during 1999, 2000, and 2001 (personal communication from Connie Blankenship, CoC, to Maria Hewitt, March 31, 2003). The information provided is self reported on the application forms completed by institutions in advance of their on-site survey (Table 6-5). At least some level of supportive care was available in the reporting sites, for example, social workers were available in 99 percent of programs, psychologists were available in 91 percent of programs, and the ACS Reach to Recovery was available in 90 percent of programs.

Association of Community Cancer Centers Standards (ACCC) ACCC is a membership organization that includes 650 medical centers, hospitals, oncology practices, and cancer programs. The organization estimates that its members provide services to 40 percent of all new cancer patients in the United States (http://www.accc-cancer.org/about/, accessed January 24, 2003). The provision of psychosocial services is necessary to meet ACCC cancer program standards (Box 6-2) (http://www.accc-cancer.org/pubs/Standardstemp.html, accessed January 22, 2003). The ACCC revised its Standards for Psychosocial Services based on the NCCN standards (1999) and clinical practice guidelines to note that psychosocial services should be provided by several kinds of professionals, all of whom should have training or experience in the psychosocial problems of patients with cancer (Standard 1). Standard 2 outlines the need for a multidisciplinary committee to tailor the standards to the needs of each clinical setting and to monitor programs to ensure accountability for undertaking recommendations and changes. Unlike the CoC, there is no formal review of compliance to these standards.

National Cancer Institute-designated cancer centers The Cancer Centers Program of the NCI supports cancer research programs in 61 institutions across the United States (Figure 6-1) (http://www3.cancer.gov/cancercenters/description.html). Although the support from NCI is mainly limited to support of research infrastructure, all clinical and comprehensive cancer centers also provide clinical care and services for cancer patients. Three types of centers are supported through the Cancer Centers Program:

1. Generic cancer centers have a narrow research that may focus, for example, on basic sciences;
2. Clinical cancer centers usually integrate strong basic science with strong clinical science; and
3. Comprehensive cancer centers integrate strong basic, clinical, and prevention, control, and population sciences.

As shown by the map, large areas of the United States particularly the midsection of the country, are not near an NCI-designated cancer center.

BOX 6-2
Standards for Psychosocial Services, Association of
Community Cancer Centers Standards for Cancer Programs

Standard I

Psychosocial services are provided by several disciplines in order to address the range of problems that patients and their families have as a consequence of cancer and its treatment. The disciplines are represented by social workers, nurses, psychologists, and psychiatrists, who are trained and skilled in the identification of psychological and social problems and are able to work with the primary oncology team and assure triage of the patient to the appropriate resources for assistance and/or treatment.

Standard II

Psychosocial services, provided by the professional outlined above, will follow clinical practice guidelines that are both consensus and empirically derived.

A. Psychosocial services include, but are not limited to:
  1. Social work services
    a) Patients and their families are evaluated and managed for practical problems such as those which are illness-related as well as concrete needs such as housing, food, financial assistance, school, employment, language and cultural barriers.
    b) Patients and their families are evaluated and managed for their psychosocial problems, including family conflict/isolation, treatment decisions, quality of life issues and transitions in care, advance directives, domestic violence, coping/communication, and functional changes.
  2. Mental health services
    a) Patients and their families are referred, evaluated and managed for psychological/ psychiatric problems and disorders, including dementia, delirium (encephalopathy), mood disorders, adjustment disorders, anxiety disorders, substance abuse and personality disorders.
  3. Pastoral counseling services

B. A multidisciplinary committee should be established to assume responsibility for the quality of psychosocial services given, implementation of standards of care and quality assurance projects to assure that distressed patients are identified and treated promptly and appropriately.

C. The multidisciplinary committee should be responsible for assuring that qualified and trained professionals in each discipline are available to provide the multidisciplinary services, or that they are accessible by consultation.

D. The multidisciplinary committee should develop methods for rapid screening of patients for distress, an algorithm to trigger referral for psychosocial services and to assure that the professionals utilize clinical practice guidelines developed for their discipline.

E. Institutions, through their multidisciplinary committees, should undertake the educational efforts to inform staff and patients of the fact that psychosocial services are part of the total care provided and inform them of the procedures to obtain care.

SOURCE: http://www.accc-cancer.org/pubs/Standardstemp.html, accessed January 22, 2003.

A few studies have examined the availability of supportive care services in these cancer centers. Surveys of NCI clinical and comprehensive cancer centers conducted in the early 1990s indicate that virtually all of the responding cancer centers offered group support programs (Presberg and Levenson, 1993; Coluzzi et al, 1995, Gruman and Convissor, 1995). In a more recent study conducted in 2000, about half of the NCI-designated comprehensive cancer centers (18 of 37 centers) had professionally led support groups for post-treatment cancer survivors (all 37 NCI-designated centers participated) (Tesauro et al., 2002).

At the October 2002 NCPB workshop, a psychologist from the Comprehensive Cancer Center of Wake Forest University/Baptist Medical Center (an NCI-designated center) described its psycho-oncology program (R. McQuellon, workshop presentation, October 2002; McQuellon et al., 1996). The program provides individual and family counseling (inpatient and outpatient), support groups, new patient orientation, patient education, case consultation, veteran patient consultation, volunteer hospitality, and breast cancer risk assessment. Also available to patients are psychiatry, pastoral counseling, physical therapy, and other resources of the hospital/medical school. To facilitate access to these services, resources have been located near outpatient treatment areas, for example in the hematology and oncology, radiation oncology clinics, and breast care center. The psychosocial needs of about 2,000 hospitalized cancer patients and nearly 5,000 individuals seen in outpatient clinics are met by 4 professional staff. The program is heavily dependent on a group of trained volunteers (about 20 per week participate in care) to extend services. Financial support comes largely through an annual fund raiser (60 percent), Wake Forest/Baptist Medical Center (20 percent), grants (10 percent), fee for service (5 percent), and donations (5 percent). According to the program director, this reliance

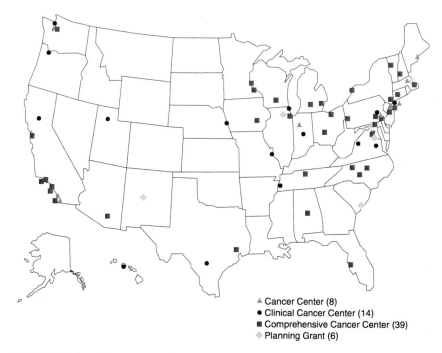

▲ Cancer Center (8)
● Clinical Cancer Center (14)
■ Comprehensive Cancer Center (39)
◈ Planning Grant (6)

FIGURE 6-1 NCI-supported cancer centers.
SOURCE: http://www3.cancer.gov/cancercenters/description.html,
accessed January 24, 2003.

on private donations and volunteer support is typical of such hospital-based
programs.

Psychosocial services for cancer patients have become more constrained
due to increasing financial pressures in the health-care setting. Social work
departments have contracted as hospital resources have diminished, and in
many clinical settings these services only exist through philanthropic support. Under these circumstances, it is only the most needy patients who
receive attention for the psychosocial issues associated with their breast
cancer experience.

Community-Based Support

There are psychosocial services for women with breast cancer available
through voluntary organizations, many of them at no cost. Table 6-6 describes some of the programs that are available nationally. Among the services these programs offer are peer support, individual counseling by tele-

TABLE 6-6 Selected National Community-based Psychosocial Resources

Program Name, Sponsor	Services and Availability	Content of Services	Patient Eligibility
Reach to Recovery, American Cancer, Society (ACS) (www.cancer.org)	• One-on-one peer support and education (in-person or by telephone) Available nationwide	• Emotional support from cancer survivor • Educational materials for patient and family • Assistance obtaining prostheses	Women facing breast cancer diagnosis, patients. Self or doctor referral.
I Can Cope, ACS	• Series of classes taught by doctors, nurses, social workers, and other health care professionals or community representatives • Focus on reliable information, peer support, and practical coping skills Available nationwide	• Diagnosis, treatment, side effects of treatment • Emotions and self-esteem, cancer and intimacy • Communication skills • Community resources, financial concerns • Pain management • Nutrition	Cancer patient and/or family. Self or doctor referral.
Look Good … Feel Better, ACS, Cosmetic, Toiletry, and Fragrance Association Foundation, and the National Cosmetology Association (www.lookgoodfeelbetter.org)	• Information and hands-on instruction on makeup and skincare and suggestions for using wigs, turbans, and scarves. Available nationwide	• Teaching women how to cope with the appearance related side- effects of cancer • Enhancing appearance and make-over • Learning to use wigs, hair pieces, turbans, etc.	Patient concerned about appearance-related side effects of cancer
The Wellness Community, Donations from individuals, corporations, or foundations	• Weekly cancer support groups • Diagnosis specific support groups • Family/caregiver groups • Bereavement groups • Online support groups • Nutrition/exercise, mind/body programs • Physician lectures • Stress reduction workshops Available in 22 locations throughout the U.S.	• Emotional support • Coping strategies • Relaxation/visualization training • Cancer information/education • Cognitive-behavioral techniques • Exercise techniques • Nutritional guidance • Principles of Patient Active Concept (combo of psychology and PNI)	Cancer patient and/or family
Cancer Care	• One-on-one counseling • Group Therapy • Cancer information/education Available nationwide by telephone	• Emotional support and encouragement • Psychological counseling from social worker • Teleconferences for cancer information • Group peer support via telephone or internet • Financial advice and assistance	Cancer patient

(continued)

TABLE 6-6 (*Continued*)

Program Name, Sponsor	Services and Availability	Content of Services	Patient Eligibility
Cancer Hope Network	• One-on-one peer support via telephone or in person Available nationwide by telephone, or in person at some locations	• Emotional support and encouragement from cancer survivor	Cancer patient
ACOR (Association of Cancer Online Resources)	• Group discussion and peersSupport • Information Available nationwide via the Internet	• E-mail list-servs, networks, and chatrooms for specific cancersites and common interests monitored by healthcare • Information Resources	Cancer Patient and/or family professionals
Other groups (Y-Me, Bosom Buddies, Sisters Network, YWCA, Circle of Life, TOUCH)	• Group therapy Available in regions nationwide	• Emotional support • Group psychotherapy • Coping strategies	Cancer patient and/or family

phone, information on nutrition and exercise, and assistance with appearance, for example, wigs and breast prostheses. This section of the report highlights programs represented at the October 2002 NCPB workshop, those offered by the American Cancer Society, the Wellness Community, and a few programs that focus on the needs of Hispanic and African American women with breast cancer.

American Cancer Society Programs The American Cancer Society sponsors several programs for women with breast cancer (see Table 6-6). The Reach to Recovery program, offered since 1960, provides peer support to women with breast cancer. Initially designed for women after mastectomy in hospitals, the program is now offered largely in the community. Attempts are made to match peer counselors with women with cancer by age, type of procedure, and cancer stage. There were 75,000 to 80,000 visits made by 16,000 trained volunteers in 2000. Road to Recovery is an outgrowth of this program that provides rides to individuals with cancer who need transportation to treatment. There are no national estimates of how many people use this program; however, in Massachusetts about 35,000 trips were made in recent years as part of this program.

Since 1989, the Look Good...Feel Better (LGFB) Program has provided assistance with makeup, skincare, and other aspects of appearance (e.g., consultation on wigs, turbans). The program is co-sponsored by the Cosmetic, Toiletry, and Fragrance Association Foundation and the National Cosmetology Association. In recent years the LGFB program has reached 43,000 women. A magazine and catalogue called "tlc," or Tender Loving Care, combines articles and information about products for women coping with cancer treatment (e.g., wigs, mastectomy forms and products, hats and headcoverings, bathing suits, and lingerie) (www.tlccatalog.org, accessed April 15, 2003).

The I Can Cope program started as a series of classes for individuals with cancer, but has been adapted for use for discussion groups and most recently as a Web-based interactive program. The Cancer Survivors Network is an ACS-sponsored website to support online interaction between cancer survivors. Participants can create a personal website, post pictures, poems and other expression, and engage in online discussions in English, Spanish, and Chinese. A health-care navigator program is under development by ACS that will direct individuals to resources within their community.

The Wellness Community The Wellness Community, founded in 1982, provides free education and support services to individuals with cancer and their families (see Table 6-6). The founding principle of the Wellness Community is that patients who participate in recovery improve the quality of their lives and may enhance the possibility of recovery. In 2002, 25,000 patients made 150,000 visits to Wellness Community Programs located in 22 sites across the country (Wellness Community Fact Sheet, undated). Among those served were 8,000 women with breast cancer, 3,000 of whom joined support groups (Mitch Golant, workshop presentation, 2002). All programs are facilitated by health care professionals, including social workers, psychotherapists, nurses, and psychologists, and all programs and training curricula are uniform throughout the country. Its newest program, The Virtual Wellness Community, includes online support groups, Webcasts, mind/body exercises, and information (see Figure 6-2). Evaluations of programs are ongoing in collaboration with investigators at Stanford University and the University of California at San Francisco (Lieberman et al., 2003). A comparison of face-to-face and online support services, an examination of provider best practices, and analyses of outcomes associated with interventions are among the research activities that are underway.

Community-based support targeted to racial and ethnic minority groups A number of psychosocial support programs are targeted to members of racial and ethnic minority groups. La Vida, a program to meet the needs of Hispanic women in the District of Columbia, was described at the October

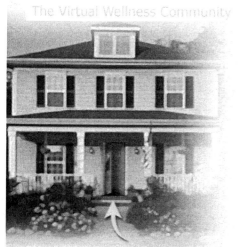

FIGURE 6-2 The virtual wellness community.
SOURCE: http://www.thewellnesscommunity.org.

2002 NCPB workshop. Established in 1996, La Vida offers support groups, crisis intervention, and peer support to breast cancer survivors. Because many women served are poor, uninsured, and speak Spanish, La Vida provides "patient navigation" services to help women make appointments and get appropriate follow-up care, assistance with health insurance applications and claim translation, and social supports (assistance with transportation, babysitting). Support groups focus on stress reduction, education (e.g., nutrition), and the implications of cancer for families. La Vida is creating a national psychosocial support resource directory for Hispanic women with breast cancer. To date, 63 programs have been identified, many in California and New York (Hinestrosa, workshop presentation, October 2002). The most pressing needs of Hispanic women identified by programs surveyed thus far are related to poor access to health care, information, psychosocial support, and difficulties navigating the health care system.

Sister's Network was founded in 1993 to address the needs of African American women with breast cancer (www.sistersnetworkinc.org, accessed April 15, 2003). The only national African American breast cancer survivors organization in the United States, Sisters network has 35 affiliate chapters across the country. Over 2,000 members are involved in breast health training, attending conferences, and serving on various national boards and review committees. Chapters offer individual and group support, community education, advocacy, and research-related activities (e.g., promoting access to clinical trials).

Support available by telephone and online Many psychosocial support services are available by phone to residents of rural areas and those living far from cancer centers, and increasingly online through the World-Wide Web. This section of the report describes three such programs: Cancer Care, The Association of Cancer Online Resources (ACOR), and CHESS (Comprehensive Health Enhancement Support System). A new resource is able to help find psychosocial and mental health services: The American Psychosocial Oncology Society (APOS; http://www.aspboa.org/patient/default.asp. There are other organized online lay information and support groups, for example, FertileHope.org, Living Beyond Breast Cancer (lbbc.org), and cancerandcareers.org, and many Internet chat rooms. There are also radio resources, for example, the Group Room weekly cancer talk radio show (and Internet simulcast) provided by Vital Options® International, which could reach those in rural and other distant areas. The potential for these resources to help survivors and to serve as collaborators in psychosocial care and research is not clear but merits investigation.

Cancer Care Since 1944, Cancer Care has provided emotional support, information, and practical help to people with cancer and their families (Cancer Care Annual Report, 2001). This nonprofit social service agency takes calls through its toll-free Counseling Line, sponsors teleconference programs, and provides support services on site in New York and via the Internet (www.cancercare.org, accessed April 15, 2003). All services are provided free of charge. With a staff of more than 50 professional oncology social workers, Cancer Care in 2001 provided services to more than 80,000 people. Among the services provided are individual and family counseling, group counseling (in-person, online, or by telephone), referrals to other resources, direct financial assistance, and teleconference programs which allow people to listen via telephone to experts in oncology or related fields discuss state-of-the-art treatment options, provide coping strategies for side effects, make recommendations on communicating with one's healthcare team, and offer advice on how best to maintain quality of life while living with cancer. Cancer care is also involved in professional education and training offering seminars, workshops, and teleconferences in all fields of oncology care. Distance learning programs are conducted entirely on the website.

The Association of Cancer Online Resources (ACOR) ACOR provides opportunities for individuals with cancer to interact with other cancer patients, therapists, or doctors through chat rooms, e-mail, or listserves. Psychosocial support is available through listserves dedicated to breast cancer, cancer-related depression, and caregivers. Another feature of ACOR is the provision of information about cancer from sources deemed to be credible (www.acor.org, accessed April 15, 2003).

CHESS (Comprehensive Health Enhancement Support System) CHESS provides information, social support, and decision-making assistance via a personal computer and modem that are placed in patients' homes. Women of all ages and varied socioeconomic backgrounds have successfully used the program to become active participants in their care following a diagnosis of breast cancer. CHESS allows participants to talk anonymously with peers, question experts, learn where to obtain help and how to use it, read stories about people who have survived similar crises, read relevant articles, monitor their health status, consider decision options, and plan how to implement decisions (Gustafson et al., 1993; Shaw et al., 2000). Support group use is the most popular aspect of CHESS. CHESS support groups are monitored by a facilitator. Several major medical centers and health plans are involved in CHESS research dissemination (http://chess.chsra.wisc.edu/chess/consortium/consortium_members.htm, accessed April 15, 2003).

American Psychosocial Oncology Society (APOS) Members of APOS include professionals from all disciplines who are involved in providing psychosocial and mental health services for cancer patients and their families. Established in 1986, APOS has recently addressed the information gap for patients whose psychosocial needs are not met by the services of the advocacy organizations and who are in need of more formal mental health services. The APOS Referral Directory (available online at www.apos-society.org, accessed April 15, 2003) and their toll-free number (1-866-APOS-4-HELP) provide patients and their families with information about qualified professionals with skills in psycho-oncology and who are located in their community. In addition, APOS offers a core curriculum in psycho-oncology, free online, to professionals who wish to ensure their basic skills in the psychosocial care of patients. APOS presently serves as backup to CancerCare, The Wellness Community, and the National Coalition of Cancer Survivors (NCCS).

SUMMARY

Advances in breast cancer diagnosis and care have changed the composition of women with breast cancer and the way in which they receive care. Widespread use of mammography has, for example, led to women being diagnosed at younger ages, which likely has increased the need for psychosocial services because younger people, in general, report higher rates of mental problems, and their mental health service use tends to be high.

There have been dramatic shifts in the site of breast cancer care, from the hospital to outpatient settings, making access to psychosocial support services more difficult because psychologists, social workers, and nurses, the mainstays of psychosocial care, are usually based in hospitals. While evidence is limited, it appears unlikely that most women with breast cancer receive hospital care of any duration. There are only about 150,000 hospitalizations for breast cancer each year, with two-thirds of these hospitalizations for mastectomies. And among women hospitalized for breast cancer care, relatively few stay in the hospital longer than 2 days.

Most contemporary breast cancer care takes place during nearly 5 million ambulatory care visits made annually, most of these to private physicians' offices. Here, only 5 percent of breast cancer-related visits include psychosocial care. Contact with nurses who might be expected to provide some supportive care appears to be limited during visits to physicians' offices, with fewer than 40 percent of visits bringing women seeking breast cancer care into contact with a registered nurse, nurse practitioner, or physician assistant.

Use of psychosocial services may be limited because the delivery of breast cancer care has become so complex, involving multiple treatment modalities and providers. As women go from office to office for consultation and treatment, there may be no coordinator of care and no one responsible for making the patient aware of psychosocial services that are available. Comprehensive breast centers have emerged that put providers and services "under one roof," but there are no estimates of the number of women receiving care in these settings.

The involvement of oncology providers in post-treatment follow-up care has been questioned by findings, largely outside the United States, that specialized surveillance has no benefit for survival or patient satisfaction. Long term follow-up of women with breast cancer may eventually move to the hands of primary care providers, who may not have extensive experience in cancer-related psychosocial issues or the expected long-term treatment effects with psychosocial consequences.

Collaborative practice is a promising approach to providing psychosocial services to the vast majority of women with breast cancer who receive their care in ambulatory care settings. This approach involves integrating a psychologist (usually in private practice) into the outpatient oncology practice team; however, current reimbursement for mental health services cannot fully support a salary for such a person. Managed care programs that improve satisfaction with breast cancer care by enhancing educational materials and supportive care also show promise. Although a minority of women appear to be getting breast cancer care in hospital-based settings, these programs are important sites of training and research. Many hospital-based programs have standards in place to assure the provision of at least some level of psychosocial support. Hospital-based programs, however, even at comprehensive cancer centers appear to have unstable support for their programs, relying extensively on philanthropy and volunteer staff. There are many free, community-based psychosocial programs available and increasingly services are accessible by telephone and the Internet. Little is known regarding their use, and few have been formally evaluated.

There are few estimates with which to gauge how often women with breast cancer use psychosocial services, but generally use appears to be low, with up to 30 percent of women reporting some level of service. Psychosocial service use seems to decline into the survivorship period, with some studies suggesting that between 10 and 15 percent of long-term breast cancer survivors use psychosocial services.

REFERENCES

American Cancer Society. 2001. *Breast Cancer Facts & Figures 2001–2002*. Atlanta: American Cancer Society.

American Cancer Society. 2002. *Cancer Facts & Figures 2002*. Atlanta: American Cancer Society.

Case C, Johantgen M, Steiner C. 2001. Outpatient mastectomy: Clinical, payer, and geographic influences. *Health Serv Res* 36(5):869–884.

Coluzzi PH, Grant M, Doroshow JH, Rhiner M, Ferrell B, Rivera L. 1995. Survey of the provision of supportive care services at National Cancer Institute-designated cancer centers. *J Clin Oncol* 13(3):756–764.

Curry C, Cossich T, Matthews JP, Beresford J, McLachlan SA. 2002. Uptake of psychosocial referrals in an outpatient cancer setting: Improving service accessibility via the referral process. *Support Care Cancer* 10(7):549–555.

Donaldson MS. 1998. Accountability for quality in managed care. *Jt Comm J Qual Improv* 24(12):711–25.

Ferrell BR, Grant MM, Funk BM, Otis-Green SA, Garcia NJ. 1998. Quality of life in breast cancer survivors: Implications for developing support services. *Oncol Nurs Forum* 25(5):887–895.

Frost MH, Arvizu RD, Jayakumar S, Schoonover A, Novotny P, Zahasky K. 1999. A multidisciplinary healthcare delivery model for women with breast cancer: Patient satisfaction and physical and psychosocial adjustment. *Oncol Nurs Forum* 26(10):1673–80.

Ganz PA, Desmond KA, Leedham B, Rowland JH, Meyerowitz BE, Belin TR. 2002. Quality of life in long-term, disease-free survivors of breast cancer: A follow-up study. *J Natl Cancer Inst* 94(1):39–49.

Geiger AM, Mullen ES, Sloman PA, Edgerton BW, Petitti DB. 2000. Evaluation of a breast cancer patient information and support program. *Eff Clin Pract* 3(4):157–165.

Gruman J, Convissor R. 1995. *Psychosocial Services in Cancer Care: A Survey of Comprehensive Cancer Centers.* Washington, DC: The Center for the Advancement of Health.

Grunfeld E, Fitzpatrick R, Mant D, Yudkin P, Adewuyi-Dalton R, Stewart J, Cole D, Vessey M. 1999. Comparison of breast cancer patient satisfaction with follow-up in primary care versus specialist care: Results from a randomized controlled trial. *Br J Gen Pract* 49(446):705–710.

Grunfeld E, Mant D, Yudkin P, Adewuyi-Dalton R, Cole D, Stewart J, Fitzpatrick R, Vessey M. 1996. Routine follow up of breast cancer in primary care: Randomised trial. *Br Med J* 313(7058):665–669.

Gustafson D, Wise M, McTavish F, Taylor J, Wolberg W, Steward J, Smalley R, Bosworth K. 1993. Development and pilot evaluation of a computer-based support system for women with breast cancer. *Journal of Psychosocial Oncology* 11(4):69–93.

Hewitt M, Breen N, Devesa S. 1999. Cancer prevalence and survivorship issues: Analyses of the 1992 National Health Interview Survey. *J Natl Cancer Inst* 91(17):1480–1486.

Hewitt M, Rowland JH. 2002. Mental health service use among adult cancer survivors: Analyses of the National Health Interview Survey. *J Clin Oncol* 20(23):4581–4590.

Landon BE, Wilson IB, Cleary PD. 1998. A conceptual model of the effects of health care organizations on the quality of medical care. *JAMA* 279(17):1377–1382.

Lerner BH. 2001. *The Breast Cancer Wars: Hope, Fear, and the Pursuit of a Cure in Twentieth-Century America.* New York: Oxford University Press.

Lieberman MA, Golant M, Giese-Davis J et al. 2003. Electronic support groups for breast carcinoma: A clinical trial of effectiveness. Cancer 97(4):920–925.

McQuellon RP, Hurt GJ, DeChatelet P. 1996. Psychosocial care of the patient with cancer: A model for organizing services. *Cancer Practice* 4(6):304–311.

National Breast Cancer Coalition. *Guide to Quality Breast Cancer Care.* 2nd ed. Washington, DC: National Breast Cancer Coalition.

Plass A, Koch U. 2001. Participation of oncological outpatients in psychosocial support. *Psycho-oncology* 10(6):511–520.

Presberg BA, Levenson JL. 1993. A survey of cancer support groups provided by National Cancer Institute (NCI) clinical and comprehensive centers. *Psycho-oncology* 2:215–217.

Rabinowitz B. 2002. Psychosocial issues in breast cancer. *Obstet Gynecol Clin North Am* 29(1):233–247.

Rosselli Del Turco M, Palli D, Cariddi A, Ciatto S, Pacini P, Distante V. 1994. Intensive diagnostic follow-up after treatment of primary breast cancer. A randomized trial. National Research Council Project on Breast Cancer follow-up. *JAMA* 271(20):1593–1597.

Shaw BR, McTavish F, Hawkins R, Gustafson DH, Pingree S. 2000. Experiences of women with breast cancer: Exchanging social support over the CHESS computer network. *J Health Commun* 5(2):135–159.

Simmons J. 1998. AAHP identifies best practices for breast cancer. *Qual Lett Healthc Lead* 10(9):13–14.

Sorensen M, Liu ET. 1995 With a different voice: Integrating the psychosocial perspective into routine oncology care. *Breast Cancer Res Treat* 35(1):39–42.

Tesauro GM, Rowland JH, Lustig C. 2002. Survivorship resources for post-treatment cancer survivors. *Cancer Pract* 10(6):277–283.

The GIVIO Investigators. 1994. Impact of follow-up testing on survival and health-related quality of life in breast cancer patients. A multicenter randomized controlled trial. *JAMA* 271(20):1587–1592.

Trief PM, Donohue-Smith M. 1996. Counseling needs of women with breast cancer: What the women tell us. *J Psychosoc Nurs Ment Health Serv* 34(5):24–29.

U.S. Department of Health and Human Services. 2000. *Mental Health: Culture, Race, and Ethnicity: A Supplement to Mental Health: A Report of the Surgeon General.* Rockville, MD: U.S. Department of Health and Human Services, Substance Abuse and Mental Health Services Administration, Center for Mental Health Services, National Institutes of Health, National Institute of Mental Health.

Worden JW, Weisman AD. 1980. Do cancer patients really want counseling? *Gen Hosp Psychiatry* 2(2):100–103.

7

Barriers to Appropriate Use of Psychosocial Services

Although there is a general consensus that psychosocial services are needed and valuable, less is known about why services are not widely offered or used. Individuals may face barriers to receipt of psychosocial services because they do not have access to care, because they lack either health insurance or coverage that includes mental health services, or because they do not ask for help because of stigma. Among the barriers imposed by providers and systems of care are: patient–provider miscommunication, failure to implement clinical practice guidelines, inexperience with assessment for psychosocial distress and rapid screening tools, poor coordination and fragmentation of complex care, a lack of provider familiarity with community resources, and limited systems of quality assurance and accountability. This chapter reviews available evidence regarding these barriers to receipt of appropriate psychosocial care.

ACCESS TO CARE

The link between poor access to care and poor health outcomes is well established (IOM, 2001; IOM, 2002), but the reasons for inadequate access are not well understood. Some of the connections are intuitive and obvious: women without health insurance have breast cancer detected at later stages and have poorer survival rates than women with insurance (Ayanian et al., 1993; Lee-Feldstein et al., 2000; Roetzheim et al., 2000, 1999). People who lack health insurance are also less likely to receive mental health services (Landerman et al., 1994).

One in seven adult women in the United States lacks health insurance, which creates a general barrier to getting medical care of any kind (U.S. Census Bureau, 2002). Some other barriers to receiving appropriate care are less obvious. Non-financial barriers that may prevent people from "getting to the door" of a health-care provider include geography (travel distance), language, fear and distrust of health care providers, and difficulties getting through appointment or "gatekeeper" systems. Once "in the door," other barriers to access may surface when attempting to navigate the system: for example, getting from a primary care provider to a specialist. This is especially problematic for referral to mental health and psychosocial services. Within the system, providers may lack information about the diagnosis and management of distress, have difficulty communicating with patients or understanding their problems due to cultural differences, or have insufficient staff to adequately explore patients' psychosocial needs and provide referral to needed services. The cancer care system is complex, and for breast cancer, it may involve the surgeon, radiologist, and oncologist at different times (see Chapter 5 for a description of breast cancer care). Consequently, various barriers that serve to limit access may surface during each phase of care. These barriers to optimal care are themselves a potential source of psychosocial distress for many women (Hinestrosa, workshop presentation, 2002).

Access, as defined by the Institute of Medicine (IOM, 1993), is the timely use of personal health services leading to the best possible health outcomes. This definition of access implies the use of health services, the quality of such services, and the degree to which access has been achieved. The test of equity of access involves first determining whether there are systematic differences in use and outcomes among groups in United States society and, if there are, the reasons for these differences (IOM, 1993). Some of the factors that have been investigated as possibly affecting access to mental health services include:

- Health insurance coverage and type of coverage;
- Cost, including health insurance and out-of-pocket costs;
- Attributes of the health care delivery system (e.g., geographic distribution of cancer care facilities, lack of service coordination; separation of medical and behavioral (mental) health in different and unrelated contracts);
- Attributes of individuals (lack of knowledge or misperceptions about mental health services; linguistic or cultural attributes); and
- Attributes of health-care providers (e.g., lack of knowledge about mental health resources; communication styles).

This section of the report describes these barriers in the context of access to mental health services among women with breast cancer.

Health Insurance Coverage and Type of Coverage

Women with breast cancer are more likely than other women to be insured, because as many as 45 percent of newly diagnosed cases occur among women age 65 and older who generally are covered by Medicare (in 2001, an estimated 46 percent of incident cases and 59 percent of women dying of cancer were covered by Medicare). Nevertheless, of the 203,500 women diagnosed with invasive breast cancer in 2002, an estimated 16,350 women, or 8.0 percent of women with breast cancer and 6.1 percent of women who died of cancer, would have been expected to be uninsured (Table 7-1). Nationally, 14 percent of adult women were uninsured in 2001 (U.S. Census Bureau, 2002).

The diagnosis of cancer can, in itself, lead to a loss of health insurance coverage or to higher insurance premiums. In 1992, 7 percent of cancer survivors who were insured prior to their diagnosis reported that their health

TABLE 7-1 Estimates of Health Insurance Coverage Among Women with Breast Cancer (diagnoses and deaths), United States, 2001

Health Insurance Coverage[a]	US Female Population (age 18+)		Breast Cancer Diagnoses		Breast Cancer Deaths	
	Number (in 1,000s)	%	Number	%	Number	%
Total	108,752	100.0	203,500	100.0	39,600	100.0
Private or government insurance	93,462	85.9	187,151	92.0	37,171	93.9
Private insurance	77,577	71.3	140,550	69.1	26,319	66.5
Employment-based	66,036	60.7	106,388	52.3	18,390	46.4
Government insurance						
Medicaid	9,697	8.9	18,196	8.9	3,775	9.5
Medicare	21,480	19.8	93,930	46.2	23,474	59.3
Military[b]	3,305	3.0	7,984	3.9	1,667	4.2
No health insurance[c]	15,291	14.1	16,350	8.0	2,429	6.1

[a]Categories are not mutually exclusive.
[b]Includes CHAMPUS (Comprehensive Health and Medical Plan for Uniformed Services)/ Tricare, Veterans, and military health care.
[c]Estimates are of women without health insurance coverage for the entire year.
NOTE: Age-specific insurance rates among U.S. women age 18 and older were applied to incident breast cancer cases and deaths, stratified by age.
SOURCES: Insurance rates are from the U.S. Census Bureau, Current Population Survey, Annual Demographic Supplements, Income Statistics Branch/HHES Division, January 30, 2003. Estimates of the number of incident breast cancer cases and deaths are from Cancer Facts & Figures 2002. Estimates of the age distribution of breast cancer incident cases and deaths are from SEER.

insurance changed following their cancer diagnosis (e.g., 5 percent said that their insurance costs increased (Hewitt et al., 1999). Congress tried to remedy this problem in 1996, enacting the Health Insurance Portability and Accountability Act (Kennedy-Kassebaum Act) to improve the portability and continuity of health insurance coverage in private insurance markets and among employer-sponsored group health plans. The act limits the ability of insurers to deny or discontinue coverage because of preexisting conditions such as cancer. The increased cost of premiums for portable insurance products and difficulties in implementing the law, however, have limited the value of these protections for consumers (U.S. General Accounting Office, 1997).

If individuals are uninsured and not eligible for Medicaid, medical expenses related to cancer may force them to "spend down" to become eligible for Medicaid—that is, to deplete their assets until they meet eligibility criteria. Alternatively, individuals who are disabled by cancer for a period of 2 years may become eligible for Medicaid coverage through the Supplemental Security Income (SSI) program. Some hospitals are obligated to provide some charity care to the uninsured (i.e., under the Hill-Burton Act of 1946). State and federal programs provide free cancer screening and sometimes cover the expense of treatment for the uninsured (e.g., the state option to provide Medicaid coverage for women diagnosed through the Centers for Disease Control and Prevention [CDC] National Breast and Cervical Cancer Early Detection Program) (http://www.cdc.gov/cancer/nbccedp/law106-354.htm, accessed April 17, 2003).

More than half the states operate high-risk insurance pools to help provide coverage to individuals with serious medical conditions who have been denied private health insurance in the individual market (Achman and Chollet, 2001). The insurance provided through these state risk pools (also known as Guaranteed Access Programs) generally costs more than regular insurance, and in some states there are long waiting lists or the programs are closed to new applicants altogether. More than 153,000 individuals are currently covered by state risk pools (DHHS, 2002). Many charitable organizations (e.g., Cancer Care, American Cancer Society) provide free services or financial assistance to individuals with cancer who lack the means to pay for their care. These programs and services cannot substitute for adequate insurance coverage for cancer care, but they can ease the financial burden for small numbers of individuals in need.

Cost, Including Health Insurance and Out-of-Pocket Costs[1]

Health insurance coverage may not adequately protect individuals from the high costs associated with cancer treatment and may not cover mental

---

[1]Much of this section of the report is based on *Mental Health: A Report to the Surgeon General*, 1999.

health services. Some policies have high deductibles (e.g., some catastrophic policies may contain a deductible as high as $15,000 or more), and copayments or coinsurance over the course of cancer treatment can be substantial. Relatively few studies specific to cancer exist regarding the magnitude of the financial burden associated with out-of-pocket costs, but available evidence suggests that it is substantial (Sofaer et al., 1990). Unlike the great majority of employer-provided insurance plans, Medicare does not cap beneficiaries' total payments for cost sharing (AARP, 1997). Medicare HMOs typically have lower cost sharing than the traditional Medicare program and may offer additional benefits such as outpatient prescription drug coverage, but they may impose certain restrictions on use of specialty providers (AARP, 1997). Relatively few Medicare beneficiaries are enrolled in HMOs (12 percent as of 2003) (http://cms.hhs.gov/healthplans/statistics/mmcc/, accessed April 18, 2003).

Before 1990, most mental health care was covered by indemnity plans that used benefit limits and patient cost sharing to control service use and spending. By the late 1990s, managed care was the norm in health service delivery, covering an estimated 56 percent of Americans. With the growing complexity of care, it can be difficult to distinguish one type of managed care plan from another, but major types of such plans include:

- Health maintenance organizations (HMO) provide all medical services on a prepaid, per capita basis. Medical staff members may be salaried, but increasingly HMOs have developed networks of physicians—so-called Independent Practice Associations, or IPAs—who are paid on a fee-for-service basis and function under common management guidelines.
- Preferred Provider Organizations (PPOs) are managed care plans that contract with networks of providers to supply services. Providers are typically paid on a discounted fee-for-service basis. Enrollees are offered lower cost-sharing to use providers on the "preferred" list but can use non-network providers at a higher out-of-pocket cost.
- Point-of-Service (POS) plans are managed care plans that combine features of prepaid (or capitated) and fee-for-service insurance. Enrollees can choose to use a network provider at the time of service. A significant copayment typically accompanies use of non-network providers. Although few plans are purely of one type, an important difference between a PPO and POS is that in a PPO plan, the patient may select any type of covered care from any in-network provider, while in a POS plan, use of in-network services must be approved by a primary care physician.

Increasingly, mental health services are being provided by managed behavioral health organizations, which are estimated to cover approximately 200 million Americans (IOM, 1997; Goff, 2002). Often mental health services are covered in a separate contract between the payer (insurer or employer) and a behavioral health provider. These so-called "carve-out" managed behavioral health care arrangements allow payers to isolate mental health services from overall insurance risk and have mental health care services managed separately from general health care (Box 7-1). This separation is generally acceptable for physically healthy individuals. However, this arrangement is highly disadvantageous to patients with a life-threatening or chronic illness who require psychiatric/psychological consultation for related mental disorders (e.g., confusion/delirium from disease or medication or severe anxiety or depression). The separation of care delivery can lead to fragmentation of services across medical and behavioral health providers.

Managed care may also serve as a barrier to appropriate psychosocial services when mental health providers who are trained in psycho-oncology and management of distress in patients with cancer are not available within the behavioral health plan's service network. Concerns have been raised that mental health providers in networks often do not have expertise in psycho-oncology (Wellisch, IOM workshop, October 2002).

BOX 7-1
Carve-Out Managed Behavioral Health Care

Many HMOs and other health plans carve out mental health care for administration by a managed behavioral health company. This arrangement permits a larger range of services than can be provided within the health plan and permits the application of specific cost controls to behavioral health care. Carve-outs generally have separate budgets, provider networks, and financial incentive arrangements. Covered services, utilization management techniques, financial risk, and other features vary depending on the particular carve-out contract. The employee as a plan member may be unaware of any such arrangement. These separate contracts delegate management of mental health care to specialized vendors known as managed behavioral health care organizations.

There are two general forms of carve-outs:
- In payer carve-outs, an enrollee chooses a health plan for coverage of health care with the exception of mental health and must enroll with a separate carve-out vendor for mental health care.
- In health plan subcontracts, administrators of the general medical plan arrange to have mental health care managed by a carve-out vendor; the plan member does not have to take steps to select mental health coverage.

SOURCE: U.S. Surgeon General's Report, 1999.

There is a range of management controls currently applied to enrollees in managed care plans (e.g., utilization review). Some are concerned that excessively restrictive cost containment strategies and financial incentives to providers and facilities to reduce specialty referrals, hospital admissions, or length or amount of treatment contribute to lowered access and quality of mental health care (U.S. Department of Health and Human Services, 1999). Despite these significant concerns, raised repeatedly by mental health professionals, particularly consultation-liaison psychiatrists who work with the medically ill, the actual impact of these policies has received relatively little systematic study. There are currently no benchmark standards for access to specialized mental health services for medically ill patients, making assessment of access difficult. Some evidence suggests that, in the general population, the use of mental health care increases after managed behavioral health care is implemented in private insurance plans (Goldman et al., 1998). This is, in part due to shifts from in-hospital to outpatient mental health care.

Most Medicare beneficiaries have coverage of outpatient health services, including mental health services, through Medicare Part B. Medicare beneficiaries are much less likely than individuals covered by private insurance or Medicaid to be in a managed care plan. An estimated 88 percent of beneficiaries are covered under the traditional Medicare fee-for-service program. Mental health services reimbursed by Medicare include psychiatric diagnostic or evaluative interview procedures, individual psychotherapy, group psychotherapy, family psychotherapy, psychoanalysis, psychological testing, and pharmacologic management (DHHS, 2001). Practitioners who can provide mental health services to Medicare beneficiaries include: physicians, clinical psychologists, clinical social workers, nurse practitioners, clinical nurse specialists, and physician assistants (Code of Federal Regulations, Title 42, Part 410). Under Medicare, professional fees are based on a relative value scale. Psychologists and social workers are paid on a percentage markdown from psychiatrists (Frank, 2000). Under traditional Medicare, beneficiaries pay 50 percent of Medicare's allowed fee for outpatient mental health therapy. Most Medicare Plus Choice plans also require some cost-sharing for these services (Gold and Achman, 2001).

Coverage of mental health benefits under Medicaid is complex, because of the program's variation in coverage by state. Mandated benefits under Medicaid include general hospital inpatient care, physician services, outpatient services in general hospitals, nursing home care, and prescription drugs. States have had the freedom to choose a number of optional benefits, for example, non-physician services, services provided in freestanding outpatient clinics, and case management. States have often limited costs and coverage through their reimbursement policies. Fees to professionals are commonly set well below market levels of reimbursement, which limits the supply of physician services to Medicaid beneficiaries (Frank, 2000). State Medicaid programs are increasingly delegating management of mental health services to managed behavioral health care organizations (Frank, 2000).

Reimbursement of the treatment of psychosocial services for women with breast cancer through public and private insurers may be facilitated by the development of six reimbursement codes for psychological services to patients with physical health diagnoses (APA, undated memo; http://www.apa.org/practice/cpt_2002.html, accessed April 17, 2003) (see Box 7-2). The new CPT codes, which became effective January 1, 2002, cover behavioral, social, and psychophysiological procedures for the prevention, treatment, or management of physical health problems. These codes, for the first time, permit reimbursement for treatment by a psychologist without the need for a mental health diagnosis (in fact, they cannot be used for treating patients with a psychiatric diagnosis). Types of assessment and intervention services that will be covered by the codes include patient adherence to medical treatment, symptom management, health-promoting behaviors, health-related risk-taking behaviors, and overall adjustment to physical illness. For private and third-party insurance plans, the services will likely be treated under the physical illness benefits, and thus not be relegated to behavioral health "carve out" programs.

BOX 7-2
New Health And Behavior CPT Codes And Associated
Medicare Reimbursement Rates

CPT Code	Service	Approximate Medicare Payment (in dollars)	
		15 min (1 unit)	1 hour (4 units)
96150	Assessment-initial	$26	$106
96151	Re-assessment	26	103
96152	Intervention: individual	25	98
96153	Intervention: group (per person)	5	22
96154	Intervention: family w/patient	24	96
96155	Intervention: family w/o patient	23	93

SOURCE: APA, undated memo; http://www.apa.org/practice/cpt_2002.html, accessed April 17, 2003.

There have been many efforts to bring coverage of services for mental illness on a par with that for somatic illness. The Mental Health Parity Act of 1996 (PL 104-204) has improved insurance coverage for mental illnesses, but many gaps remain (www.nami.org/update/parity96.html). Implemented in 1998, this legislation focused on only one aspect of the inequities in mental health insurance coverage: "catastrophic" benefits. It prohibited the use of lifetime and annual limits on coverage that were different for mental and somatic illnesses. The law does not mandate coverage and applies only to employers that offer mental health benefits. It also does not affect rules for service charges, such as co-payments, deductibles, and out-of-pocket payment limits. A growing number of states have parity legislation, but some states have targeted their legislation narrowly to include only people with severe mental disorders.

The experience of a pilot project to incorporate psychosocial support services into an outpatient medical oncology practice illustrates some of the problems encountered in insurance coverage (Sellers, 2000). The project placed a medical family therapist for 20 hours a week in a multi-specialty practice in Seattle. After 6 months of this collaborative practice, the providers reviewed the financial costs and levels of reimbursement for psychosocial care. In this practice, 60 percent of patients receiving psychosocial services had some form of behavioral health coverage and of these 30 percent were Medicare patients. The analysis showed that insurance reimbursements covered 60 percent of the program cost and that external funding would be needed to support the service. The following problems with insurance coverage were noted:

• Because of frequent changes in insurance carriers and plans, behavioral health benefit review was needed for each new patient prior to a visit.
• The amount of time and effort required to track down a relatively small number of reimbursement dollars was not cost effective.
• Medicare reimbursement was relatively low, roughly half of non-Medicare reimbursement.
• For Medicare reimbursement, patients could not see the psychosocial provider on the same day as a physician visit.

Attributes of the Health Care Delivery System

How breast cancer care is organized and delivered can greatly affect access to mental health care services (see also Chapter 6). There is limited information on the extent to which women's breast care is coordinated and organized to facilitate the identification and management of psychosocial distress. One important study in this area found breast cancer care sites in New York City to lack comprehensive systems to ensure care coordination

(Bickell and Young, 2001). While this study's findings may not be applicable to other geographic areas, it suggests an important link between care coordination and the provision of support services.

As part of their study of institutional approaches to coordinate care for women with early-stage breast cancer, Bickell and colleagues completed in-depth semi-structured interviews at six hospitals with providers of breast cancer care and their support staff. Systematic use of patient support programs, such as patient educators and navigators, were perceived to be valuable in coordinating care. Three of the six sites had patient support programs, which all provided:

- a systematic method to identify patients;
- education about breast cancer including treatment options and counseling;
- calls to patients to remind them of upcoming appointments; and
- navigators to bring patients to appointments or enable them to attend appointments, for example, by arranging for child care or transportation.

Two of the three programs were staffed with trained volunteers. Physicians found the programs to be extremely valuable because they provided services that were otherwise missing at the sites or supplemented services, thereby reducing physicians' work-load. The patient education and counseling provided were viewed as improving patient's understanding and ability to make informed treatment decisions. Also valued were practical social and financial support, such as assistance with (Bickell, workshop presentation, 2002):

- navigation through the care system,
- forms to get home health aides,
- arranging transportation and child care,
- completing insurance forms, and
- applying for compassionate drug programs.

Particularly helpful was having systematic case finding to identify new patients and e
nsure that the need for supportive care services was assessed and offered. In some cases, women were approached by a person at preadmission testing so that a connection was made to a person who would contact them later. Other programs placed volunteers at key sites, for example, the breast clinic, mammography clinic, and radiation therapy and infusion suites. According to institutional staff, physician "buy-in" was crucial to program success. Physicians tended to be initially resistant, but later came to rely on

services (Bickell, workshop presentation, 2002). In general, barriers to program coordination included:

- lack of physician referral;
- the fragmentation of care (dispersed offices);
- lack of hospital support (i.e., reliance on philanthropy);
- difficulty in finding/keeping committed volunteers, especially in poor communities; and
- reaching speakers of languages other than English.

Findings from this study of breast cancer care delivery are consistent with the emerging chronic disease model of care (Wagner et al., 1996; Von Korff et al., 1997). The chronic disease model posits that through more productive interactions between patients and provider teams, functional and clinical outcomes can be improved. The model calls for improvements in coordinated delivery systems including connecting health systems with community resources to support patients in a meaningful way (www.Improvingchroniccare.org). Research and demonstration projects to evaluate this model of care are being supported by the Robert Wood Johnson Foundation.

The most extensive effort to improve psychosocial care at a population level has been in Australia where a National Breast Cancer Center has undertaken review of evidence-based research for psychosocial interventions and developed the findings into recommendations and clinical practice guidelines. National efforts have involved oncologists, mental health professionals, and breast cancer advocacy groups to change current practices through demonstration projects and education (Redman et al., 2003).

Attributes of Individuals

Lack of knowledge or misperceptions about mental health services are among the most significant barriers to receipt of appropriate care. According to a recent survey, only 55 percent of Americans understand depression is a disease and not a state of mind that a person can snap out of (NMHA, 2001). The 1999 Surgeon General's report on mental illness identified stigma as a major barrier to addressing the nation's mental health needs. Stigma can be defined as a label that sets a person apart from others and links that person to undesirable characteristics. People tend to reject and avoid stigmatized people. The stigma associated with mental illness may be declining with the growing acceptance of depression and other conditions as treatable health problems. Despite this, patients with a life-threatening illness like cancer often express their reluctance to request psychological help because they feel it would be a sign of moral weakness or that they would be labeled by others as "crazy."

There has been a dramatic increase in the number of people treated for depression in the last 15 years. Between 1987 and 1997, the rate of outpatient treatment for depression increased from 0.73 per 100 persons in 1987 to 2.33 in 1997 (Olfson et al., 2002). The advent of better tolerated antidepressants, expanded availability of third-party payment, advertising on the part of the pharmaceutical industry, public health campaigns to educate the public about depression and reduce its stigma, and the development of more rapid and efficient procedures for diagnosing depression in clinical practice are among the factors thought to contribute to this trend (Olfson et al., 2002). Lower rates of treatment were found among black and Hispanic individuals, those with less education, and those without health insurance. These lower rates of treatment are largely attributable to poor access to mental health care, but they can also be traced to culturally bound attitudes about mental health and related services. According to one study, fear and stigma associated with seeking emotional support were among the barriers to treatment participation identified among African American cancer patients participating in focus groups (Matthews et al., 2002a). Culture influences many aspects of mental health including how patients from a given culture express and manifest their symptoms, their style of coping, their family and community supports, and their willingness to seek treatment (U.S. Department of Health and Human Services, 2000).

Educating the public about the availability and usefulness of mental health services is a general strategy to improve acceptance and reduce the stigma associated with mental health care. Another strategy that is clinically effective with cancer patients is to integrate their psychosocial care into their total care, so that they do not experience a "disconnect" and hence do not perceive their psychological care as a separate, potentially stigmatized aspect of care. Conducting a psychosocial assessment routinely with all new breast cancer patients is one way to integrate it into medical care and reduce the perceived stigma of being "singled-out." In addition, efforts are needed to improve the cultural competency of mental health providers to address some of the culturally based misapprehensions regarding mental health.

Attributes of Health-Care Providers

A lack of awareness on the part of breast cancer care providers of psychosocial needs and available resources, problems in patient–provider communication, and the absence of clear direction on how to distinguish "normal" and expected distress from significant distress that should be referred for evaluation by psycho-oncologists are among the factors that inhibit health-care providers in their delivery of optimal psychosocial services.

Lack of Awareness of Community Resources

There are many support services available to women with breast cancer, but evidence suggests that one barrier to their use is a lack of awareness on the part of physicians and other health-care providers of psychosocial services in their community. A survey sponsored in 2001 by the American Cancer Society (ACS) assessed awareness, attitude, and referral to community-based supportive care programs among 2000 physicians, nurses, and social workers who were active members of their respective oncology associations (Matthews et al., 2002b). Awareness of the programs was relatively high, with 77 to 79 percent of respondents aware of three of the most prominent American Cancer Society programs (i.e., I Can Cope, Reach to Recovery, and the ACS Cancer Information Database toll free number). Somewhat fewer, 49 to 59 percent, reported referring patients to these programs, and 55 to 63 percent said that they found them helpful. Social workers in the study were more likely to know about, recommend, and regard program or services as helpful relative to nurses and physicians. A lack of provider referral is often mentioned as a reason for not using psychosocial services (Eakin and Strycker, 2001). According to a study conducted in Montreal, Quebec, relatively few women (42 percent) who had used professionally provided support services had learned about them from their oncologist (Edgar et al., 2000).

Problems in Patient–Provider Communication

A basic psychosocial support for women with breast cancer is their relationship to physicians who provide them with full information, who are willing to answer questions and show respect for the "human" side of illness. Psychosocial distress among patients may not be addressed in practice because of problems in patient–provider communication, and efforts are underway to improve oncologists' communication skills (Schapira, 2003; Fallowfield et al., 2001; Baile et al., 1999) (see also Chapter 4 for a discussion of the education and training of psychosocial service providers). Some problems can be traced to the tendency for patients to wait for physicians to inquire about their coping or distress, or to inquire about support groups or a mental health referral. Physicians may assume that patients will ask for such help if it is needed. This "don't ask, don't tell" policy is even more pervasive in busy outpatient clinics (Holland, 1999). Evidence of this kind of miscommunication comes from a study conducted in the Netherlands where patients and oncologists were found to be willing to discuss a wide range of quality of life issues, but had competing expectations as to who should initiate such discussions (Detmar et al., 2000). In their study of 274 patients receiving palliative chemotherapy and the ten physicians who cared for them, almost all patients were willing to address their emotional functioning and daily activities, but a sizable share (25 percent) of patients were only willing to discuss these issues at the initiative of their physician. This was especially true for older and less well-educated patients. All of the physicians, however, indicated that they generally defer to their patients in initiating discussions of psychosocial issues. This study also found some resistance to discussing psychosocial issues, with 20 percent reporting no interest in discussing their family and social life.

Overcoming communication problems is a promising approach to improving psychosocial care, with attention to recognizing distress and awareness of cultural factors in coping with illness. Enhanced communication often improves patients' psychological adjustment, and conversely, interventions that lower distress and modify coping style will often enhance communication (Lerman et al., 1993). A high degree of physician-initiated communication has been associated with increased patient satisfaction in the context of discussing treatment options for breast cancer (Liang et al., 2002).

A program to enhance doctors' communication skills is an integral part of the national strategy in Australia to improve breast cancer psychosocial care (Redman et al., 2003; Butow, 1995). Increasing the recognition and management of depression through communication education programs has shown promise among primary care providers (Gerrity et al, 1999; Roter et al., 1995), indicating that such an approach holds promise for improving psychosocial care among cancer care providers.

Lack of Widespread Adoption of Clinical Practice Guidelines

Efforts to improve the provision of psychosocial services for women with breast cancer have recently focused on implementing clinical practice guidelines. Clinical practice guidelines are "systematically developed statements to assist practitioner and patient decisions about appropriate health care for specific clinical circumstances" (IOM 1990). Guideline recommendations are ideally based on high-level evidence (i.e., clinical trials and meta-analyses). Guidelines are available for the treatment of breast cancer, follow-up care post-treatment, management of cancer-related psychosocial distress, and more generally for the assessment and management of mental disorders such as depression. This section of the report reviews the status of these guidelines and their potential to improve the management of psychosocial distress for women with breast cancer.

The most widely used American breast cancer clinical practice guidelines do not address the management of psychosocial distress. The National Comprehensive Cancer Network (NCCN), a coalition of major cancer centers (Figure 7-1), has published guidelines for breast cancer treatment and

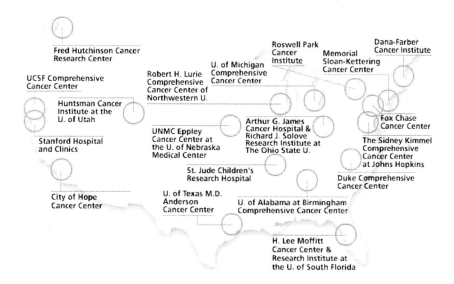

FIGURE 7-1 Institutional members of the National Comprehensive Cancer Network.
SOURCE: http://www.nccn.org/, accessed April 17, 2003.

for cancer-related fatigue, pain, distress, and palliative care (Benedetti et al., 2000; Carlson et al., 2000; Levy et al., 2001; McGivney et al., 2000; Mock et al., 2000; NCCN, 1999). In 1999, NCCN established a multidisciplinary panel to develop management and clinical practice guidelines for mental health, social work, and pastoral counselors (NCCN, 1999) (Box 7-3). Developed by a multidisciplinary panel, the NCCN psychosocial distress guideline is intended for use in busy outpatient oncology practices to quickly identify patients who are distressed, by use of a rapid screening tool, and to provide an algorithm for triage to psychosocial support services. The NCCN guideline has been endorsed by several organizations: American Psychosocial Oncology Society; Oncology Nursing Society; American Society of Oncology Social Work; Professional Chaplains' Organization; American College of Surgeons, Commission on Standards for Cancer Care; and the American Community Cancer Centers (Holland et al., 2001).

Guidelines developed in countries such as Australia, Canada, and Scotland have attempted to incorporate the management of psychosocial concerns into their cancer-related clinical practice guidelines (Table 7-2). The potential need to provide support and counseling with additional visits for some women, for example, is noted in the guidelines for follow-up after treatment for breast cancer published by The Canadian Steering Committee

---

BOX 7-3
Standards of Care for Distress Management

• Distress should be recognized, monitored, documented, and treated promptly at all stages of disease
• All patients should be screened for distress at their initial visit, at appropriate intervals and as clinically indicated.
• Screening should identify the level and nature of the distress.
• Distress should be assessed and managed according to clinical practice guidelines.
• Multidisciplinary institutional committees should be formed to implement standards for distress management.
• Educational and training programs should be developed to ensure that health-care professionals and clergy have knowledge and skills in the management of distress.
• Mental health professionals and clergy experienced in psychosocial issues in cancer should be available as staff members or by referral in a timely manner.
• Medical care contracts must include reimbursement for the management of distress.
• Clinical health outcomes measurement must include assessment of the psychosocial domain, e.g., cost-effectiveness, quality of life, and patient satisfaction.
• Patients and families should be informed that management of distress is an integral part of total medical care
• Quality of the management of distress should be included in institutional continuous quality improvement (CQI) projects.

SOURCE: NCCN (1999).

---

on Clinical Practice Guidelines for the Care and Treatment of Breast Cancer (Canadian Medical Association, 1998). The Canadian guideline states that "psychosocial support should be encouraged and facilitated" (Canadian Medical Association, 1998). The Scottish Intercollegiate Guidelines Network (SIGN), Guideline on Breast Cancer in Women calls for specific action on the part of oncology caregivers in the section on psychosocial aspects of care (SIGN guideline, section 16):

• "All professionals involved in the management of patients with breast cancer should have a high index of suspicion regarding the presence of psychological and psychiatric problems."
• "Patients with significant psychological problems should be assessed by a liaison psychiatrist or clinical psychologist."

TABLE 7-2 Selected Clinical Practice Guidelines for the Management of Psychosocial Distress

Guideline	Description	Status
National Comprehensive Cancer Network (NCCN) Guidelines for the Management of Psychosocial. Distress, US, 1997 (www.nccn.org)	Stand-alone guideline for the management of psychosocial distress (not site specific).	Adopted by several professional organizations, no data on adoption or use.
Canadian Association of Psychosocial Oncology (CAPO), National Psychosocial Oncology Standards for Canada, 1999 (www.capo.ca/finalstandards.cfm)	Standards for the delivery of psychosocial services, research, and education in oncology (not site specific).	CAPO has examined personnel needs and has appealed to provincial government for assistance in adopting standards.
Scottish Intercollegiate Guidelines Network (SIGN), Guideline on Breast Cancer in Women, 1998 (http://www.sign.ac.uk/guidelines /published/index.html)	Breast cancer guideline incorporates consideration of psychological and psychiatric problems.	Applied within the National Health Service in Scotland. Responsibility for implementation rests with each individual NHS Trust.
Australian National Health and Medical Research Council, Psychosocial Clinical Practice Guidelines: Information, Support, and Counseling for Women With Breast Cancer, 1999 (http://www.nbcc.org.au/)	Specific psychosocial guideline on breast cancer.	Extensive experience with adoption of psychosocial guidelines into breast cancer care.

- "Patients should be given appropriate information over a period of time, since what they may wish, or need to know, may vary over time."

This strategy of incorporating consideration of psychosocial concerns into clinical guidelines encourages the integration of psychosocial services into routine care.

Australia has the most extensive experience in the adoption of psychosocial guidelines, and in many respects, can serve as a model. Their guideline, "Psychosocial Clinical Practice Guidelines: Information, Support, and Counseling for Women With Breast Cancer" was published in 1999 and has subsequently been adopted as the standard of care in major health service delivery programs (Redman et al, 2003). An initiative to provide training in communications to clinicians involved in breast cancer care is underway, and the Royal Australian College of Physicians is in the process of implementing an approach to compulsory communication skills training for its medical oncology trainees (Redman et al., 2003). All trainees are strongly encouraged to undertake communication skills training, which is provided free of charge, and participation is compulsory for some trainees depending on skill level. The employment of specialist breast nurses is being promoted to improve patient education, satisfaction, and care coordination (Parle et al., 2001). In addition, an audit of care is being conducted, through a population-based survey of women with early breast cancer, to assess whether women's receipt of information and supportive care is in line with guideline recommendations (Redman et al., 2003). National efforts are underway to educate advocacy groups and health professionals about psychosocial issues in breast cancer and to influence health policy through a coalition of consumer advocates and professionals.

A number of issues are unresolved in the area of guideline development. It is unclear, for example, whether psychosocial guidelines need to be tumor specific. Generic guidelines for the management of psychosocial distress may be needed, with special modules to address site-specific issues (e.g., body image, sexuality) (Winn, workshop presentation, October 2002).

There are many general mental health guidelines available for the management of common psychiatric conditions such as depression. The National Guideline Clearinghouse, a repository of evidence-based clinical practice guidelines maintained by the Agency for Healthcare Research and Quality, the American Medical Association, and the American Association of Health Plans includes 94 mental disorder-related guidelines, but none is specific to cancer (http://www.guideline.gov/index.asp, accessed January 23, 2003). The only cancer-specific psychosocial guidelines are those from NCCN, Australia, Canada, and Scotland.

The American Society of Clinical Oncology (ASCO) has issued 17 clinical practice guidelines; however, none addresses psychosocial issues (http://www.asco.org/ac/1%2C1003%2C_12-002130%2C00.asp, accessed April 18, 2003). ASCO has a communication initiative underway for practicing oncologists and trainees that addresses some of the related issues, for example, communication skills in delivering bad news and implications of cultural diversity on practice. Programs addressing how and what to tell children when a parent has cancer are being developed. For example, a unique program at Massachusetts General Hospital (called PACT – Parenting at Challenging Times) has five trained child psychologists and psychiatrists available to provide free consultation and psycho-education to adults undergoing cancer treatment, and a national Internet program, KIDS KONNECT, has been established. The development and dissemination of guidelines alone has minimal effect on clinical practice, but a growing body of evidence indicates that when guideline development includes providers, and when guidelines are implemented with systems in place to give providers information about their practice and remind them to use the guidelines, the quality of care can improve. Also recognized as essential to guideline implementation is up-front involvement of leaders from the health professions and representatives of patients in the guideline development process (IOM, 2001; Smith and Hillner, 2001).

Guidelines can be effective in aligning care with evidence-based standards and can also influence insurers in their coverage policies. For example, reimbursement for psychosocial assessments prior to bone marrow transplantation has been easier to obtain from insurers following the publication of the American Society of Blood and Marrow Transplantation guideline that recommends a psychiatric consultation as part of the transplant work-up (Richard McQuellon, Associate Professor and Director, Psychosocial Oncology and Cancer Support Programs, Wake Forest University/Baptist Medical Center, personal communication to Maria Hewitt, November 4, 2002). Although bone marrow transplantation is not recommended for women with advanced breast cancer, these guidelines have facilitated the use of psychosocial services among those for whom the intervention is appropriate.

Ideally, clinical practice guidelines not only give providers the guidance they need to deliver interventions, they also lay out a plan for the integration of services into the delivery of care. Such a plan for the integration of psychosocial services into oncology practice is outlined in Figure 7-2. The essential steps according to this scheme include screening patients for distress as they

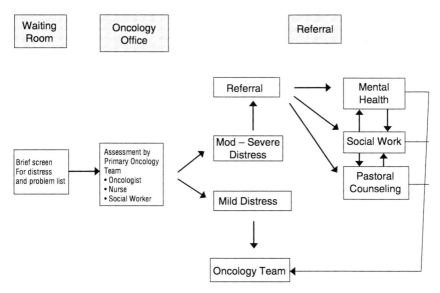

FIGURE 7-2 The integration of psychosocial services into oncology practice.
SOURCE: Holland, workshop presentation, October 2002.

wait for their appointments using a simple self-report. Concerns raised by the assessment are addressed during the clinical encounter, and as necessary according to the assessment, patients are referred to the appropriate psychosocial service, which is determined by the nature of the problems. Oncology providers remain an integral part of the process insofar as they continue the evaluative and treatment process at subsequent appointments. The roles of mental health, social work, and pastoral care providers in assessing need and providing psychosocial services are delineated in Table 7-3.

The NCCN guidelines on psychosocial distress were developed in 1997, and research to assess their value is ongoing. However, there is little available information on the extent of their use, their feasibility, and their potential to improve the quality of care and reduce psychosocial distress. A validation study in four institutions has been completed to test the use of the Distress Thermometer and Problem List (Jimmie Holland, personal communication to Maria Hewitt, 2003). Needed are well-designed research studies to investigate the value of guidelines. The NCCN guidelines are not specific to type of cancer, and questions remain regarding the need for specific modules to address some of the issues unique to certain types of cancer, for example, to address sexuality and body image in breast cancer, in particular. Other questions remain regarding their implementation, for example, which assessment tools should be used and how the assessment might be carried out in busy oncology practices. How psychosocial guidelines can be integrated into guidelines that direct the treatment of the different sites of cancer also needs to be addressed.

The American Psychological Association has developed a template for constructing psychological intervention guidelines that stresses the importance of both efficacy (internal validity) and clinical utility (external validity) (Barlow and Barlow, 1995). Important aspects of clinical utility include:

• Feasibility, whether patients find the guideline acceptable, ease of adoption and use;
• Generalizability, whether the guidelines are applicable across cultural groups, ages, and other patient characteristics;
• Costs and benefits, including both costs to individuals and society.

Lack of Accepted Methods of Clinical Assessment[2]

While guidelines call for the recognition of psychosocial distress in patients, they generally do not provide specific guidance on how to go about

---

[2]This section of the chapter is based on a background paper written for the Board by Patricia A. Ganz, M.D., Jonsson Comprehensive Cancer Center, UCLA Schools of Medicine and Public Health, Los Angeles, CA (www.iom.edu/ncpb).

TABLE 7-3 NCCN Distress Management Guideline (Version 1. 1999)

Expertise	Areas to evaluate	Interventions
Mental health	• Distress • Behavior/symptoms • Psychiatric history/medications • Pain syndromes • Body image/sexuality • Ethical dilemmas	Guideline- directed treatment • Adjustment disorders • Major depression • Delirium • Anxiety disorders • Dementia • Substance use • Personality disorders • Supportive psychotherapy and follow-up • Community resource mobilization • Cognitive-behavioral therapy • Problem-solving teaching • Advocacy and family/patient • Education/support group sessions • Resource lists
Social work	Social needs • Family dysfunction • Social isolation/conflict • Decision-making, quality of life issues • Advance directive • Domestic violence Practical needs • Illness-related needs assessment • Basic needs including housing, food, finance assistance programs, transportation • Employment/school/career concerns	
Pastoral care	• Isolation from religious community • Grief • Guilt • Hopelessness • Concerns about death and afterlife • Conflicted or challenged belief systems • Loss of faith • Concerns with meaning/purpose of life • Concerns about relationship with deity • Conflict between religious beliefs and recommended treatment • Ritual needs	• Spiritual counseling • Referral to mental health as needed

SOURCE: Adapted from NCCN, 1999.

identifying individuals in need of intervention. Effective assessment strategies for psychosocial distress are needed because symptoms and concerns of women with breast cancer frequently go undetected in both the oncology setting and in primary care. One study of 2,300 cancer patients in 34 hospitals across Britain found that while more than a third of cancer patients (all types) could have benefited from some type of psychological help, the specialists treating them only spotted the symptoms in 29 percent of these distressed patients (Fallowfield et al., 2001). Patients with overt symptoms of distress were the most likely to be identified. In a United States-based study of 1,109 patients seen in 25 ambulatory oncology clinics (treated by 12 oncologists), physicians' perceptions of depressive symptoms in their patients were correlated with patient's ratings, but physicians tended to underestimate the level of depressive symptoms in the most severely depressed patients. The authors concluded that screening instruments and the use of brief follow-up interviews would help to systematically identify patients who are depressed (Passik et al., 1998).

Routinely asking all women about psychosocial distress during visits for care using validated screening instruments could effectively focus limited health care resources on individuals who are most likely to need them. Despite the intuitive appeal of such an approach, it has rarely been adopted, and when it has, the outcome of screening has not been evaluated. The oncology group at Johns Hopkins has been screening patients with the Brief Symptom Inventory (BSI) for over a decade (Zabora et al. 1990); however, there has been limited reporting of the impact it has made on clinical care and practice at that institution.

It is important to distinguish screening from assessment. As described by Zabora, "Screening is a rapid method to prospectively identify potential patients who may experience significant difficulty in their attempts to cope and adapt to their diagnoses and treatments. Screening is a predictive model. Assessment seeks to accomplish a series of tasks in the early phases of a relationship with a patient. These tasks include an estimate of the severity of the patient's distress, definition of the initial course of action, development of a dynamic understanding of the patient, the establishment of a diagnosis, and the first step in the development of a therapeutic relationship" (Passik et al., 1998; Zabora, 1998).

A major impediment to the adoption of screening is the limited clinical experience with the many assessment tools that have been developed in research settings (see Chapter 3 for a description of these instruments). While many clinical trials support the value of psychosocial interventions, there have been no studies demonstrating that systematic screening of women with breast cancer for psychosocial distress has led to improved health and quality of life. The potential impact of screening on the use of mental health and community services is also needed to help gauge the adequacy of the supply of support services. Applied research in this area is in progress and is sorely needed (Holland, workshop presentation, October 2002).

In the Board's review of the literature, only one study was found that attempted to screen for anxiety and depression in breast cancer patients in the clinical setting as part of a quality assurance project (Payne et. al., 1999). In that study, three different instruments were evaluated (Hospital Anxiety and Depression Scale [HADS], the Brief Symptom Inventory [BSI], and a single-item visual analog scale) (see Chapter 3 for descriptions of these assessment tools). All three instruments were effective in identifying women with psychosocial distress, but the authors concluded that the HADS seemed to be the simplest and most practical tool to use in this setting (Payne et al. 1999). Some screening instruments have been adapted so that they can be administered in waiting rooms using touch screens on computers. Scored results are available immediately to providers so that they can discuss results during the scheduled visit (Cull et al., 2001). The results of psychosocial assessments may be of some value and interest to women who are interested in charting their reactions to their disease and treatment.

In choosing a screening instrument, clinicians need to assess whether they want to focus on psychiatric disorders such as anxiety and depression (e.g., as measured in HADS), or whether they want to assess broader quality of life concerns such as symptoms (e.g., fatigue, pain), social issues (e.g., relationships and family concerns), and practical problems (e.g., problems working, paying for care) (e.g., as measured in the CARES instrument or the NCCN distress thermometer).

Despite the lack of evidence for the benefits of screening for psychosocial distress in the cancer context, there is widespread agreement that clinicians should at least be screening their patients for depression which is a prevalent, treatable, condition in the general population, and of higher prevalence among individuals with chronic illness such as cancer. The U.S. Preventive Services Task Force, for example, issued guidelines in 2002 recommending that primary care physicians routinely screen their patients for depression using any one of a number of validated screening instruments (http://www.ahrq.gov/clinic/uspstf/uspsdepr.htm) (Pignone et al., 2002; Williams et al., 2002). The Task Force concluded that screening for depression can improve outcomes, particularly when screening is coupled with system changes that help ensure adequate treatment and follow-up (Pignone et al., 2002).

A past history of depression or prior psychological difficulties places individuals at higher risk of psychosocial distress and early referral of such patients for additional support following a diagnosis of breast cancer may be indicated. In addition, younger women, women with other comorbid conditions, and women with limited social support should be carefully assessed for the additional distress they may experience in association with the cancer diagnosis.

A stepped care approach can be envisioned so that individuals with mild distress could be treated by oncology providers, moderately distressed patient referred to community resources, and severely distressed patients referred to psychologists and psychiatrists. This model has been adapted from the widely used WHO Analgesic Ladder for pain management (Figure 7-3).

The inclusion of a nursing or mental health specialist as part of the care team in larger practices such as comprehensive breast care programs can facilitate both screening and the provision of services (Sorensen and Liu, 1995). In these settings, early contact with a mental health professional is routine which destigmatizes use of services and facilitates referral for individual or group counseling. While this approach may not be feasible in all practice settings, use of the screening tools described earlier in all patients could alert the practicing physician to patients who need appropriate referrals. In a study of the effect of counseling by a nurse specialist on recovery among breast cancer patients following mastectomy conducted in the late 1970s, the nurse's regular monitoring of women's progress facilitated the recognition and subsequent referral of three-quarters of women who needed psychiatric help (Maguire et al., 1980).

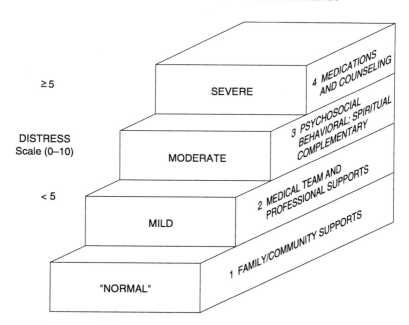

DISTRESS LADDER:
MANAGEMENT BY STANDARDS & PRACTICE GUIDELINES

FIGURE 7-3 Stepped care approach to managing psychosocial distress.
SOURCE: Holland, workshop presentation, October 2002

Psychosocial needs change over the cancer care trajectory, so that reassessment is necessary during and after treatment or during the recovery phase. The assessment must be sensitive to the changes in psychosocial needs. Survivorship issues like sexual problems, distress related to body image, cognitive function, and lymphedema may only emerge following treatment. Assessments must take into consideration the context of a woman's age and social situation. Family, career, sexual, and reproductive issues may be at the forefront of concerns for younger women. Women in midlife may, in addition, have concerns related to menopause, while elderly women may have distinct concerns regarding other chronic health conditions. Some issues not of concern around the time of diagnosis may emerge later as sources of distress, for example, body image. How often an assessment is done may depend on the planned schedule of visits for follow-up for women with breast cancer. Who performs the assessment may vary depending on whether women are followed by their oncology or primary care provider.

There is a fear that screening will result in identifying so many women that they cannot be given the psychosocial services needed. Where routine screening has been adopted, for example, at the Johns Hopkins Oncology Center, this has not occurred. In fact, screening all patients helps deploy available services to those most in need and allows referral of others to groups and community resources. Assistance to the primary oncology team in identifying patients who are distressed, by means of a screening tool, can also provide a triage algorithm to use for referral to specialized psychosocial services. This has proved to be the case in pain management which has improved by asking patients to rate their pain on a scale of 1 to 10, and using any score above 5 as indication for a pain consultation. The NCCN distress thermometer follows the same algorithm.

Inadequate Quality Assurance and Accountability

There is no one system to assure the quality of cancer care, but several programs in place could potentially serve to improve access to psychosocial services. As described in Chapter 6, there are two sets of standards that address cancer-related quality of care, those of the American College of Surgeons' (ACoS) Commission on Cancer (CoC), and those of the Association of Community Cancer Centers (ACCC). Of the two, the standards of the CoC affect more individuals with cancer because an estimated 82 percent of new cases of cancer are seen in the 1,428 hospitals approved by the CoC. Staffing and programmatic needs are outlined in these standards to ensure, at a minimal level, the capacity to provide psychosocial service.

The American Cancer Society (ACS) has launched an ambitious community-based Quality of Life initiative aimed at cancer patients and their caregivers and families. The provision of psychosocial services is an important component of its initiative (Box 7-4).

BOX 7-4.
American Cancer Society Nationwide Objectives to Improve
the Quality of Life (QoL) of Cancer Patients and
their Caregivers and Families

QOL Goal: Measurable improvement in the quality of life (physical, psychological, social, and spiritual) from the time of diagnosis and for the balance of life of all cancer survivors by the year 2015.

PHYSICAL ASPECTS OF QUALITY OF LIFE
• Physical Effects: By 2015, provide appropriate care for symptom control, emphasizing pain, fatigue, rehabilitation, and side effects of treatment based upon an appropriate care plan using uniform standards of care for 90% of cancer survivors.
• Pain Control: By 2015, provide appropriate care for the control of pain based upon an appropriate care plan using uniform standards of care for 90% of cancer survivors. By 2005, 75% of health care systems will have institutionalized quality standards for the management of pain.
• Physical Appearance: By 2015, the negative impact of cancer on physical appearance and body image will be substantially reduced in 75% of those affected cancer survivors.

SOCIAL ASPECTS OF QUALITY OF LIFE
• Social Support: By 2005, the number of cancer survivors, their families, and caregivers who participate in appropriate ACS patient support programs or are referred to other community programs will increase by at least 50%.
• By 2005, 60% of survivors, their families, and caregivers will be aware of and have knowledge about American Cancer Society quality of life education and support services.

PSYCHOLOGICAL AND SPIRITUAL DOMAINS
• Psychological, Emotional, Spiritual Effects: By 2015, 90% of cancer survivors and families and caregivers of those affected by cancer will receive appropriate care or appropriate referral to services for identified psychological, emotional, and spiritual problems and/or needs.
• Provider Education: By 2015, 90% of health care providers will assess psychological, emotional, and spiritual needs of cancer survivors and families and caregivers of those affected by cancer and provide appropriate care or appropriate referral to services.

SOURCE: B. Teschendorf, October workshop, 2002.

Achieving these national goals will involve actions at the 17 ACS Divisions throughout the country (B. Teschendorf, IOM workshop, 2002). To aid in implementation, assessments of community resources are taking place and a database is being created, by state, within each Division. The database will be used for referral and as a navigation tool. Certain areas will aim to be designated as "Communities of Excellence" through the setting of specific goals and the measurement of their achievement. Working with advocates and consumers, some communities might elect to focus on pain, social support, or other areas within the broad set of quality of life measures. Worksites provide another opportunity to implement the ACS goals. ACS is planning a program for large employers to ease the transition of cancer survivors back to work.

Other cancer advocacy organizations have promoted an awareness of psychosocial services as a part of quality cancer care. The National Breast Cancer Coalition (NBCC), for example, has published a Guide to Quality Breast Cancer Care for consumers that identifies social and support services as part of comprehensive care (NBCC, 2002). The National Coalition for Cancer Survivorship (NCCS) has published quality imperatives (Box 7-5) that include the need for psychosocial services (see principle 5 below) and

---

BOX 7-5 Quality Cancer Care: Declaration of Principles, National Coalition for Cancer Survivorship

Principle 1 People with cancer have the right to a system of universal health care. This access should not be precluded because of preexisting conditions, genetic or other risk factors, or employment status.

Principle 2 Quality cancer care should be available in a health care system whose standards and guidelines are developed in consideration of treating the whole person with cancer. Health care plans must regard the cancer patient as an autonomous individual who has the right to be involved in decisions about his or her care.

Principle 3 Standards of cancer care should be driven by the quality of care, not only by the cost of care, and should include participation in clinical trials and quality of life considerations.

Principle 4 All people diagnosed with cancer should have access to and coverage for services provided by a multidisciplinary team of care providers across the full continuum of care. Health care plans should be held accountable for timely referral to appropriate specialists when symptoms of cancer or its recurrence may be present.

Principle 5 People with cancer should be provided a range of benefits by all health care plans that includes primary and secondary prevention, early detection, initial treatment, supportive therapies to manage pain, nausea, fatigue and infections, long-term follow-up, psychosocial services, palliative care, hospice care, and bereavement counseling.

Principle 6 People with histories of cancer have the right to continued medical follow-up with basic standards of care that include the specific needs of long-term survivors.

Principle 7 Long-term survivors should have access to specialized follow-up clinics that focus on health promotion, disease prevention, rehabilitation, and identification of physiologic and psychosocial problems. Communication with the primary care physician must be maintained.

Principle 8 Systematic long-term follow-up should generate data that contribute to improvements in cancer therapies and decreases in morbidity.

Principle 9 The responsibility for appropriate long-term medical care must be shared by cancer survivors, their families, the oncology team, and primary care providers.

Principle 10 The provision of psychosocial services must be safeguarded and promoted. Persons diagnosed with cancer should receive psychosocial assessments at critical junctures along the continuum of cancer care to determine availability of needed support and their ability to seek information and to advocate on their own behalf.

Principle 11 Psychosocial research is integral to comprehensive cancer care and, as such, psychosocial outcome measures should be included in all future clinical trials. The importance of this research and its application and transfer to oncology care plans should be recognized and encouraged.

Principle 12 Cancer survivors, health care providers and other key constituency groups must work together to increase public awareness; educate consumers, professionals, and public policy makers; develop guidelines and disseminate information; advocate for increased research funding; and articulate for and promote survivors' rights.

SOURCE: NCCS, 1995.

has created a cancer survivorship tool kit to help patients advocate for care that meets these quality standards (http://www.canceradvocacy.org/).

With nearly half (45 percent) of new cases of breast cancer occurring among women age 65 or older, the Medicare program has an interest in ensuring the delivery of quality care to its beneficiaries. The agency overseeing the Medicare program, the Centers for Medicare and Medicaid Services (CMS), has systems in place to monitor quality of care, but assessments to date on cancer-related care have focused on breast cancer screening (IOM, 2002). Assessments of the delivery of psychosocial care are hampered by the lack of validated measures of quality. The National Quality Forum (NQF) is a not-for-profit membership organization created in 2000 to develop and implement a national strategy for healthcare quality measurement and reporting (http://www.qualityforum.org/, accessed April 18, 2003). In 2002 the NQF formed a Cancer Care Quality Measures Steering Committee to reach consensus on a core set of quality measures. Breast cancer is one of the focus areas of this activity, as well as symptom management and palliation.

There is more experience with quality of care measurement for breast cancer care, relative to other types of cancer care (IOM, 2000). The Foundation for Accountability (FACCT), for example, developed a set of breast cancer quality indicators which included satisfaction with care, and quality of life as measured by the Cancer Rehabilitation Evaluation System (CARES) instrument (see Chapter 3 for a description of this instrument). The Providence Health System uses FACCT to assess breast cancer care within its 17 member institutions (located from California to Alaska) (http://www.providence.org/Oregon/Programs_and_Services/Research/CORE/performance, accessed April 18, 2003). More direct measurement of the provision of psychosocial care within systems of care have not yet been performed, but could likely be incorporated into assessments of satisfaction of care. In a review of quality-of-care measure that could be used to assess oncology practice, Mandelblatt and colleagues suggest that rates of clinical assessment of the need for psychological support services (both group and individual) could be documented and serve as a process measure of rehabilitative care (Mandelblatt et al., 1999). Evaluations of the feasibility and value of such quality of care assessments are needed.

SUMMARY AND RECOMMENDATIONS

Many barriers need to be overcome to meet the psychosocial needs of women with breast cancer. Lack of access to health care is a general societal problem in America. An estimated 8 percent of women with breast cancer lack health insurance coverage, and many more have inadequate health insurance coverage for even basic health care needs. Health insurance coverage often provides poor coverage of mental health benefits or imposes restrictions on benefits through high out-of-pocket payments or limits on care. At the individual level, the stigma associated with seeking mental health care can inhibit use of services, but such stigma may be waning with the well-publicized successes of the treatment of common disorders like depression.

Health-care providers can serve as barriers to appropriate psychosocial care if they fail to acknowledge such issues in the course of providing cancer care or if they do not refer patients to available services. Implementing clinical practice guidelines that incorporate assessment and treatment of psychosocial distress is a promising strategy to overcome many of these barriers. While there is limited evidence on the use and effectiveness of such guidelines in reducing psychosocial distress and improving quality of life of women with breast cancer, the guidelines have established the first standards for care in this "soft" area of clinical work. As such, these guidelines have provided the first benchmarks against which to monitor psychosocial care and services.

At present there is little evidence that psychosocial interventions are integrated into routine breast cancer care. In general, the oncology nurse and social worker serve as front line staff to identify patients in need of psychosocial services. Guidelines are available to help clinicians identify and manage individuals with cancer who are distressed, but the Board could identify no studies of their use. Perhaps a demonstration project could explore this. Certain organizations, for example, the American College of Surgeons' Commission on Cancer, have developed standards to ensure the availability of psychosocial services, but a consideration of such standards is usually outside of the scope of ongoing quality assurance programs.

To overcome the range of barriers to delivering psychosocial services to women with breast cancer, the Board recommends that:

1. Breast cancer care clinicians, such as oncologists and other medical professionals, responsible for the care of women with breast cancer should incorporate planning for psychosocial management as an integral part of treatment. They should routinely assess and address psychosocial distress as a part of total medical care. Validated assessment tools are available to screen for psychosocial distress and especially for anxiety and depression. Quality of life instruments also can be used to identify function (psychological, social, physical, sexual) and to facilitate discussion of patient concerns, and serve as a basis for referral. Financial considerations may dictate that in most instances screening is carried out using simple, rapid tools such as the Distress Thermometer or Hospital Anxiety and Depression Scale (HADS).

2. *Providers of cancer care should meet the standards of psychosocial care developed by the American College of Surgeons' Commission on Cancer and follow the National Comprehensive Cancer Network's (NCCN) Clinical Practice Guidelines for the Management of Distress.* Education about psychosocial needs and services should be undertaken through collaboration between professional organizations and advocacy groups.

3. *The NCI, the American Cancer Society (ACS), and professional organizations (e.g., American Society of Clinical Oncology, American College of Surgeons, American Association of Colleges of Nursing, American Psychosocial Oncology Society, American Society of Social Work, American Society for Therapeutic Radiology and Oncology, Oncology Nursing Society) need to partner with advocacy groups (e.g., National Breast Cancer Coalition, National Alliance of Breast Cancer Organizations, Wellness Community, NCCS) to focus attention on psychosocial needs of patients and resources that provide psychosocial services in local communities and nationally.*

Organizations with effective outreach to cancer constituencies should be assisted in making resource directories available to providers and patients; these directories would identify the range of supportive services, from the free services of advocacy groups to services provided by mental health professionals.

Translational research is also needed to test interventions to overcome barriers to the provision of effective psychosocial care within practice settings. The current status of psychosocial research and the Board's recommendations for research action are discussed in Chapter 8.

REFERENCES

Achman L, Chollet D. 2001. *Insuring the Uninsurable: An Overview of State High-Risk Health Insurance Pools.* Mathematica Policy Research, Inc. Princeton, NJ. [Online]. Available: http://www.mathematica-mpr.com/3rdlevel/uninsurablehot.htm [accessed March 21, 2003].

American Association of Retired Persons (AARP), Public Policy Institute and the Lewin Group. 1997. *Out-of-Pocket Health Spending by Medicare Beneficiaries Age 65 and Older: 1997 Projections.*

Ayanian JZ, Kohler BA, Abe T, Epstein AM. 1993. The relation between health insurance coverage and clinical outcomes among women with breast cancer. *N Engl J Med* 329(5):326–331.

Baile WF, Kudelka AP, Beale EA, Glober GA, Myers EG, Greisinger AJ, et al. 1999. Communication skills training in oncology: Description and preliminary outcomes of workshops on breaking bad news and managing patient reactions to illness. *Cancer* 86:887–897.

Barlow DH, Barlow DB. 1995. Practice guidelines and empirically validated psychosocial treatments: Ships passing in the night? *Behavioral Healthcare Tomorrow* May/June 25–29, 76.

Benedetti C, Brock C, Cleeland C, Coyle N, Dube JE, Ferrell B, Hassenbusch S 3rd, Janjan NA, Lema MJ, Levy MH, Loscalzo MJ, Lynch M, Muir C, Oakes L, O'Neill A, Payne R, Syrjala KL, Urba S, Weinstein SM. 2000. NCCN practice guidelines for cancer pain. *Oncology (Huntingt)* 14(11A):135–150.

Bickell NA, Young GJ. 2001. Coordination of care for early-stage breast cancer patients. *J Gen Intern Med* 16(11):737-742.

Butow PN, Dunn SM, Tattersall MHN. 1995. Communication with cancer patients: Does it matter? *J Palliat Care* 11:34–38.

Canadian Medical Association - Steering Committee on Clinical Practice Guidelines for the Care and Treatment of Breast Cancer. 1998. Follow-up after treatment for breast cancer. *Canadian Medical Association Journal* 158:565–570.

Carlson RW, Anderson BO, Bensinger W, Cox CE, Davidson NE, Edge SB, Farrar WB, Goldstein LJ, Gradishar WJ, Lichter AS, McCormick B, Nabell LM, Reed EC, Silver SM, Smith ML, Somlo G, Theriault R, Ward JH, Winer EP, Wolff A. 2000. NCCN practice guidelines for breast cancer. *Oncology (Huntingt)* 14(11A):33–49.

Cull A, Gould A, House A, Smith A, Strong V, Velikova G, Wright P, Selby P. 2001. Validating automated screening for psychological distress by means of computer touchscreens for use in routine oncology practice. *Br J Cancer* 85(12):1842–1849.

Department of Health and Human Services, CMS. 2002. *HHS to Help States Create High-Risk Pools to Increase Access to Health Coverage*. Press release, November 26, 2002. [Online]. Available: www.hhs.gov/news/press/2002pres/20021126a.html [accessed January 31, 2003).

Department of Health and Human Services. 2001. *Medicare Part B Payments for Mental Health Services*. Philadelphia: Department of Health and Human Services.

Detmar SB, Aaronson NK, Wever LD, Muller M, Schornagel JH. 2000. How are you feeling? Who wants to know? Patients' and oncologists' preferences for discussing health-related quality-of-life issues. *J Clin Oncol* 18(18):3295–3301.

Eakin EG, Strycker, LA. 2001. Awareness and barriers to use of cancer support and information resources by HMO patients with breast, prostate, or colon cancer: patient and provider perspectives. *Psycho-oncology.* 10(2):103-113.

Edgar L, Remmer J, Rosberger Z, et al. 2000. Resource use in women completing treatment for breast cancer. *Psycho-oncology.* 9(5):428-438.

Fallowfield L, Ratcliffe D, Jenkins V, Saul J. 2001. Psychiatric morbidity and its recognition by doctors in patients with cancer. *Br J Cancer* 84(8):1011–1015.

Frank RG. 2000. The creation of Medicare and Medicaid: The emergence of insurance and markets for mental health services. *Psychiatr Serv* 51(4):465–468.

Gerrity MS, Cole SA, Dietrich AJ, et al. 1999. Improving the recognition and management of depression: Is there a role for physician education? *J Fam Pract* 48(12):949–957.

Goff VV. 2002. Depression: A decade of progress, more to do. *NHPF Issue Brief* (786):1–14.

Gold M, Achman L. 2001. Trends in premiums, cost-sharing, and benefits in Medicare+Choice health plans, 1999–2001. *Issue Brief (Commonw Fund)* 460:1–6.

Goldman W, McCulloch J, Sturm R. 1998. Costs and use of mental health services before and after managed care. *Health Aff (Millwood)* 17(2):40–52.

Hewitt M, Breen N, Devesa S. 1999. Cancer prevalence and survivorship issues: Analyses of the 1992 National Health Interview Survey. *J Natl Cancer Inst* 91(17):1480–1486.

Holland JC. 1999. Update: NCCN practice guidelines for the management of psychosocial distress. *Oncology* 13(11A):459–507.

Holland JC, Jacobsen PB, Riba MB. 2001. Distress management. *Cancer Control* 8(6):88–93.

Institute of Medicine. 1990. *Clinical Practice Guidelines: Directions for a New Program*. Washington, DC: National Academy Press.

Institute of Medicine. 1993. *Access to Health Care in America*. Washington DC: National Academy Press.

Institute of Medicine. 1997. *Managing Managed Care: Quality Improvement in Behavioral Health*. Washington, DC: National Academy Press.

Institute of Medicine. 2000. *Enhancing Data Systems to Improve the Quality of Cancer Care*. Washington, DC: National Academy Press.

Institute of Medicine. 2001. *Coverage Matters: Insurance and Health Care*. Washington, DC: National Academy Press.

Institute of Medicine. 2002. *Care Without Coverage: Too Little, Too Late*. Washington, DC: National Academy Press.

Institute of Medicine. 2002. *Leadership by Example: Coordinating Government Roles in Improving Healthcare Quality*. Washington, DC: National Academy Press.

Landerman LR, Burns BJ, Swartz MS, Wagner HR, George LK. 1994. The relationship between insurance coverage and psychiatric disorder in predicting use of mental health services. *Am J Psychiatry* 151(12):1785–1790.

Lee-Feldstein A, Feldstein PJ, Buchmueller T, Katterhagen G. 2000. The relationship of HMOs, health insurance, and delivery systems to breast cancer outcomes. *Med Care* 38(7):705–718.

Lerman C, Daly M, Walsh WP, Resch N, Seay J, Barsevick A, Birenbaum L, Heggan T, Martin G. 1993. Communication between patients with breast cancer and health care providers. Determinants and implications. *Cancer* 72(9):2612–2620.

Levy MH, Weinstein SM, Carducci MA. 2001. NCCN: Palliative care. *Cancer Control* 8(6 Suppl 2):66–71.

Liang W, Burnett CB, Rowland JH, Meropol NJ, Eggert L, Hwang YT, Silliman RA, Weeks JC, Mandelblatt JS. 2002. Communication between physicians and older women with localized breast cancer: Implications for treatment and patient satisfaction. *J Clin Oncol* 20(4):1008–1016.

Maguire P, Tait A, Brooke M, et at. 1980. Effect of counseling on the psychiatric morbidity associated with mastectomy. *Br Med J*. 281(6253):1454-1456.

Mandelblatt JS, Ganz PA, Kahn KL. 1999. Proposed agenda for the measurement of quality-of-care outcomes in oncology practice. *J Clin Oncol* 17(8):2614–2622.

Matthews AK, Sellergren SA, Manfredi C, Williams M. 2002a. Factors influencing medical information seeking among African American cancer patients. *J Health Commun* 7(3):205–219.

Matthews BA, Baker F, Spillers RL. 2002b. Healthcare professionals' awareness of cancer support services. *Cancer Pract* 10(1):36–44.

McGivney WT, McGinnis L, Gansler TS. 2000. The NCCN/American Cancer Society partnership. *Oncology (Huntingt)* 14(11A):213–216.

Mock V, Atkinson A, Barsevick A, Cella D, Cimprich B, Cleeland C, Donnelly J, Eisenberger MA, Escalante C, Hinds P, Jacobsen PB, Kaldor P, Knight SJ, Peterman A, Piper BF, Rugo H, Sabbatini P, Stahl C. 2000. NCCN Practice Guidelines for Cancer-Related Fatigue. *Oncology (Huntingt)* 14(11A):151–161.

National Breast Cancer Coalition. 2002. *Guide to Quality Breast Cancer Care*. 2nd edition. Washington, DC: National Breast Cancer Coalition.

National Comprehensive Cancer Network. 1999. NCCN practice guidelines for the management of psychosocial distress. *Oncology (Huntingt)* 13(5A):113–147.

NCCN. 2003. Clinical Practice Guidelines for Management of Distress. *Journal of the NCCN*.

National Coalition for Cancer Survivorship. 1995. *Imperatives for Quality Cancer Care: Access, Advocacy, Action, and Accountability*. Silver Spring, MD.

National Mental Health Association. 2001. *Americans Say Depression is a Disease "Not a State of Mind," but Stigma and Policy Impede Treatment*. Alexandria, VA.

Olfson M, Marcus SC, Druss B, Elinson L, Tanielian T, Pincus HA. 2002. National trends in the outpatient treatment of depression. *JAMA* 287(2):203–209.

Parle M, Gallagher J, Gray C, Akers G, Liebert B. 2001. From evidence to practice: factors affecting the specialist breast nurse's detection of psychological morbidity in women with breast cancer. *Psycho-oncology* 10(6):503–510.

Passik SD, Dugan W, McDonald MV, Rosenfeld B, Theobald DE, Edgerton S. 1998. Oncologists' recognition of depression in their patients with cancer. *J Clin Oncol*

16(4):1594–1600.

Payne DK, Hoffman RG, Theodoulou M, Dosik M, Massie MJ. 1999. Screening for anxiety and depression in women with breast cancer. *Psychosomatics.* 40(1):64–69.

Pignone MP, Gaynes BN, Rushton JL, Burchell CM, Orleans CT, Mulrow CD, Lohr KN. 2002. Screening for depression in adults: A summary of the evidence for the U.S. Preventive Services Task Force. *Ann Intern Med* 136(10):765–776.

Redman S, Turner J, Davis C. 2003. Improving supportive care for women with breast cancer in Australia: The challenge of modifying health systems. *Psycho-oncology* 12(6):521–531.

Roetzheim RG, Gonzalez EC, Ferrante JM, Pal N, Van Durme DJ, Krischer JP. 2000. Effects of health insurance and race on breast carcinoma treatments and outcomes. *Cancer* 89(11):2202–2213.

Roetzheim RG, Pal N, Tennant C, Voti L, Ayanian JZ, Schwabe A, Krischer JP. 1999. Effects of health insurance and race on early detection of cancer. *J Natl Cancer Inst* 91(16):1409–1415.

Roter DL, Hall JA, Kern DE, et al. 1995. Improving physicians' interviewing skills and reducing patients' emotional distress. A randomized clinical trial. *Arch Intern Med* 155(17):1877–1884.

Schapira, L. Communication skills training in clinical oncology: The ASCO position reviewed and an optimistic personal perspective. *Crit Rev Oncol Hematol* 46(1):25–31.

Sellers T. 2000. A model of collaborative healthcare in outpatient medical oncology. *Families, Systems & Health* 18(1):19–33.

Smith TJ, Hillner BE. 2001. Ensuring quality cancer care by the use of clinical practice guidelines and critical pathways. J Clin Oncol 19(11):2886–2897.

Sofaer S, Davidson BN, Goodwan RD, et al. 1990. Helping Medicare beneficiaries choose health insurance: The illness episode approach. *Gerontologist* 30(3):308-315.

Sorensen, M, Liu, ET. 1995. With a different voice: Integrating the psychosocial perspective into routine oncology care. *Breast Cancer Res Treat* 35(1):39–42.

U.S. Census Bureau. 2002. *Health Insurance Coverage: 2001.* Washington DC: U.S. Department of Commerce, Economics and Statistics Administration.

U.S. Department of Health and Human Services. 2000. *Mental Health: Culture, Race, and Ethnicity: A Supplement to Mental Health: A Report of the Surgeon General.* Rockville, MD: U.S. Department of Health and Human Services, Substance Abuse and Mental Health Services Administration, Center for Mental Health Services, National Institutes of Health, National Institute of Mental Health.

Von Korff M, Gruman J, Schaefer JK, Curry SJ, Wagner EH. 1997. Collaborative management of chronic illness. *Annals of Internal Medicine* 127:1097–1102.

Wagner EH, Austin BT, Von Korff M. 1996. Organizing care for patients with chronic illness. *Millbank Quarterly* 74:511–544.

Williams JW Jr, Pignone M, Ramirez G, Perez Stellato C. 2002. Identifying depression in primary care: A literature synthesis of case-finding instruments. *Gen Hosp Psychiatry* 24(4):225–237.

Zabora JR. 1998. Screening Procedures for Psychosocial Distress. In: Holland JC, Breitbart W, eds. *Psycho-Oncology.* New York: Oxford University Press. Pp. 653–661.

Zabora JR, Smith-Wilson R, Fetting SH, et al. 1990. An efficient method for psychosocial screening of cancer patients. *Psychosomatics.* 31(2):192-196.

8

Research

The National Cancer Policy Board, in an effort to understand how resources for research are applied to questions regarding psychosocial services for women with breast cancer, undertook a review of the status of research. Such a review provides only a snapshot as of 2003, but it does give an indication of the prominence and priority of psychosocial subjects as components within the field of breast cancer research, and a sense of the emphasis on different concerns and services within psychosocial breast cancer research. With these understandings, the Board was able to suggest ways in which a research program could be structured in the future to support better responses to psychosocial needs of women with breast cancer.

This chapter first describes publication trends in breast cancer-related research and then summarizes major sources of support for research within the following organizations:

Federally Sponsored Research
  Department of Health and Human Services
  National Institutes of Health (National Cancer Institute, National
  Institute of Nursing Research)
  Department of Defense

Privately Sponsored Research
  American Cancer Society
  Foundations (e.g., Komen Foundation, Avon Foundation)

Although these organizations are not the only sponsors of breast cancer-related psychosocial research, they represent the major funding sources
for such research. Excluded from this review is research supported by health
plans, insurers, pharmaceutical companies, and other private organizations.
Much of the research in these settings is proprietary. The chapter concludes
with the Board's identification of priority areas for research and recommendations to increase research opportunities.

STATUS OF BREAST CANCER-RELATED RESEARCH

Publications

Evaluating trends in research publications is one way to assess the level
of activity within a discipline. A resource for tracking such studies in the
National Library of Medicine (NLM) Medline bibliographic database,
which stores information about individual citations including index terms
used to characterize each article (articles are indexed according to a dictio-
nary of medical subject headings called MESH terms).

The volume of breast cancer-related psychology research articles appears to have almost tripled from 1990 to 2000 (from 150 to 431 citations),
but throughout the period such articles represent a small fraction of breast
cancer-related research, less than 7 percent according to Medline searches
(Figures 8-1 and 8-2). These trends reflect publications in English, but not
limited to articles written by United States investigators. Figures 8-1 and 8-
2 therefore reflect trends in the general medical literature, not necessarily
trends in the United States. These trends must be interpreted with caution
because they may reflect changes in the way MESH headings are applied to
index the literature rather than real increases in breast cancer-related psychological research.

Research Support

A more direct way to assess the status of United States-based breast
cancer-related psychosocial research is to describe topics of investigation
and levels of research spending. There is no one comprehensive source of
information on research support; as part of its review, the Board relied on
the following sources:

• Listings of research projects provided by some organizations (e.g.,
National Cancer Institute);
• The federal listing of research projects (CRISP);
• Review of agency web sites (e.g., Department of Defense); and

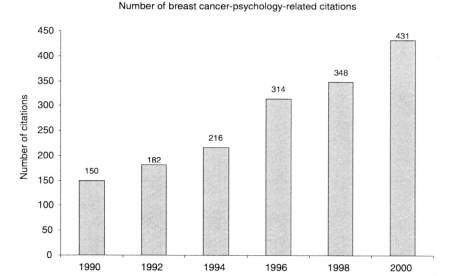

Number of breast cancer-psychology-related citations

FIGURE 8-1 PubMed citations for breast cancer psychological research, 1990–2000. Citations were identified in the National Library of Medicines's PubMed database using the MESH term "breast neoplasms," and the MESH subheading "psychology." Only articles published in English are counted.

- Informal contacts with agency representatives known to be involved in research (e.g., foundations).

Despite the best efforts of the Board, the description of the nation's breast cancer-related psychosocial research portfolio that follows may under- or overestimate the actual level of research. Some research activities may have been missed because of limitations of research tracking systems. The review is limited to currently active research projects for most organizations.

Federally Sponsored Research

National Cancer Institute, Office of Cancer Survivorship

The main locus of cancer-related psychosocial research support within the Department of Health and Human Services (DHHS) is the National Cancer Institute (NCI). Table 8-1 describes the NCI's overall budget request for 2004, which includes $46 million for cancer survivorship research as detailed in Table 8-2 (0.7 percent of the total FY 2004 budget request). Cancer survi-

Percent of breast cancer-related citations pertaining to psychology

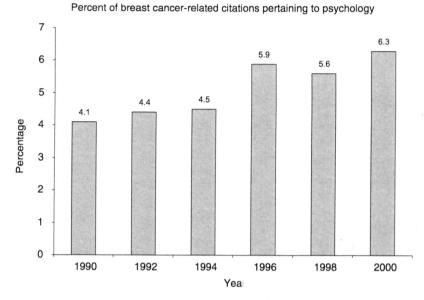

FIGURE 8-2 PubMed citations for psychology related breast cancer research as a percentage of all breast cancer-related research, 1990–2000. Percentages were calculated as the number of psychology-related breast cancer citations (as described in Figure 8-1) divided by the number of citations categorized under the MESH term "breast neoplasms." Only articles published in English are counted.

vorship research has been designated by NCI as an "Extraordinary Opportunity for Investment." A research initiative focused on long-term survivors was announced in 2003, providing $20 million to support awards for studies of individuals who are five years or more beyond cancer diagnosis (http://grants1.nih.gov/grants/guide/rfa-files/RFA-CA-04-003.html, accessed April 14, 2003).

NCI's work on survivorship is administered through its Office of Cancer Survivorship (OCS), which was established in 1996 to promote research and to provide information to cancer patients, their families, health-care providers, advocates, and the research community (http://dccps.nci.nih.gov/ocs/, accessed April 18, 2003). OCS grants relating to breast cancer are shown in Table 8-3. About half of these are on psychosocial or quality of life subjects.

National Cancer Institute, Office of Behavioral Research

Psychosocial research is also supported through the NCI's Office of Behavioral Research (BRP). Research supported in this office ranges from

TABLE 8-1 NCI's Budget Request for Fiscal Year 2004 (in thousands)

Fiscal Year 2003 President's Budget	$ 4,637,869
Increase to core budget	294,014
Capacity building increase	
Enhancing investigator-initiated research	69,887
Expanding the capacity of centers, networks, and consortia	79,530
National clinical trials program in treatment and prevention	340,100
Developing bioinformatics for cancer research	88,000
Subtotal capacity building	577,517
Discovery and application increase	
Genes and the environment	51,800
Signatures of the cancer cell and its microenvironment	41,200
Molecular targets of prevention and treatment	54,800
Cancer imaging and molecular sensing	78,700
Cancer communications	39,750
Subtotal discovery and application	266,250
Public health emphasis increase	
Improving the quality of cancer care	27,000
Reducing cancer-related health disparities	61,350
Cancer survivorship	46,000
Research on tobacco and tobacco-related cancers	76,000
Subtotal public-health emphasis	210,350
Total FY 2004 budget request	5,986,000

SOURCE: The Nation's Investment in Cancer Research: A Plan and Budget Proposal for Fiscal Year 2004, Prepared by the Director of the National Cancer Institute.

basic behavioral research to research on the development, testing and dissemination of disease prevention and health promotion interventions in areas such as tobacco use, screening, dietary behavior and sun protection. The BRP programs support five areas (http://www.dccps.nci.nih.gov/brp/index.html):

• *Applied Cancer Screening Research.* Facilitates and supports effectiveness trials and related social and behavioral research to promote the use of effective cancer screening tests, as well as strategies for informed decision making regarding all cancer screening technologies, in both community and clinical practice.

• *Basic Biobehavioral Research.* To serve as a national model for promoting, sponsoring, and supporting basic biobehavioral research and training.

• *Health Communication and Informatics Research.* To advance communication and information science across the cancer continuum—prevention, detection, treatment, control, survivorship, and end of life. Communication and information science systematically examines the fundamental processes and effects of human and mediated communication.

• *Health Promotion Research.* Coordinates research on non-tobacco behavioral prevention of cancer in the areas of diet, physical activity, en-

TABLE 8-2 Cancer Survivorship Component of NCI's Budget Request for Fiscal Year 2004 (in millions)

Research – biological, physical, psychological, and social response to disease, treatment and recovery	$9.50
Physiologic and psychosocial effects on post-treatment survivors	3.00
Late effects case studies	5.00
Socio-cultural, behavioral, emotional, and spiritual factors	1.50
Intervention research – to reduce cancer-related late morbidity and mortality	12.00
Research of cost-effective medical, educational, and psychosocial interventions	9.00
Development of interventions for families, minorities, and medically underserved	3.00
Development of assessment tools for quality of life and post-treatment care	5.50
New instruments for quality of life assessment (e.g., toxicity criteria for late effects)	2.00
Screening tools for high risk physical, psychosocial, or behavioral outcomes	2.00
Use of applied/theoretical statistics to establish criteria for clinically significant changes	0.50
Collaboration with other NIH institutes to develop measures to evaluate co-morbidities	1.00
Enhance NCI's capacity to track outcomes for cancer survivors	5.50
Expansion of data collection on health-related outcomes for survivors in SEER registries	1.00
Development of infrastructure for clinical trials groups to follow patients long-term	2.00
Establishment of separate registry for pediatric cancer survivors	2.50
Development and dissemination of new interventions and best practice guidelines	3.50
Best practice guidelines for follow-up care and surveillance for survivors	1.25
Support studies to test adoption and impact of best practices in post-treatment care	1.50
Develop/disseminate curricula and standards for delivery of effective psychosocial care	0.75
Expansion of scientific base for understanding the biologic mechanisms in adverse late effects	9.00
Funding of pre-clinical studies examining incidence/mechanism of late effects treatment	3.00
Support research that seeks to investigate the neuropsychologic impact of cancer therapy	6.00
Management and support	1.00
Total	46.00

SOURCE: The Nation's Investment in Cancer Research: A Plan and Budget Proposal for Fiscal Year 2004, Prepared by the Director of the National Cancer Institute.

ergy balance, virus exposure, and sun exposure.

• *Tobacco Control Research.* To reduce cancer incidence and mortality caused by tobacco use through a comprehensive research program. To provide recommendations to the scientific and public health communities by synthesizing and disseminating research findings.

A selection of some of the grants from this office that have focused on psychosocial research is displayed in Table 8-4.

TABLE 8-3 Selected Current Breast Cancer-related Survivorship Research, Office of Cancer Survivorship, NCI

- Facilitating positive adaptation to breast cancer
- Center for psycho-oncology research
- Breast cancer survivors, physical activity, and quality of life
- Bone marrow transplant (BMT) survivors study
- Young breast cancer survivors—population based cohort
- Quality of life in adult cancer survivors
- Menopausal symptom relief for women with breast cancer
- Breast cancer and function in aging women
- Quality of life of older long-term cancer survivors
- Quality of life intervention in breast cancer survivors
- Insomnia intervention for breast cancer survivors
- Psychological well being in long-term cancer survivors
- African American breast cancer survivor quality of life
- Characteristics of long-term breast cancer survivors
- Adjustment to breast cancer
- Home-based moderate exercise for breast cancer patients
- The economic consequences of cancer survival
- Breast cancer treatment outcomes in older women
- Psychosocial treatment effects on cancer survival
- Return to work in cancer survivors: A pilot study
- Enhancing long-term survival after BMT
- Biobehavioral and supportive needs during high dose TMT
- Enhancing recovery from blood and marrow transplantation
- Cognitive effects of breast cancer treatment
- Impact of maternal breast cancer on children
- Quality of life and relationships after BMT

SOURCE: http://dccps.nci.nih.gov/ocs/portfolio.asp, accessed April 18, 2003.

Department of Defense

Beginning in FY 1992, the U.S. Congress directed the Department of Defense (DoD) to manage several appropriations for an extramural grant program directed toward specific research initiatives. The United States Army Medical Research and Materiel Command (USAMRMC) established the office of the Congressionally Directed Medical Research Programs (CDMRP) to administer these funds. Between FY 1992 and 2003, $1.37 billion has been appropriated by Congress to DoD for research on breast cancer. In addition, $7.0 million was generated in sales of the U.S. Postal Service's first-class stamp (Public Law 105-41, Stamp Out Breast Cancer Act [H.R. 1585]). The CDMRP strives to identify gaps in funding and provide award opportunities that will enhance program research objectives without duplicating existing funding opportunities.

TABLE 8-4 Selected Grants from NCI's Office of Behavioral Research, FY 2001 and 2002[1]

Project Title
Fatigue, Sleep and Circadian Rhythms in Breast Cancer
Psychological Intervention for Women with Breast Cancer
The End-of-Life Family Workshop
Pain Assessment via Role-Play Internet Simulation
Health Promotion for Women at Risk for Breast Cancer
Breast Cancer Risk-Tailored Messages for More Women
Self-Advocacy and Empowerment for People with Cancer
We Can Cope—Family Support When A Parent Has Cancer
Vicarious Dissonance, Attitude Change & Identity
Web-Based Support for Informal Caregivers in Cancer
Culturally Targeted Health Information Network
Spiritually-Based Breast Cancer Communication
Cognitive Behavioral Aspects of Cancer Related Fatigue
Breast Cancer Patients Relatives—Response Over Time
Interactive CD-ROM for Coping With Breast Cancer
Quality of Life, Ethnicity, and Breast Cancer Survivors
Hormones, Quality of Life & Breast Cancer Support Groups

[1]The list contains grants carried over from prior fiscal years (FY 2001 and prior) and new grants awarded in FY 2002.
SOURCE: NCI website, accessed on 2/27/03: http://dccps.nci.nih.gov/brp/research.asp.

The Breast Cancer Research Program (BCRP) has sponsored over 2,800 awards for peer-reviewed breast cancer research at the community, state, and national level (Table 8-4). The BCRP divides the awards into three categories:

1. research (basic and clinical),
2. infrastructure, and
3. training and recruitment.

In addition, an Innovator Award was initiated in FY01 that grants $5 million to individuals engaged in "visionary research." Within the BCRP, psychosocial research awards fall within the category of "Biobehavioral Sciences." A total of 35 of the 105 biobehavioral awards of the BCRP pertain to psychosocial issues (Table 8-5).

TABLE 8-5 BCRP Study Awards with Psychosocial Component

Name of Research Study	Institution	$ Amount	Fiscal Year
Evaluation of a Peer-Staffed Hotline for Families who Received Genetic Testing for Risk of Breast Cancer	Univ. of Pennsylvania	$79,250.00	2000
Assisting Survivors in Meeting Challenges at end of Treatment: A Problem Solving Approach	Univ. of Pennsylvania	$79,250.00	2000
Hatha Yoga and Breast Cancer: Integrating a Mind/Body Intervention During Adjuvant Chemotherapy	Columbia Univ.	$81,725.00	2000
A Longitudinal Study of Emotional Distress and the Use of Complementary Alternative Medicine in Women with Breast Cancer	Univ. of Hawaii	$66,000.00	2000
Breast Cancer Protective Behaviors among Low-income, Ethnically Diverse Women: The Role of Biopsychosocial. Factors	Florida State Univ.	$22,000.00	2000
Spirituality-Based Intervention for African American Women with Breast Cancer	Wayne State Univ.	$334,599.00	1999
Interdisciplinary Research Training in Breast Cancer	Yale Univ.	$749,432.00	1999
Medical Decision-Making about Breast Cancer among African Americans: Evaluating the Roles of Beliefs, Knowledge, Medical Care Access, and Social Support	Univ. of Texas at Houston	$73,513.00	1999
Internet Support and Information for Women with Breast Cancer	Univ. of Alabama at Birmingham	$61,519.00	1999
Stress and Immunity Breast Cancer Project	Ohio State Univ.	$808,568.00	1998
Identifying Quality of Life and Psychosocial Risk Factors and Their Sociocultural Mediators in African American, Filipino, Latino, and White Breast Cancer Survivors	UCLA	$761,421.00	1998
Postdoctoral Training Program in Biobehavioral Breast Cancer Research	Mount-Sinai (NY)	$782,413.00	1998
Psychological Distress, Cognitive Bias, and Breast Cancer Surveillance Behavior in Women Tested for BRCA1/2 Mutation	Mount Sinai (NY)	$125,737.00	1998
The Effect of Emotional Disclosure Interventions on Psychological and Physical Well-Being of Breast Cancer Patients	Virginia Commonwealth University	$44,622.00	1998

(continued)

TABLE 8-5 *(Continued)*

Name of Research Study	Institution	$ Amount	Fiscal Year
The Development and Evaluation of an Innovative Internet-Based Breast Cancer Psychosocial Intervention	Stanford Univ.	$327,015.00	1998
Inherited Susceptibility to Breast Cancer in Healthy Women: Mutations in Breast Cancer Genes, Immune Surveillance and Psychological Distress	Sloan-Kettering	$481,210.00	1997
Psycho-Endocrine-Immune Profile: Implications for Quality of Life in Breast Cancer Patients	Loyola University - Chicago	$325,626.00	1997
Development of an Integrated Program of Health related Quality of Life Research for the National Surgical Adjuvant Breast and Bowel Project (NSABP).	Univ. of Pittsburgh	$227,876.00	1996
Social Support and Endocrine Function: A Randomized Trial with Breast Cancer Patients	Ohio State Univ.	$82,932.00	1996
Preventive Psychosocial Intervention for Young Women with Breast Cancer	Univ. of Pittsburgh	$292,243.00	1996
Stress and Coping in Genetic Testing for Cancer Risk	Univ. of Michigan	$837,296.00	1995
Effects of Psychosocial Intervention in Women Following Breast Cancer Diagnosis	Univ. of Rochester	$149,991.00	1995
Delays and Refusals in Treatment for Breast Cancer among Native American and Hispanic Women with Breast Cancer	Univ. of New Mexico	$72,043.00	1995
Psychobehavioral Impact of Genetic Counseling and Breast Cancer Gene Testing in Healthy Women of African Descent	Sloan-Kettering	$579,581.00	1995
Psychological Intervention for Women with Breast Cancer	Ohio State Univ.	$86,896.00	1993 & 94
Enhancing Positive Reactions to Breast Cancer Risk Appraisal	Hutchinson Cancer Center	$597,673.00	1993 & 94
The Effects of a Comprehensive Coping Strategy on Clinical Outcomes in Breast Cancer Bone Marrow Transplant Patients and Primary Caregiver	Johns Hopkins Univ.	$783,572.00	1993 & 94

Effects of Meditation-Based Stress Reduction in Younger Women with Breast Cancer	Univ. of Massachusetts	$799,843.00	1993 & 94
Psycho Educational Group Intervention for Women at Increased Risk for Breast Cancer	Strang Cancer Center	$799,837.00	1993 & 94
The Effects of Brief Psychotherapy on Coping with Breast Cancer	North Dakota State Univ.	$143,510.00	1993 & 94
Incidence and Psychophysiology of Post-Traumatic Stress Disorder in Breast Cancer Victims and Witnesses	Harvard Univ.	$724,375.00	1993 & 94
Knowledge and Beliefs of Breast Cancer Among Elderly Puerto Rican Women	Univ. of Puerto Rico	$771,159.00	1993 & 94
An Evaluation of A Peer Support Program to Improve Quality of Life With Breast Cancer	Kaiser Foundation	$595,732.00	1993 & 94
Emotional Processing and Expression in Breast Cancer Patients: Effects on Health and Psychological Adjustment	Univ. of Kansas	$145,839.00	1993 & 94
A Community Study of Psychological Distress and Immune Function in Women with Family Histories of Breast Cancer	Sloan-Kettering	$200,000.00	1993 & 94

SOURCE: Department of Defense Breast Cancer Research Program: Search Awards Database, http:Hcdmrp.army.mil/cgi-bin/search/search-bcrp.pi, accessed November 21, 2002.

Privately Funded Research

Private philanthropic organizations have been major sponsors of breast cancer research. This section of the report reviews the research activity of the American Cancer Society, the Avon Foundation, the Susan G. Koman Foundation, and the Bristol Myers Squibb Foundation.

American Cancer Society

The American Cancer Society (ACS) is the largest non-government funder of cancer research in the United States and supports psychosocial and behavioral research. In FY 2001–2002, approximately 20 percent of the total research program was devoted to these areas (see Table 8-6).

The ACS intramural research program includes a Behavioral Research Center which is conducting two large population-based surveys of cancer survivors at a cost of $2 million for the pilot phases. The first is the "Study of Cancer Survivors-Incidence." This survey of up to 100,000 cancer survivors is underway in a pilot phase and is designed as a 10-year prospective study of survivors enrolled within the first year after diagnosis of any one of

TABLE 8-6 ACS Extramural and Intramural Funding in Selected Priority Areas*: FY 2001-2002 (in thousands)

Area of Research	$ Awarded
Total	102,415
Prevention	13,648
Nutrition	4,013
Tobacco control	3,141
Other prevention	6,494
Detection	6,051
Treatment	22,849
Psychosocial and behavioral	20,471
Poor and underserved	10,780
Childhood cancer	4,257
Environmental carcinogenesis	909
Epidemiology	6,112
Cause/etiology	36,637
Major organ sites	
Breast	27,312
Leukemia	14,000
Colon/rectum	14,990
Lung	12,711
Lymphoma	5,534
Prostate	8,071
Ovary	5,108
Melanoma	4,679
Pancreas	7,845
Brain/nervous system	2,165

*Not mutually exclusive categories: e.g., a grant that is both prevention and detection is counted twice, as is a grant that studies both breast and prostate cancers. A grant emphasizing nutrition in breast and prostate cancer is counted in full in all three places. Dollar amounts are rounded off to the nearest $1,000.
SOURCE: American Cancer Society http://www.cancer.org/docroot/RES/content/ RES_7_3_Funding_By_Research_Area.asp, accessed May 1, 2003

the ten most common cancers (i.e., prostate, female breast, lung, colorectal, urinary bladder, non-Hodgkin's lymphoma, skin melanoma, uterine, kidney, ovarian). A population-based sample is being selected from area cancer registries in sufficient numbers to provide state-level estimates. The major aim of the survey is to examine the behavioral, psychosocial, treatment, and support factors that influence quality of life and survival of cancer patients. The survey includes a number of measures related to psychosocial well-being including problems in daily living, physical and mental health functioning, and problems with work.

The second survey is the "Study of Long-Term Cancer Survivors-Prevalence." This survey is a cross-sectional study of 6,000 long-term survivors (i.e., those who are 5, 10, 15 years beyond diagnosis) of six cancers (prostate, breast, colorectal, bladder, melanoma, uterine). There will be 1,000 respondents for each type of cancer.

The ACS is also conducting surveys of cancer survivors and oncology providers regarding complementary therapies (e.g., acupuncture, visualization, yoga) to determine their extent of use among people with cancer and providers attitudes toward them.

Avon Foundation

Avon Products, Inc., a manufacturer of cosmetics, founded the Avon Breast Cancer Crusade in 1993 to support breast cancer research and to improve access to care, especially among medically underserved women. With $250 million raised since its inception, the program supports programs for breast cancer in the United States and in 50 countries around the world. Originally designed to provide education, screening, and breast exam services to the underserved community, Avon expanded the crusade in 2000 by funding:

- Community outreach and referral programs.
- Support services for breast cancer patients and survivors, including financial assistance for biopsies for uninsured women, counseling, transportation, and childcare
- Educational seminars that teach the "science" of breast cancer and methods of effective advocacy.
- Medical research on breast cancer.

Selected programs that support psychosocial care are shown in Table 8-7.

Avon also collaborates with the National Cancer Institute "Progress for Patients" award program. The purpose of the program is to accelerate and expand translational research in breast cancer. Funding goes directly to United States scientists who compete for the awards. Avon Foundation dollars support direct costs of early phase breast cancer clinical trials and other studies in prevention, diagnosis, and treatment, including studies focusing on the needs of minority and other medically underserved patients. The NCI supports other costs of managing the program and the peer review process.

The Susan G. Komen Breast Cancer Foundation

The Susan G. Komen Breast Cancer Foundation is one of the nation's largest private funders of breast cancer research, awarding more than 700 grants totaling $90 million since its inception in 1982. The Komen

TABLE 8-7 Selected Programs Supported by the Avon Breast Cancer Crusade

Program	Amount awarded through October 2002 (in millions)
Avon Foundation Comprehensive Breast Evaluation Center, Massachusetts General Hospital. • Funding brings the hospital's leading edge breast cancer screening, diagnostic, and research capabilities to one location; it also supports a high risk breast evaluation center, new research projects in breast cancer genetics and biology, expands ongoing research and enhances access to clinical care and breast cancer treatment for women in community-based health care centers.	$12.2
Cancer Care, Inc. (NY) • New York City-based Cancer Care has established the national "AVONCares" Program for Medically Underserved Women, which provides financial assistance for breast cancer clinical diagnostic services; transportation and an escort to and from treatment and diagnostic workups; and elder- or childcare while undergoing breast cancer treatment or diagnostics. Women assisted by the "AVONCares" program are able to receive Cancer Care's other services, including professional counseling, education and information, breast prostheses and wigs.	$11.2
National Breast Cancer Coalition • Support to develop leadership skills among cancer advocates and to develop *A Guidebook to Quality Breast Cancer Care*: a consumer guide that helps women define quality breast care and secure access to evidence-based and patient-centered treatment and care.	4.0
Y-Me National Breast Cancer Organization (US) • Funds support expansion of the Y-Me support of Latino, Chinese and Vietnamese women. The programs educate these underserved women and link them directly to screening; assist women who have abnormal screening results in obtaining proper follow-up care; provide translation services; expand the Y-Me husband/partner hotline; and expand the Y-Me teen program, which trains high school seniors in early detection and encourages them to educate their families and neighbors.	2.5
The Cleveland Clinic (OH) • Funds support community outreach and care for the underserved and improved clinical facilities in the Women's Health Pavilion.	2.1

Food & Friends (DC)	1.0

- Organization runs a delivery service of meals and groceries to women with breast cancer to ensure that women suffering from breast cancer, along with their families, have access to better nutrition, reduced stress and improved outlook. The program also provides nutritional education and counseling. The Avon funding will cover delivery of more than 1,500 meals a week to women referred by numerous community partners and construction of the Avon Foundation Kitchen at the organizations' new facility opening October 2003.

"Rise Sister Rise'" of Breast Cancer Resource Committee (DC) .7

- National implementation of a model support group program for African-American women recovering from breast cancer.

Inova Health System Foundation/Fairfax Hospital (VA) .6

- Funds support maximizing relationship between the Women's Center and Fairfax Hospital Cancer Center, focusing on Asian and Hispanic women who are medically underserved. Women are taught to understand early detection, risk reduction, how to obtain access to clinical screening, diagnostic and treatment services, including clinical trials.

Boston Medical Center (MA) .5

- Funds support a comprehensive breast cancer screening and diagnostic program targeted to women challenged by language, cultural and economic barriers. The Women's Health Group at BMC launched the Avon Foundation Breast Health Initiative linking clinicians, outreach/inreach workers, advocates, and researchers in order to better serve women in poor, urban communities, thereby improving the rate of undetected breast cancer and overall health outcomes.

Stroger Hospital of Cook County/Hektoen Institute for Medical .5
Research (IL)

- Funds bring state-of-the-art quality breast oncology care to minority-underserved populations in their own communities through participation in NCI-approved clinical trials that specifically recruit for minority participation; extend and promote these research opportunities with emphasis on the particular needs of the community served, promoting outreach and education; focus on prevention and control as methods for reducing breast cancer incidence, morbidity and mortality, with special emphasis on involvement and education of patient advocacy groups, women's support groups, and primary care physicians.

Karmanos Cancer Institute (MI) .5

- Funds support three related projects: the Community Resource Liaison Project, designed to make clinical trials more readily available to underserved women; the Mobile Detection Center, which will travel around Michigan throughout the year, increasing access for mammography screening; and the Image Checker, which converts film screen to digital images and identifies areas of suspicion.

(continued)

TABLE 8-7 *(Continued)*

Program	Amount awarded through October 2002 (in millions)
Univ. of Miami/Sylvester Cancer Center (FL) • Funds are enhancing the infrastructure of the breast clinic at Jackson Memorial Hospital, a public hospital that serves the poor in Miami, in particular, women born in Latin America and the Caribbean and African Americans.	.5
Moores Univ. of Calif. At San Diego Cancer Center (CA) • Funds enable the Cancer Center to expand its efforts to build on existing programs in community outreach, clinical cancer genetics, diet intervention and state of the art breast care with underserved populations.	.5
Univ. of Texas Southwestern Medical Center/Parkland Hospital (TX) • Funding supports the Avon Foundation Breast Cancer Program, focusing on facilitating easier access to care and clinical trials for the medically underserved, and identifying and monitoring women in populations at greater risk for breast cancer.	.5

SOURCE: Accessed from Avon website at www.avoncompany.com/women/avoncrusade/services/beneficiaries_factsheet.shtml), accessed Feruary 20, 2003.

Foundation's Research Program is funded by 25 percent of all funds raised by Komen affiliates and Komen Race for the Cure events across the United States, as well as by certain private and corporate donations.

In addition to research programs, Komen Affiliates throughout the United States fund community-based breast health education and breast cancer screening and treatment projects (STEP) for the medically underserved. In order to ensure that they are funding programs that address the specific unmet breast health needs of their communities, Komen Affiliates work with local medical experts and community leaders to conduct comprehensive community needs assessments. These profiles are then used to establish local grant application and review processes. From 1998 to 2002 $97 million was awarded through the STEP program. Selected psychosocial programs supported through the program are shown in Table 8-8.

A Population Specific Program of the Komen Foundation funds innovative projects studying the prevention and control of breast cancer within certain at risk populations (Table 8-9). The focus of the program is to support research designed to assess and identify unique needs,

TABLE 8-8 Selected Programs Supported through the Susan G. Komen Breast Canceroundation, 2000-2002 Psychosocial STEP Grants and Funding

Grant Program	Institution	Komen Affiliate
Educational Support Program for Women with Breast Cancer	The Wellness Community	South Florida
Outreach Services for Women with Breast Cancer	Center for Hope, Inc.	Greater New York City
Cancer Patient Matching and Support	Cancer Hope Network	North New Jersey
Psychosocial Support for Latino Women with Breast Cancer	The Wellness Community	Los Angeles County
Art and Educational Therapy Pilot Program	. Presbyterian Healthcare Services	Central New Mexico
Complementary Alternative Medicine, Education & Advocacy for Breast Cancer	Charlotte Maxwell Complementary Clinic	San Francisco Bay Area
LatinaSHARE: Medical/Community Outreach and Mentoring Project	SHARE: Self-Help for Women with Breast or Ovarian Cancer, Inc.	Greater New York'City
Psychosocial Support Services for Breast Cancer Patients	The Wellness Community	San Diego
Counseling for Breast Cancer Patients	UNC Lineberger Comprehensive Cancer Center	NC Research Triangle Area
Breast Cancer Education and Support Project	Cancer Care, Inc.	New Jersey Race for the Cure®
Year 2001 Casting for Recovery Retreats	Casting for Recovery	Vermont
A Healing Journey Pre-Operative	St. Mary's Foundation Robert Wood Johnson	Greater Evansville, IL New Jersey Race for the
Education/Complementary Therapy Consultation	University Hospital Foundation	Cure®
Outreach to the Underserved Check It Out	Gilda's Club Nashville St. Louis Chapter of Hadassah	Greater Nashville St. Louis
Breast Cancer in Young Women: Establishing an Outreach and Mentoring Program	Washington University School of Medicine	St. Louis

(continued)

TABLE 8-8 *(Continued)*

Grant Program	Institution	Komen Affiliate
Group Therapy for Newly Diagnosed African American Breast Cancer Patients	Wake Forest University Baptist Medical Center	North Carolina Triad
Psychosocial Support for Latino Women with Breast Cancer	The Wellness Community	Los Angeles County
Support Services for Breast Cancer Patients with a focus on Underserved Populations	The Wellness Community	San Diego
Casting for Recovery 2002,	Casting for Recovery	Vermont
Cancer Patient Matching and Support	Cancer Hope Network	North New Jersey
LatinaSHARE: Medical and Community Outreach and Mentoring Project	SHARE: Self-Help for Women with Breast or Ovarian Cancer, Inc.	Greater New York City
WomensCare Center Breast Health Program	St. Rose Dominican Hospital and St. Rose Dominican Health	Las Vegas
Breast Health Resource Guide	Orange County Breast Cancer Coalition	Orange County
Counseling for Breast Cancer Patients	UNC Lineberger Comprehensive Cancer Center	NC Triangle Area
Support for Life: Women Focused on Recovery	The Wellness Community	Phoenix
Complementary Alternative Medicine, Psychosocial Support, Advocacy, and Education for Low Income Women with Breast Cancer	The Charlotte Maxwell Complementary Clinic	San Francisco Bay Area
WINGS	WINGS	San Antonio
Breast Cancer Registry, Psychosocial Screening, and Improvement of Compliance and Reduction of Distress	Barbara Ann Karmanos Cancer Institute	Detroit Race for the Cure®
Breast Health Education for Nurses Breast Cancer Support and	Intermountain Health Care Cancer Care	Salt Lake City Connecticut
Education Project for Underserved Women		
Education and Psychosocial Support for Women with Breast Cancer	Cancer Wellness Organizations of Metropolitan Chicago Area	Chicago

SOURCE: http://www.komen.org/grants/step/stepresults.asp, accessed February 20, 2003.

RESEARCH 217

TABLE 8-9 The Susan G. Komen Breast Cancer Foundation 2001
Population Specific Grants

Grant	Institution	Amount (in US$)
Health Care Experiences of Lesbians with Breast Cancer	Boston University	$120,638
Variation in Stage at Diagnosis in Breast Cancer Across California: Effects of Race/Ethnicity and Rural/Urban Residence	Public Health Institute	$128,867
Influence of Behavioral Factors on Breast Cancer Risk and Survival	Howard University	$215,168
African American Lesbian Breast Cancer Screening Study	Mautner Project for Lesbians with Cancer	$237,847
Korean American Breast Health Project in Maryland	The Johns Hopkins University	$249,442
Breast Cancer Control: Needs and Practices of African American Women and their Providers	University of Southern Mississippi	$248,483
Genetic Epidemiology of Breast Cancer in African Americans	Wayne State University	$249,493
Impact of Culture on Breast Cancer Screening in Chinese American Women	Georgetown University	$249,998
Project Hoffnung: Delivering Hope with Culturally Appropriate Breast Health to Amish and Mennonite Communities	University of Utah College of Nursing	$249,969
"Comadre A Comadre" A One-on-one Peer Support Project for Hispanic Women with Breast Cancer	University of New Mexico	$250,000
Not Yet Well: the Self Management of Post-treatment Symptoms by Breast Cancer Survivors	University of California, Los Angeles	$248,183

(continued)

TABLE 8-9 (Continued)

Grant	Institution	Amount (in US$)
The Helping Path, Four Directions: A California Indian Breast Cancer Education	University of California, Los Angeles	$247,065
Lay Health Advisors to Promote Breast Cancer Screening Among Asian Americans	University of Michigan	$250,000
	Total	$2,945,153

SOURCE: Accessed from website: http:Hwww.komen.org/grants/awards/O I awards.asp?id=1, accessed February 20, 2003.

trends, barriers and solutions to breast health care among populations such as African American, Asian American, Native Hawaiian and Pacific Islanders, Hispanic/Latina, Native American, Lesbian, Low Literacy, Breast Cancer Survivors, Women with Disabilities, and other defined communities. Areas of interest include cancer prevention and control, behavioral science research, epidemiology, and health service delivery programs. Komen gives preference to applicants who demonstrate collaboration with a community-based organization. This program offers funding of up to $250,000 (combined direct and indirect costs) over a 2- or 3-year period.

Bristol Meyers Squibb Foundation

The Bristol Meyers Squibb Foundation has sponsored a demonstration project (currently in its second phase) to bring more psychosocial services to patients and their families at a local level. A second goal is to test the feasibility of training master's level counseling psychologists in psychosocial oncology in order to increase the cadres of professionals available to patients in smaller communities.

To date, 150 psychologists in Florida have been given face to face and online training in psychosocial counseling in oncology. A current plan is to explore the development of this group further in an effort between the American Psychosocial Oncology Society (APOS) and the Bristol Meyers Squibb Foundation in which APOS will provide a core online curriculum and an examination to those who wish to add qualifications in psychosocial oncology. Counselors in Employment Assistance Programs and family service organizations, already trained in counseling should be rather easily trained in psychosocial issues in oncology. If so, the demonstration will have been able to increase the number of psychosocial oncology counselors with a wider geographic distribution who can be reached through the APOS Referral Directory and toll-free number, along with the traditional psychosocial oncology professionals (www.apos-society.org; 1-866-APOS-4-HELP).

SUGGESTIONS FOR FUTURE RESEARCH PRIORITIES

Relative to other areas of research in breast cancer, psycho-oncology is still in its infancy. Just over 20 years have elapsed since the first randomized psycho-oncology trial in breast cancer was reported by Maguire in 1980 (Maguire et al., 1983), and for this report Goodwin was able to find and review a total of 31 randomized trials in women with breast cancer in the literature (see Chapter 5). These trials cover a broad spectrum of interventions (relaxation/hypnosis with or without imagery, group interventions involving structured or unstructured groups, supportive–expressive therapy, cognitive–behavioral therapy, mind–body–spirit interventions, psycho-educational interventions and/or peer discussion, as well as individual interventions involving telephone counseling, specialized nursing interventions, cognitive–behavioral therapy and problem-solving skills training). The reported trials have enrolled from 24 to 312 women, and the interventions evaluated have ranged from 75 minutes to lifelong. Some general conclusions can be drawn regarding the effectiveness of these psychosocial interventions in breast cancer. For example, there is fairly consistent evidence that relaxation/hypnosis/imagery interventions are beneficial in a variety of acute care settings, particularly in the short-term. Furthermore, there is growing evidence of the efficacy of a variety of group and individual interventions, using different strategies for different periods of time at different points along the breast cancer trajectory.

Despite this, many unresolved questions remain which should be the focus of future research activities. Based on discussions at its workshop, the analysis of Goodwin in her commissioned paper, and its own deliberations reviewing the trials presented and analyzed in Chapter 5, the Board was able to formulate some suggestions for areas of needed research and priorities. Along with some brief comments on the relevance of psychosocial research in other than breast cancer and on indexing, coordination, and collaboration issues, these suggestions are discussed below. The Board believes that much of value can be learned building on the base of the existing trials.

Determining Relative Benefits of Different Interventions

Most of the reported randomized trials have compared an active intervention to a no-treatment control group, an attention control group, or a control group that passively received educational materials. Few have compared different active interventions. As a result, there is little information available regarding whether one intervention is better than others and, if so, whether such interventions are more effective in all settings, and with all types of patients, or whether specific interventions are more effective with specific groups of patients. With some types of interventions, such as relaxation/imagery, the approach to the intervention does not appear to be as important as the fact that the intervention was delivered. In other types of interventions, for example, individual interventions, the specific approach appears to be critical in determining benefits of the intervention. Furthermore, although there is early evidence that group interventions (of a variety of types) are beneficial in both early stage and advanced breast cancer, it is unclear whether one type of group intervention is better than others, what the optimal duration of such intervention should be, whether the type or duration of the intervention should be tailored to individual patient characteristics or phase of illness, and, if that is the case, what those characteristics are. Existing research suggests that the psychological profile of the patient may be one such characteristic (Goodwin et al., 2001; Hosaka et al., 2000a, 2001b, 2000b, 2000c).

Additional research to directly compare different interventions that have been shown to be effective in breast cancer (e.g., expressive–supportive group therapy versus cognitive–behavioral group therapy) is important in order to determine the relative effectiveness of these interventions overall and in subgroups of interest (e.g., distressed versus non-distressed). Ideally, this research should be conducted in early stage and advanced breast cancer separately as it is possible that effects may differ. Similarly, group interventions should be compared to individual interventions and efforts made to identify the benefits of different components of the more complex interventions (e.g., the contribution of relaxation and imagery to a cognitive–behavioral intervention). In this comparative research, outcome measures should be selected that target attributes likely to be influenced by the intervention (e.g., psychological status—mood, traumatic stress symptoms, coping—as well as overall quality of life, patient satisfaction, and cost-effectiveness). Given the current evidence of a variety of benefits of psychosocial interventions in breast cancer, the use of no-treatment control arms may become increasing difficult for ethical reasons; this will enhance the likelihood of comparative research in future.

Determining Optimal Timing and Duration of Psychosocial Interventions

In general, randomized trials of relaxation/hypnosis have tended to involve short interventions (one session to 6 months), whereas interventions in early stage breast cancer have been somewhat longer (4 weeks to 3 or 4 months), and interventions in women with metastases have been the longest (6 months to the end of life). However, none of the randomized trials to date has evaluated the effect of duration of the intervention on the magnitude and persistence of psychosocial benefits or on cost-effectiveness. Randomized trials to evaluate the optimal duration of intervention will be important, and these trials should be conducted separately in early stage and late stage breast cancer, as it appears likely the optimal duration of the intervention differs according to the disease stage. Within each phase of illness, research is also needed to identify the optimal timing of psychosocial interventions.

Identifying Patient Characteristics Associated with Intervention Benefits

A number of the published trials have suggested that psychological benefits vary according to patient characteristics. For example, Goodwin et al. found that psychological benefits of supportive–expressive therapy in metastatic breast cancer were limited to women who were distressed at the time the intervention began (Goodwin et al., 2001). Similar differential effects in subgroups of women have been reported by others, although there is little evidence that predictors of benefit are consistent across studies (Hosaka et al., 2000c, 2001a, 2001b, 2000b). Many of the predictors will likely be psychosocial in nature (e.g., presence of acute distress, underlying psychosocial illness or adjustment disorder, personality traits, social and family support). However, some may involve demographic characteristics (e.g., age, social status) or medical factors. For example, relaxation/imagery has been shown to be effective in early-stage breast cancer, but the single trial in women with metastases yielded no benefit (Arathuzik, 1994).

Although these results should not be interpreted as proof of benefit only in early disease, they point to the need for more formal evaluation in the metastatic setting. Because it is possible that some women may benefit more from certain interventions and, indeed, that certain interventions may benefit certain types of women to a greater extent than others, research is desirable to further examine the patient characteristics that are predictive of greatest benefit of psychosocial interventions in breast cancer. Some of this research might involve re-analysis of existing trials, but it is likely that new trials will also be necessary. One of the goals of this research should be to determine whether some women do not require psychosocial intervention, in the same way that some women do not require adjuvant chemotherapy.

Understanding the Role of Nursing Interventions

A considerable number of randomized trials, predominantly in early stage breast cancer, have evaluated nursing interventions. There is some evidence of benefit for these nursing interventions. However, these studies all evaluated different interventions, some used small sample sizes, and some of the studies had significant methodologic limitations. Because nurses are so intimately involved in the care of breast cancer patients, better understanding is needed of the precise benefits of specialized nursing interventions on the psychosocial status of women with breast cancer and how these interventions are best integrated into a more comprehensive psychosocial intervention program.

Evaluating Peer Support/Peer Discussion Groups

Peer support groups have gained widespread acceptance among women with breast cancer. However, there is little clear evidence of benefit, and the single randomized trial that evaluated facilitated peer discussion failed to identify any psychological benefits (Helgeson et al., 2000, 1999). Although many testimonials exist as to the benefits of individual peer support (Cella and Yellen, 1993), formal evaluation of the benefit of this support is lacking. Given the nature and widespread availability of peer support, the use of randomized designs may be challenging; however, evaluation using the strongest methodology possible is needed.

Evaluating Novel Interventions

There is growing interest among breast cancer patients and their families in the potential benefits of non-traditional, complementary and alternative medicine approaches to psychosocial support. These approaches include Internet chat groups and peer support groups, as well as a variety of non-traditional therapies, many of which focus on helping patients distract themselves from their breast cancer experience or turn their focus to other areas of their lives. Such interventions include yoga, reflexology, reiki, t'ai chi, music therapy, and art therapy. Because these interventions are of great interest to patients, and because they are often pursued by patients with little evidence of benefit apart from anecdotal testimonials, formal evaluation of their benefit in the setting of randomized trials would be useful. Such trials could include wait list control groups if resistance to randomization is encountered. The importance of research in this area is highlighted by the observations of Targ and Levine that a complex mind–body–spirit group intervention was at least equivalent to a standard psychoeducational support group intervention and that it led to enhanced satisfaction, fewer dropouts, and greater spiritual integration.

Addressing the Needs of Breast Cancer Survivors

Only one randomized trial of a purely psychosocial intervention was conducted in breast cancer survivors, and it did not address the psychosocial needs of breast cancer survivors (Fogarty et al., 1999). Instead, it used them as a convenience sample to evaluate the benefits of an enhanced compassion videotape. Research into survivorship issues is just beginning, but it is an important area involving millions of people. This research should be facilitated, and, as problems are identified, targeted interventions should be developed and tested to address the unique needs of this large population.

Addressing Family Issues

Only a small number of the randomized trials reported to date have involved partners or family members of breast cancer patients. Yet it is widely recognized that these individuals are often greatly affected by the illness of the breast cancer patient and that they may suffer significant emotional distress that may continue long after the breast cancer patient dies. The Board believes that research should be pursued to identify the psychosocial needs of this population and to develop interventions to ameliorate their psychological distress.

Addressing Cultural/Minority Issues

None of the randomized trials in the United States addressed cultural and/or minority issues. Although there is some evidence from some countries outside of the United States that psychosocial interventions may have similar effects in different cultures, the influence of cultural and/or minority background requires further investigation (Fukui et al., 2000; Hosaka et al., 2000a, 2001a, 2001b, 2000b, 2000c). Specifically, descriptive research should be carried out to examine the unique needs of different cultures and/ or minority groups, followed by development of interventions that target these unique needs.

Developing Appropriate Measures of Psychosocial Outcomes

Many of the randomized trials reported to date have used a fairly consistent group of well studied psychosocial questionnaires, including the Profile of Mood States, the Impact of Events Scale, the Beck Depression Inventory, and the State Trait Anxiety Index. However, many others have used novel instruments, some of which are not well validated or are not well known. Furthermore, the standard psychosocial measurement instruments do not address all of the outcomes that are of interest in psychosocial intervention trials in breast cancer. A critical review is needed to identify domains and attributes that are not well addressed by well characterized questionnaires commonly used in breast cancer psychosocial intervention studies (e.g., cognitive functioning), to identify instruments used in other settings that measure those attributes, and to identify areas where there should be development of new instruments. The importance of different psychosocial outcomes should be prioritized (to the extent possible), and the magnitude of psychosocial benefit that is clinically important should be explored. This research might involve a consensus conference to identify a small number of clearly defined outcomes that could be used across a broad spectrum of trials so that the results of trials are more readily compared, followed by targeted research studies.

Translation of Research Findings to Community Practice

There is considerable evidence of efficacy of some types of psychosocial interventions in breast cancer; however, the extent to which these interventions are used in clinical practice is unclear. Therefore, the current use of psychosocial interventions in breast cancer in academic and private medical practice should be evaluated. This evaluation should address access to, and utilization of, relaxation/hypnosis, peer support, and novel forms of support discussed above as well as more traditional group and individual interventions. An assessment of barriers to more widespread use of psychosocial interventions in breast cancer may be useful. Such barriers include (but are not limited to) cost, patient acceptability, physician acceptability, availability and preferences of psychosocial practitioners, logistical barriers to delivery, and knowledge of (or belief in) the effectiveness of psychosocial interventions. Evaluations are needed of psychosocial interventions implemented in "real world" settings, in which cost and integration into breast care in various community settings are assessed (Redman et al., 2003).

Applicability of Findings from Other Research to Women With Breast Cancer

In addition to the psychosocial research conducted in breast cancer patients reviewed here, there is also a large body of literature describing psychosocial research in other cancer types and in patients with other serious illnesses. The extent to which the results of this research in other settings are generalizable to women with breast cancer is not clear. A critical review of the published literature in other illnesses, focusing predominantly on other cancers, could provide evidence of generalizability, or lack of generalizability, of psychosocial research findings in these other settings to breast cancer.

Tracking Results of Psycho-oncology Studies

Indexing of psycho-oncology studies is inconsistent and may be delayed depending on the journal used. Because these trials may be published in journals related to different disciplines, they are often difficult to find, even in exhaustive literature searches. Encouragement of a more standardized and timely approach to indexing would be helpful. A prospective registry of psychosocial intervention trials would facilitate tracking of ongoing studies and assist in planning of new intervention trials.

These research priorities will be addressed most effectively if the psycho-oncology research community works together to build on the strengths of previous research and to ensure that future research provides clinically meaningful information. Unless there is a compelling reason to study entirely new intervention approaches, the comparative research outlined above should compare two or more therapies that have previously been shown to be effective; the most effective therapy can then be used in subsequent comparative work. Similarly, if one or more patient characteristics are identified as being predictive of benefit in one intervention study, future studies should examine those characteristics (as well as others if desired) in an attempt to replicate the earlier finding and contribute to a body of knowledge regarding predictors of benefit. This approach may be facilitated by more widespread conduct of multicenter trials of psychosocial interventions, a move away from many of the single-center studies that have been reported to date. In order to facilitate this broader type of research, it may be necessary to establish psychosocial intervention research networks, similar to those that exist for evaluation of other breast cancer treatments (chemotherapy, radiation, surgery). These collaborative networks might be "free standing," but the benefits of integrating these networks into already established clinical trials groups should also be explored.

To continue progress in the research base that is necessary for sound development of interventions to address psychosocial, psychiatric, and quality of life issues in breast cancer, the Board recommends:

1. Research sponsors (e.g., NCI, ACS) and professional organizations (e.g., American Society of Clinical Oncology, American College of Surgeons, American Association of Colleges of Nursing, American Psychosocial Oncology Society, American Society of Social Work, American Society for Therapeutic Radiology and Oncology, Oncology Nursing Society) need to support efforts in collaboration with advocacy groups (e.g., National Breast Cancer Coalition; National Alliance of Breast Cancer Organizations) to enhance practice environments to promote coordinated, comprehensive, and compassionate care. Rigorous evaluations are needed of the cost and effectiveness of delivery models that show promise in improving access to psychosocial support services. These might include:

• Collaborative practices in which a psychologist or other mental health provider forms a partnership with an office-based oncology provider to make psychosocial services available within the oncology practice;

- Comprehensive breast cancer centers that generally integrate supportive care into a "one-stop-shopping" model of clinical practice;
- Breast cancer nurse managers who provide case management, education, and supportive care within oncology practices;
- Novel models of psychosocial services, such as ICAN project, in phase 2 demonstration, which utilizes master's level counselors who receive a core curriculum in psychosocial oncology;
- Demonstration projects to test the effectiveness of clinical practice guidelines on the management of psychosocial distress in improving psychosocial outcomes;
- Development of measures of quality of cancer care that pertain to supportive care (including psychosocial services). Measures might include provider assessment of psychosocial concerns, the provision of information regarding community supportive care resources, and satisfaction with care.

In general, investigators working in this field should recognize that studies in the past would in many cases have been stronger if they had been on other than selected patients mostly in tertiary settings, or had not been unblinded, with small sample size, of insufficient power, of short duration, and the like. Future study designs should try to minimize such weaknesses.

2. Research sponsors (e.g., NCI, ACS) should continue to support basic and applied psycho-oncology research. This might include:
- Further development of simple, rapid screening tools for identifying the patient with distress in outpatient offices and training of primary oncology teams in diagnosis of distress that exceeds the "expected" and when referral to supportive services should be made;
- Studies that assess the relative effectiveness of various psychosocial interventions, using population-based patient samples of adequate size, the timing and duration of interventions, and innovative and inexpensive modes of administration (e.g., Internet-based approaches);
- A consensus conference to develop a battery of standard instruments for outcome measures to permit comparison of data from studies carried out by different research groups;
- Organization of a psychosocial clinical trials group in which a network of researchers could address key questions in multicenter studies that would allow access to large, population-based samples;
- Clinical trials of psychosocial interventions that are conducted within routine breast cancer care in which cost and quality of life are outcome measures;
- A registry of ongoing psychosocial research/trials to assist researchers in identifying and tracking new areas of study

3. *The NCI should support a special study to ascertain the use of, and unmet need for, cancer-related supportive care services (including psychosocial services) in the United States. The results of such a study could provide benchmarks against which care can be measured and performance monitored. Such a study would document existing disparities in service use by age, race/ethnicity, geography, and insurance coverage.*

REFERENCES

Arathuzik D. 1994. Effects of cognitive–behavioral strategies on pain in cancer patients. *Cancer Nurs* 17(3):207–214.

Cella DF, Yellen SB. 1993. Cancer support groups: The state of the art. *Cancer Pract* 1(1):56–61.

Classen C, Butler LD, Koopman C, et al. 2001. Supportive–expressive group therapy and distress in patients with metastatic breast cancer: A randomized clinical intervention trial. *Arch Gen Psychiatry* 58(5):494–501.

Fogarty LA, Curbow BA, Wingard JR, et al. 1999. Can 40 seconds of compassion reduce patient anxiety? *J Clin Oncol* 19(17):3793–3794.

Fukui S, Kugaya A, Okamura H, et al. 2000. A psychosocial group intervention for Japanese women with primary breast carcinoma. *Cancer* 89(5):1026–1036.

Goodwin PJ, Leszcz M, Ennis M, et al. 2001. The effect of group psychosocial support on survival in metastatic breast cancer. *N Engl J Med* 345(24):1719–1726.

Helgeson VS, Cohen S, Schulz R, Yasko J. 1999. Education and peer discussion group interventions and adjustment to breast cancer. *Arch Gen Psychiatry* 56(4):340–347.

Helgeson VS, Cohen S, Schulz R, Yasko J. 2000. Group support interventions for women with breast cancer: Who benefits from what? *Health Psychol* 19(2):107–114.

Hosaka T, Sugiyama Y, Hirai K, Okuyama T, Sugawara Y, Nakamura Y. Effects of a modified group intervention with early-stage breast cancer patients. *Gen Hosp Psychiatry.* 2001a;23(3):145–151.

Hosaka T, Sugiyama Y, Hirai K, Sugawara Y. 2001b. Factors associated with the effects of a structured psychiatric intervention on breast cancer patients. *Tokai J Exp Clin Med* 26(2):33–38.

Hosaka T, Sugiyama Y, Tokuda Y, Okuyama T. 2000a. Persistent effects of a structured psychiatric intervention on breast cancer patients' emotions. *Psychiatry Clin Neurosci* 54(5):559–563.

Hosaka T, Sugiyama Y, Tokuda Y, Okuyama T, Sugawara Y, Nakamura Y. 2000b. Persistence of the benefits of a structured psychiatric intervention for breast cancer patients with lymph node metastases. *Tokai J Exp Clin Med* 25(2):45–49.

Hosaka T, Tokuda Y, Sugiyama Y, Hirai K, Okuyama T. 2000c. Effects of a structured psychiatric intervention on immune function of cancer patients. *Tokai J Exp Clin Med* 25(4–6):183–188.

Maguire P, Brooke M, Tait A, Thomas C, Sellwood R. 1983. The effect of counselling on physical disability and social recovery after mastectomy. *Clin Oncol* 9(4):319–324.

Redman S, Turner J, Davis C. 2003. Improving supportive care for women with breast cancer in Australia: The challenge of modifying health systems. *Psycho-Oncology* 12(6):521–531.

Appendix A

Meeting Psychosocial Needs of Women with Breast Cancer

National Cencer Policy Board
Institute Of Medicine
*Supported By The Longaberger Company Through
The American Cancer Society*

Monday, October 28, 2002
Describing Psychosocial Services

8:00- 8:30   Continental breakfast

8:30-9:30   Welcome and introduction (Jimmie Holland, Ellen Stovall,
and Tom Smith)

Overview: The status of mental health service delivery in the US
* Psychosocial implications of chronic illness
* Delivery of psychosocial services in the US

Speaker: Howard H. Goldman

**Overview: Psychosocial interventions for women with breast
cancer**
* Psychosocial issues throughout the breast cancer
trajectory
* Prevalence of psychosocial distress
* Types of interventions and their modes of delivery

Speaker: Jimmie Holland

9:30-10:30   **Identifying women in need of services: The effectiveness of assessment tools**
• Discussion of commissioned paper

Speaker: Patricia Ganz
Reactor: Julia Rowland

10:30-10:45   **Break**

10:45-12:30   **The effectiveness of psychosocial interventions**
• Discussion of commissioned paper

Speaker: Pamela Goodwin
Reactors: Katherine DuHamel; Gary Morrow

12:30-1:30   **Lunch available**

1:30-3:15   **Research issues: The need for applied research**
• Status of research and funding opportunities
• Methodological research issues
• Research priorities

Speaker: Barbara Andersen
Reactor: Joan Bloom

3:15-3:30   **Break**

3:30-5:30   **Delivering psychosocial interventions** (Presentations from selected programs)
Introduction: Ellen Stovall
• Psychologist in private practice, Helen Coons
• Oncologist in community-based practice, Lidia Schapira, Boston—Beth Israel Deaconess
• Managed care-based program (Breast Buddy Program), Ann Geiger, Kaiser Permanente, Southern CA
• Cancer center-based program, Richard McQuellon, Comprehensive Cancer Center of Wake Forest University

- American Cancer Society programs (Reach to Recovery, I Can Cope, Look Good . . . Feel Better Program), Bonnie Teschendorf
- Community-based program, The Wellness Community, Mitch Golant

Discussion Leader: Ellen Stovall

Tuesday, October 29, 2002
Overcoming Barriers to Access

8:00-8:30 **Continental breakfast**

8:30-10:30 **Changing provider behavior/practices**
Introduction: Tom Smith
- The structure of breast cancer care
  - What are the barriers to providing psychosocial services in the current delivery system?
  - How can care systems be designed to incorporate psychosocial service providers (e.g., multidisciplinary team approaches, links to community-based providers)?

Discussion leader: Nina Bickell

- The role of guidelines
  - What is the status of guidelines in the U.S.?
  - How should they be designed and implemented?
  - What is the potential for guidelines to change practice?

Discussion leader: Roger Winn

- Quality assurance
  - What quality assurance initiatives might be considered to improve the delivery of psychosocial services?
  - How has measurement of patient satisfaction with breast cancer care within managed care affected practice?
  - Could indicators of psychosocial care be incorporated into these efforts?
  - How can national goals for improved psychosocial care be achieved?

Discussion leaders: Ann Monroe and Bonnie Teschendorf

- Consumer roles and perspectives
  - How can consumers affect changes in practice?

Discussion leader: Christine Brunswick

10:30-10:45   Break

10:45-12:30   **Improving professional education/training**
Panel Discussion with Participants:
- Who provides (or should provide) psychosocial interventions?
- How adequate is their training?
- What new training opportunities are needed?
- How can we assess the effectiveness of training?

Panel: Roger Winn (physician perspective)
Jamie Ostroff (psychologist and research perspective)
Betty Ferrell (nursing perspective)
Carolyn Messner (social work perspective)
Discussion leader: Jimmie Holland

12:30-1:30   **Lunch available**

1:30-3:00   **Reducing individual barriers—social stigma, economic, racial, ethnic, cultural, language, and other barriers**

Speakers: Alicia Matthews
- Reducing stigma
Carolina Hinestrosa
- Reducing barriers to access in the Latina Community
Brian Smedley
- Briefing on IOM report, "Unequal Treatment: Confronting Racial and Ethnic Disparities in Health Care"
Discussion leader: Jimmie Holland

3:00-3:15   **Break**

3:15-4:45   **Addressing coverage and payment issues**
- How are psychosocial and mental health services paid for?
- How do reimbursement issues limit access to services (e.g., limits set by managed care)?
- Are there reimbursement models to emulate?

Speaker: Richard Frank (overview)

Panelists:
-Psychiatrist, David Wellisch
-American Psychological Association (APA), Rus Newman
-Centers for Medicare and Medicaid Services (CMS),
 Madeline Ulrich and Ken Simon
-Health Insurance Association of America (HIAA), Henry
 Desmarais
-American Association of Health Plans (AAHP), Carmella
 Bocchino

Discussion Leader: Ellen Stovall

4:45-5:30   **Wrap-up—Future directions, policy options,
            recommendations**

            Discussion leaders: Tom Smith and Diana Petitti

Appendix B

Summary tables and detailed descriptions of clinical trials of the effectiveness of psychosocial interventions for women with breast cancer

Table B-1   Description of randomized trials in "early" breast cancer

Table B-2   Description of randomized trials in "metastatic" breast cancer

Table B-3   Summary of the effectiveness of psychosocial interventions in breast cancer

Boxes B-4 to B-34 Detailed description of individual studies

TABLE B-1 Randomized Trials in "Early" Breast Cancer

Citation	n	Intervention(s)	Duration	Outcomes
Maguire 1980 1983	172	Individual counseling by nurse specialist vs. control	Every 2 months after surgery until woman had "adapted well"	• Nursing interventions did not reduce morbidity directly; however, it led to increased recognition of the need for psychiatric referral which, in turn, reduced psychiatric morbidity, anxiety and depression. *(follow-up to 12-18 months)*
Christensen 1983	20	Postmastectomy couple counseling vs. control	Weekly x 4 weeks	• No overall treatment effects (small sample size may have precluded identification of effects). • Adjusted analyses suggested tentative benefits in sexual satisfaction and psychological status (husbands and wives) and depression (wives). *(follow-up to 1 week post intervention)*
Bridge 1988	154	Structured relaxation vs. relaxation plus imagery vs. attention control	Weekly x 30 minutes x 6 weeks	• Overall mood and relaxation better for relaxation plus imagery than for relaxation alone. • Both better than attention control arm. *(follow-up to immediately post intervention)*
Cimprich 1993	32	"Restorative intervention" - individualized protocol to identify and practice restorative experiences	20–30 minutes 3x/week x 7 weeks	• Intervention improved attentional capacity and total attentional score. *(follow-up to immediately post intervention)*

TABLE B-1 Randomized Trials in "Early" Breast Cancer

Citation	n	Intervention(s)	Duration	Outcomes
Burton 1995	200	Psychological interview vs. interview plus 30 minutes psychotherapy (surgeon) vs. interview plus 30 minutes chat vs. control (all pre-mastectomy)	One day – 45 minute interview, 30 minute psychotherapy or chat	• Psychological interview led to lasting reduction in body image distress and reductions in overall distress, anxiety, depression, upset regarding loss of breast and enhanced fighting spirit coping. • Psychotherapy better than chat among women with stressful life events. *(follow-up for one year – controls unaware of study until end of study, did not provide baseline data)*
Maunsell 1996	259	Telephone screening of distress (with social work referral) vs. routine care	Monthly x 2 (average 7.6 minutes each)	• No significant effects. *(follow-up to 12 months)*
Marchioro 1996	36	Individual cognitive therapy focusing on problems relating to cancer therapy vs. standard care	Weekly x 50 minutes x ? duration	• Intervention improved depression and quality of life. • Some changes in personality factors were noted. *(follow-up to 9 months)*
McArdle 1996	272	Nurse specialist support vs. voluntary organization support vs. both vs. neither	Variable	• Support from nurse specialist resulted in improved somatic symptoms, social dysfunction and depression. • Nurse support significantly better than voluntary organization support.
Richardson 1997	47	Group support (non-structured, supportive) vs. imagery/relaxation group with one individual session vs. standard care	Weekly x 1 hour x 6 weeks	• Enhanced coping skills in Support ($p<0.01$) and Imagery group ($p<0.07$) vs. control. • Women in both types of groups sought more support from others. • Women in support group had greater acceptance of death. *(follow-up to immediately post intervention)*

TABLE B-1 Randomized Trials in "Early" Breast Cancer

Citation	n	Intervention(s)	Duration	Outcomes
Samarel 1992 1993 1997	228	Structured support group with coaches (family, friend, spouse) vs. structured support group without coaches vs. control	Weekly x 2 hours x 8 weeks	• Support group with coaching resulted in higher quality relationships at the end of the intervention but not 8 weeks later. • No effect on symptom distress or mood. *(follow-up to 8 weeks)*
Kolcaba 1999	53	Guided imagery audiotape vs. control	Audiotape use daily during radiation and for 3 weeks after	• Intervention significantly improved comfort. *(follow-up to 3 weeks post radiation)*
Walker 1999	96	Relaxation and guided imagery vs. standard care	Daily for 6 chemotherapy cycles	• Intervention enhanced overall HRQOL and reduced emotional repression (overall, unhappiness). *(follow-up to end of intervention)*
Wengström 1999 2001	134	Individual nursing intervention based on Orem's model for self-care vs. standard care	Weekly x 30 minutes x 5 weeks	• Intervention led to fewer distress reactions but no difference in HRQOL or toxicity. • Intervention resulted in "Stronger motivation to be emotionally involved" in those over 59 years old. *(follow-up to 3 months post intervention)*

TABLE B-1 Randomized Trials in "Early" Breast Cancer

Citation	n	Intervention(s)	Duration	Outcomes
Sandgren 2000	62	Telephone-based individual cognitive–behavioral therapy vs. assessment only	Weekly x 4, then every 2 weeks x 6 (each < 30 minutes)	• No consistent effects of the intervention over time. • Borderline effects for stress (early benefit, late detriment), anxiety and confusion (benefit), physical role functioning (early detriment) and mental health (early benefit). *(follow-up to 10 months)*
Bultz 2000	36	Psycho-educational group for partners of breast cancer patients vs. control	Weekly x 90–120 minutes x 6 weeks	• No significant effects. • Borderline improvement in mood of partner (p=0.07) and breast cancer patients (p=0.06) 3 months after intervention. *(follow-up to 3 months post intervention)*
Ritz 2000	210	Advanced practice nursing interventions (individual) vs. control	Not specified	• Intervention led to reduced uncertainty at 1, 3, 6 months (but not at 12 months). • Effect greatest in unmarried women. • Beneficial effect on mood at 1, 3 months in subgroup without a family history. *(follow-up to 12 months)*
Fukui 2000	50	Cognitive–behavioral group therapy with muscle relaxation and guided imagery vs. control	Weekly x 90 minutes x 6 weeks	• Intervention significantly improved mood, vigor and fighting spirit coping at the end of the intervention. • Effects were marginal at 6 months. • No effect on depression or anxiety. *(follow-up to 6 months)*

TABLE B-1 Randomized Trials in "Early" Breast Cancer

Citation	n	Intervention(s)	Duration	Outcomes
Helgeson 1999 2000 2001	312	Education group vs. Peer discussion group vs. Education and peer discussion group vs. control	Weekly x 60 minutes x 8 weeks	• Education group resulted in enhanced vitality, mental health and social functioning compared to peer discussion. • Education group resulted in above plus enhanced role functioning and reduced bodily pain compared to controls. • No benefits observed for peer discussion. • Effects "dissipated over time." *(follow-up for 48 months)*
Simpson 2001	89	Structured group psychotherapy vs. control (self-study)	Weekly x 60 minutes x 6 weeks	• Intervention reduced depression and severity of psychiatric symptoms and enhanced mood and HRQOL at 2 years (but not at earlier times). *(follow-up for 2 years)*
Lev 2001	53	Individual counseling plus videotape plus self-care booklet vs. control (educational booklet)	Monthly x ? minutes x 5 months	• Small to large effect sizes for HRQOL, psychiatric symptoms. • No statistical significance testing. *(follow-up to 8 months)*
Antoni 2001	100	Structured cognitive–behavioral group intervention vs. 1 day seminar (controls)	Weekly x 2 hours x 10 weeks	• No overall effects. • Intervention reduced the prevalence of moderate depression and it increased benefit finding and optimism. *(follow-up to 9 months post-intervention)*

TABLE B-1 Randomized Trials in "Early" Breast Cancer

Citation	n	Intervention(s)	Duration	Outcomes
Molassiotis 2002	71	Progressive muscle relaxation training (individual session, audio and videotapes) vs. control	Daily x 30 minutes x 6 days	• Intervention reduced total mood disturbance, duration of nausea and vomiting (trend to reduced frequency of nausea and vomiting). • No effect on intensity of nausea and vomiting. *(follow-up for 14 days)*
Allen 2002	164	Individual problem skills training vs. control	6 sessions over 4 months (2 in person, 4 by telephone)	• No overall effects. • Subgroup analysis indicated benefit in women with good baseline problem-solving ability. *(follow-up for 8 months)*
Targ 2002	181	Standard psychoeducational group vs. mind–body–spirit (CAM) group	Standard – 12 sessions x 90 minutes weekly x 12 weeks CAM – 24 sessions x 150 minutes twice weekly x 12 weeks	• Both interventions improved HRQOL and psychosocial functioning. • CAM led to greater spiritual integration and satisfaction. *(follow-up for 12 weeks)*

TABLE **B-2** Randomized Trials in "Metastatic" Breast Cancer

Citation	n	Intervention(s)	Duration	Outcomes
Spiegel 1981 1983 1989	86	Supportive–expressive group therapy vs. control	Weekly x 90 minutes x ≥ 1 year	• Intervention improved mood, reduced maladaptive coping responses and phobias. • Intervention prolonged survival (mean 36.6 vs. 18.9 months intervention vs. control). *(psychological follow-up x 12 months, survival > 10 years)*
Arathuzik 1994	24	Individual structured relaxation and visualization with or without cognitive–behavioral therapy vs. written handouts about pain distraction	1 x 75 minutes (relaxation and imagery alone)	• No effects of intervention. *(same day follow-up)*
Edelman 1999	121	Group cognitive–behavioral therapy vs. control	Weekly x 8, monthly x 3, one family session (each 2 hours)	• Intervention improved mood and reduced depression, enhanced self-esteem. • Effects present at end of intervention but not 3 or 6 months later. • No effect on survival. *(follow-up 12 months for psychological outcomes, 2 to 5 years for survival)*
Edmonds 1999 **Cunningham** 1999	66	Supportive plus cognitive–behavioral group therapy vs. home cognitive–behavioral study program	Weekly x 2 hours x 35 weeks (longer in some women) plus one weekend	• Intervention subjects experienced more anxious-preoccupied coping and less helplessness coping. • No survival effects. *(psychological follow-up x 12 months, survival to > 5 years)*

TABLE B-2 Randomized Trials in "Metastatic" Breast Cancer

Citation	n	Intervention(s)	Duration	Outcomes
Classen 2001	125	Supportive–expressive group therapy vs. control	Weekly x 90 minutes to end of life	• Intervention significantly reduced traumatic stress symptoms – enhanced mood if final assessment during the year prior to death was excluded. • Survival effects pending. *(follow-up to 12 months)*
Goodwin 2002	235	Supportive–expressive group therapy vs. control	Weekly x 90 minutes to end of life	• Intervention significantly enhanced overall mood, depression, anxiety, anger, confusion and experience of pain. • Intervention had no effect on survival. *(follow-up to end of life)*

TABLE B-3 Summary of the Effectiveness of Psychosocial Interventions in Breast Cancer

I. Relaxation/Imagery*

Citation	Phase	n	Intervention	Duration of Intervention	Effectiveness	Duration of Benefit	Duration of Follow-up
Bridge 1988	Early	154	• Relaxation (audiotape) • Relaxation/Imagery	6 weeks	• Improved mood, relaxation. • Imagery and relaxation had additive effects.	6 weeks	6 weeks
Richardson 1997	Early	47	• Relaxation/Imagery group intervention	6 weeks	• Greater acceptance of death, enhanced coping – no effect on mood.	6 weeks	6 weeks
Kolcaba 1999	Early	53	• Guided imagery audiotape	Radiation and 3 weeks after	• Improved "comfort".	3 weeks post radiation	3 weeks post radiation
Walker 1999	Early	96	• Relaxation/guided imagery (audiotape)	6 cycles of chemotherapy	• Improved overall HRQOL • Reduced emotional repression.	To end of chemotherapy	To end of chemotherapy
Molassiotis 2002	Early	71	• Progressive muscle relaxation – audio and videotape	6 days	• Improved mood, reduced duration and frequency but not intensity of nausea, vomiting.	14 days	14 days
Arathuzik 1994	Metastatic	24	• Relaxation plus visualization with or without cognitive-behavioral therapy	1 session	• No effect.	1 day	1 day

* *Does not include studies in which relaxation/hypnosis/imagery was delivered as a minor part of another intervention.*

TABLE B-3 Summary of the Effectiveness of Psychosocial Interventions in Breast Cancer

II. Group Interventions

Citation	Phase	n	Intervention	Duration of Intervention	Effectiveness	Duration of Benefit	Duration of Follow-up
Richardson 1997	Early	47	• Non-structured support group	6 weeks	• Greater acceptance of death, enhanced coping	6 weeks	6 weeks
Samarel 1992 1993 1997	Early	228	• Structured support group with or without coaches	8 weeks	• Coached groups resulted in higher quality relationships	8 weeks	16 weeks
Helgeson 1999 2000 2001	Early	312	• Education group • Education group plus peer discussion group • Peer discussion group	8 weeks	• Education group enhanced vitality, mental health, social functioning, role functioning and reduced bodily pain. • No benefits of peer discussion. • Effects "dissipated" over time.	48 months	48 months
Simpson 2001	Early	89	• Structured group psychotherapy	6 weeks	• Reduced depression and severity of psychiatric symptoms, enhanced mood and HRQOL	24 months	24 months
Targ 2002	Early (<10% metastatic)	181	• Psychoeducational group • Mind–body–spirit group (CAM)	12 weeks	• Both groups improved measures of HRQOL, psychosocial function. • CAM improved spiritual integration, satisfaction.	12 weeks	12 weeks

TABLE B-3 Summary of the Effectiveness of Psychosocial Interventions in Breast Cancer

II. Group Interventions (continued)

Citation	Phase	n	Intervention	Duration of Intervention	Effectiveness	Duration of Benefit	Duration of Follow-up
Spiegel 1981 1983 1989	Metastatic	86	• Supportive–expressive group therapy with relaxation	≥ 1 year	• Improved mood, reduced maladaptive coping responses and phobias. • Prolonged survival.	12 months	12 months
Classen 2001	Metastatic	125	• Supportive–expressive group therapy with relaxation	Indefinite	• Reduced traumatic stress symptoms • Enhanced mood if final measurement during the year prior to death excluded	12 months	12 months
Goodwin 2002	Metastatic	235	• Supportive–expressive group therapy with relaxation	Indefinite	• Improved mood, reduced experience of pain	12 months	12 months
Fukui 2000	Early	50	• Cognitive–behavioral group with relaxation and guided imagery	6 weeks	• Improved mood, vigor, fighting spirit	8 weeks	6 months**
Antoni 2001	Early	100	• Structured cognitive–behavioral group	10 weeks	• No overall effects • Reduced prevalence of moderate depression, increased benefit finding/optimism	—	9 months
Edelman 1999	Metastatic	121	• Cognitive–behavioral group	5 months	• Improved mood, reduced depression, enhanced self-esteem	5 months	11 months

** *Marginal effect at 6 months.*

TABLE B-3 Summary of the Effectiveness of Psychosocial Interventions in Breast Cancer

III. Individual Interventions

Citation	Phase	n	Intervention	Duration of Intervention	Effectiveness	Duration of Benefit	Duration of Follow-up
Edmonds 1999 Cunningham 1999	Metastatic	66	• Supportive plus cognitive–behavioral	35 weeks	• Increased anxious-preoccupied coping, reduced helplessness, coping "Little psychometric effects"	12 months	12 months
Cimprich 1988	Early	32	• Individualized intervention to restore attentional capacity	? (short-term)	• Enhanced attentional capacity	90 days	90 days
Burton 1995	Early	200	• Psychological interview • Psychological interview plus psychotherapy • Psychological interview plus chat	1 day	• Psychological interview led to lasting reduction in body image distress, overall distress, anxiety, depression, enhanced fighting spirit. • Psychotherapy beneficial among women with stressful life events.	1 year	1 year
Maunsell 1996	Early	259	• Telephone screening for distress	12 months	• No effects.	—	1 year
Marchioro 1996	Early	36	• Cognitive–behavioral counseling	? (short-term)	• Improved depression and quality of life.	9 months	9 months
Maguire 1980 1983	Early	172	• Nurse specialist counseling	"Until woman had adapted well"	• Increased recognition of need for psychiatric referral. • Psychiatric intervention reduced morbidity.	12 to 18 months	12 to 18 months

TABLE B-3 Summary of the Effectiveness of Psychosocial Interventions in Breast Cancer

III. Individual Interventions (continued)

Citation	Phase	n	Intervention	Duration of Intervention	Effectiveness	Duration of Benefit	Duration of Follow-up
McArdle 1996	Early	272	• Nurse specialist support • Voluntary organization support • Both • Neither	?	• Nurse specialist led to improved somatic symptoms, social dysfunction and depression.	12 months	12 months
Wengström 1999 2000 2001	Early	134	• Nursing intervention based on Orem's model for self-care	5 weeks	• Fewer distress reactions, stronger motivation to be emotionally involved.	3 months	3 months
Sandgren 2000	Early	62	• Telephone-based cognitive–behavioral therapy	16 weeks	• No consistent effects. • Borderline effects on stress, anxiety, confusion, physical role functioning and mental health varied over time.	10 months	10 months
Ritz 2000	Early	210	• Advanced practice nursing interventions	?	• Reduced uncertainty (especially in unmarried women). • Beneficial early effect on mood in those without a family history.	3 to 6 months	12 months
Lev 2001	Early	53	• Nurse counseling plus videotape plus self-care booklet	5 months	• No significance testing "Small to large effect sizes for HRQOL, psychiatric symptoms".	8 months	8 months
Allan 2002	Early	164	• Problem-solving skills training (2 session in person, 4 by telephone)	4 months	• No overall effects. • Subgroup analysis suggested benefit in women with good problem-solving skills.	8 months	8 months

BOX B-4 Clinical Trials of Psychosocial Interventions in Breast Cancer

Author(s):	Bridge LR, Benson P, Pietroni PC, Priest RG.
Title:	Relaxation and imagery in the treatment of breast cancer.
Journal:	*British Medical Journal* 1988; 297:1169–1172.
Category:	( ) Education ( ) **Individual Therapy** (X) **Relaxation/Hypnosis/Imagery** (..) **Group Therapy** ( ) **Behavioral Therapy/CBT** (..) **Other** _____
Setting:	UK – Middlesex Hospital, London
Study Design:	RCT (1) Relaxation (2) Relaxation plus Imagery (3) Attention control
Phase/Stage of Disease:	Stage I or II during local radiotherapy.
Number of Subjects:	154 **Dropouts:** ___15___ **Compliance:** Not stated
Intervention:	(1) Structured relaxation techniques + diaphragmatic breathing + audiotape (2) Above + imagery of peaceful scene (3) Controls encouraged to talk about themselves **# Sessions:** 30 min **Duration:** Weekly x 6
Measures:	(1) Profile of Mood States (POMS) (2) Leeds General Scales (anxiety and depression)
Time of Administration:	Pre and post-intervention.
Analysis:	ANCOVA
Results:	• Relaxation with imagery better than relaxation alone for total mood disturbance (POMS). • Both interventions arms better than attention control arm. • Same pattern for "relaxed" item in POMS. • No differences for Leeds General Scales.
Comments:	

BOX B-5 Clinical Trials of Psychosocial Interventions in Breast Cancer

Author(s):	Cimprich B.
Title:	Development of an intervention to restore attention in cancer patients.
Journal:	*Cancer Nursing* 1993; 16:83–92.
Category:	( ) Education ( ) Relaxation/Hypnosis/Imagery ( ) Behavioral Therapy/CBT (X) Individual Therapy (..) Group Therapy (..) Other
Setting:	United States – University Medical Center
Study Design:	RCT (1) "Restorative intervention (2) Control
Phase/Stage of Disease:	Newly diagnosed Stage I or II breast cancer
Number of Subjects:	32 **Dropouts:** 6 **Compliance:**
Intervention:	Restorative intervention – individualized protocol to identify experiences/practices that engage fascination or have other restorative properties – included a written contract and serial observations **# Sessions:** ? **Duration:** 20-30 minutes z 3 weeks x ? weeks
Measures:	(1) Digital Span (2) Leeds General Scales (anxiety and depression)
Time of Administration:	Baseline, 18, 60, 90 days post surgery
Analysis:	ANCOVA
Results:	• Intervention significantly improved attentional capacity (AFI) and total attentional score.
Comments:	

BOX B-6 Clinical Trials of Psychosocial Interventions in Breast Cancer

Author(s):	Maguire P, Tait A, Brooke M, Thomas C, Sellwood R.
Title:	Effect of counselling on the psychiatric morbidity associated with mastectomy.
Journal:	*British Medical Journal* 1980; 281:1454–1456.
Category:	( ) Education (X) **Individual Therapy** ( ) **Relaxation/Hypnosis/Imagery** (..) **Group Therapy** ( ) **Behavioral Therapy/CBT** (..) **Other**
Setting:	United Kingdom – University associated hospital
Study Design:	"Pseudo RCT" – randomization of weeks in a 24 month period to: (1) specialist nursing intervention versus (2) control according to week of admission for surgery. * Awareness of randomization may have influenced admission date.
Phase/Stage of Disease:	Breast cancer patients admitted for mastectomy
Number of Subjects:	172 **Dropouts:** 20 **Compliance:** 3 not stated
Intervention:	Individual counseling by RN before/after surgery in hospital and at subsequent home visits every 2 months until women had "adapted well" – focus on scar, arm morbidity, breast prosthesis, openness re: effect of surgery. **# Sessions:** Variable **Duration:** Variable
Measures:	(1) Present State Exam (interviewer administered) (2) LASA's – mood (self-report) (3) Brown-Birley Life Events Schedule (short version – interviewer administered)
Time of Administration:	(1) Postoperative, (2) three months later, (3) 12-18 months later
Analysis:	Not stated
Results:	• "Counseling failed to prevent morbidity but the nurses' regular monitoring of the women's progress led nurse to recognize and refer 76% of those who needed psychiatric help" (vs. only 15% of control group). • subsequent intervention reduced psychiatric morbidity at 12-18 months (also reduced anxiety and depression LASA scores).
Comments:	See also: Maguirre P, Brooke M, Tait A, Thomas C, Sellwood R. The effect of counselling on physical disability and social recovery after mastectomy. *Clinical Oncology* 1983; 9:319–324.

BOX B-7 Clinical Trials of Psychosocial Interventions in Breast Cancer

Author(s):	Christensen D.
Title:	Postmastectomy couple counseling: An outcome study of a structured treatment protocol.
Journal:	*Journal of Sex and Marital Therapy* 1983; 9:266–275.
Category:	( ) Education ( ) Individual Therapy ( ) Relaxation/Hypnosis/Imagery (..) Group Therapy ( ) Behavioral Therapy/CBT (X) Other Couples therapy
Setting:	United States – multiple referral sources
Study Design:	RCT (couples randomized)
Phase/Stage of Disease:	Post mastectomy
Number of Subjects:	20 couples Dropouts: _____ Compliance: _____
Intervention:	Structured couples intervention based on work by Mildred Witlen – specifies tailored to each couple's needs – focus on impact of mastectomy on couple's relationship. **# Sessions:** 4 x ? time **Duration:** Weekly x 4 weeks
Measures:	(1) Psychological Screening Inventory (PSI) (2) Beck Depression Inventory (BDI) (3) Spielberger State/Trait Anxiety Inventory (STAI) (4) Lowenberg Self-Esteem Scale (5) Sexual Satisfaction Scale (6) Locke-Wallace Marital Adjustment Test (7) Internal-External Locus of Control Scale, Revised
Time of Administration:	1 week before and 1 week after intervention
Analysis:	ANOVA
Results:	• No overall treatment effects identified. • adjusted analyses suggested tentative benefit for sexual satisfaction (husbands and wives), depression (wives), PSI (husbands and wives).
Comments:	

Box B-8 Clinical Trials of Psychosocial Interventions in Breast Cancer

Author(s):	Burton MV, Parker RW, Farrell A, Bailey D, Conneely J, Booth S, Elcombe S.
Title:	A randomized controlled trial of preoperative psychological preparation for mastectomy.
Journal:	*Psycho-Oncology* 1995; 4:1–19.
Category:	( ) Education (X) **Individual Therapy** ( ) Relaxation/Hypnosis/Imagery (..) **Group Therapy** ( ) Behavioral Therapy/CBT ( ) **Other** _____
Setting:	United Kingdom – Coventry Health Authority
Study Design:	RCT (1) Pre-operative interview (2) Pre-operative interview + 30 minutes psychotherapy (3) Pre-operative interview + 30 minutes chat (4) Routine care
Phase/Stage of Disease:	Pre-mastectomy (day before)
Number of Subjects:	_200_ **Dropouts:** _?_ **Compliance:** _80 declined intervention_
Intervention:	(1) Interview – psychologist – Present State Exam – focus on worries, concerns, beliefs (2) Interview + Psychotherapy – effect of illness on life situation, feelings (3) Interview + Chat – hobbies, holidays **# Sessions:** _1 or 2 (same day)_ **Duration:** - Pre-operative interview 45 minutes - Psychotherapy or chat 30 minutes
Measures:	(1) Present State Examination (shortened)/Interview – assessed depression, coping, stressful life events, social support, body image distress (2) Hospital Anxiety and Depression Scale
Time of Administration:	(1) Pre-intervention (except controls) (2) 3 months (3) 1 year
Analysis:	ANOVA
Results:	• Pre-operative interviews (vs. control) - lasting reduction in body image distress – reduced overall distress, anxiety, depression, upset re: loss of breast, enhanced fighting spirit coping. • Psychotherapy (vs. chat) superior among patients with stressful life events. (Interpret with caution – no baseline control data)
Comments:	• Control group not informed of study until final measurement. • No baseline data on controls; therefore, control group results may not be comparable to the intervention group at baseline.

BOX B-9 <u>Clinical Trials of Psychosocial Interventions in Breast Cancer</u>

Author(s):	Maunsell E, Brisson J, Deschênes L, Frasure-Smith N.
Title:	A randomized trial of a psychologic distress screening program after breast cancer: effects on quality of life.
Journal:	*Journal of Clinical Oncology* 1996; 14:2747–2755.
Category:	( ) Education ( ) Individual Therapy ( ) Relaxation/Hypnosis/Imagery (..) Group Therapy ( ) Behavioral Therapy/CBT (X) Other Telephone distress screening
Setting:	Canada – University affiliated hospital
Study Design:	RCT (1) Monthly telephone screening of distress (2) Routine care (includes brief social work contact at diagnosis)
Phase/Stage of Disease:	Newly diagnosed "localized or regional stage" disease
Number of Subjects:	259 **Dropouts:** 9 **Compliance:** 11.2 of 12 calls
Intervention:	Telephone screening q 28 days based on General Health Questionnaire – if score ≥ 5, patient's social worker intervened by telephone to confirm distress, ascertain cause and offer additional contact. (Screening performed by a research assistant) **# Sessions:** 12 x 7.6 minutes **Duration:** Monthly x 12
Measures:	(1) Social Support Questionnaire (2) Life Experiences Survey (3) Locke-Wallace Marital Adjustment Test (4) Psychiatric Symptom Index (5) Canada Health and Activity Limitation Survey
Time of Administration:	Baseline, 3, 12 months
Analysis:	Repeated Measures ANOVA
Results:	• No significant effects.
Comments:	

BOX B-10 Clinical Trials of Psychosocial Interventions in Breast Cancer

Author(s):	Marchioro G, Azzarello G, Checchin F, Perale M, Segati R, Sampognaro E, Rosetti F, Franchin A, Pappagallo GL, Vinante O.
Title:	The impact of a psychological intervention on quality of life in non-metastatic breast cancer.
Journal:	*European Journal of Cancer* 1996; 32A:1612–1615.
Category:	( ) Education (X) Individual Therapy ( ) Relaxation/Hypnosis/Imagery (..) Group Therapy (X) Behavioral Therapy/CBT ( ) Other _____
Setting:	Italy – setting not specific
Study Design:	RCT (1) Weekly cognitive individual therapy and bimonthly family counseling. (2) Standard care
Phase/Stage of Disease:	Newly diagnosed, non-metastatic breast cancer
Number of Subjects:	36 **Dropouts:** Not stated **Compliance:** Not stated
Intervention:	Individual cognitive psychotherapy aimed at problems related to cancer diagnosis and therapy, anxiety or depression; loss of behavioral or emotional control; altered cognitive functioning; social and role limitations. **# Sessions:** ? x 50 min **Duration:** Weekly x ?
Measures:	(1) Beck Depression Inventory (2) Functional living Index cancer (3) 16-PF – A form (personality) (4) Interx Introject Questionnaire.
Time of Administration:	Baseline, 1, 3 6, 9, months
Analysis:	Repeated measures ANOVA
Results:	• Intervention improved depression and quality of life. • Changes in personality factors noted.
Comments:	

APPENDIX B

BOX B-11 Clinical Trials of Psychosocial Interventions in Breast Cancer

Author(s):	Richardson MA, Post-White J, Grimm EA, Moye LA, Singletary SE, Justice B.
Title:	Coping, life attitudes, and immune responses to imagery and group support after breast cancer treatment.
Journal:	*Alternative Therapies in Health and Medicine.* 1997; 3:62–71.
Category:	( ) Education (X) Relaxation/Hypnosis/Imagery ( ) Behavioral Therapy/CBT ( ) Individual Therapy (X) Group Therapy ( ) Other _____
Setting:	United States – University associated cancer center
Study Design:	RCT (1) Support groups (2) Imagery/relaxation group (3) Standard care
Phase/Stage of Disease:	Stage I-III
Number of Subjects:	47 Dropouts: 0 Compliance: 8 attended < 50%
Intervention:	• Support Group – nonstructured, supportive – stress reduction, reducing feelings of isolation, enhancing self-esteem. • Imagery/Relaxation Group – relaxation, imagery, and basic breathing – audiotapes, discussion of stress, coping (one individual session). # Sessions: 6 x 1 hour Duration: Weekly x 6 weeks
Measures:	(1) Ways of Coping – Cancer (2) Life Attitude Profile (3) Functional Assessment of Cancer Treatment – Breast (4) Profile of Mood States (5) Duke UNC Functional Social Support Questionnaire (6) NK cytotoxicity (7) Cytokines (8) Beta endorphins.
Time of Administration:	Pre-test, Post-test
Analysis:	ANOVA
Results:	• Enhanced coping skills in support (p <0.01) and imagery groups (p < 0.07); women in both interventions sought more support from others. • Greater acceptance of death in support group (p < 0.01). • No difference in mood or QOL or immune parameters. • No significant differences between support and imagery groups.
Comments:	• Pilot Study

BOX B-12 Clinical Trials of Psychosocial Interventions in Breast Cancer

Author(s):	Samarel N, Fawcett J, Tulman L.
Title:	Effect of support groups with coaching on adaptation to early stage breast cancer.
Journal:	*Research in Nursing and Health* 1997; 20:15–26.
Category:	( ) Education ( ) Individual Therapy ( ) Relaxation/Hypnosis/Imagery (X) Group Therapy ( ) Behavioral Therapy/CBT ( ) Other
Setting:	United States
Study Design:	RCT - reassignment of women permitted in the 2 intervention arms (1) Support groups with coaching (2) Support group alone (3) Control Note: Some patients randomized to the intervention arms were re-randomized for logistical reasons.
Phase/Stage of Disease:	Stage I or II breast cancer surgically treated in the previous 4 months
Number of Subjects:	228 **Dropouts:** 47 **Compliance:**
Intervention:	(1) Structured support group designed to assist women to adapt in physiological, self-concept, role function and interdependent response modes – patients and a coach (2) Support group without coaches (3) No treatment **# Sessions:** 8 x 2 hours **Duration:** Weekly x 8 weeks
Measures:	(1) Symptom Distress Scale (2) Profile of Mood States (3) Inventory of Functional Status – Cancer (4) Relationship Change Scale
Time of Administration:	(1) Baseline (2) End of group intervention (3) 8 weeks later
Analysis:	Repeated measures MANOVA, ANOVA
Results:	• Support group with coaching resulted in higher quality relationships at the end of the group but not 8 weeks later. • Interventions had no effect on symptom distress, mood or functional status.
Comments:	See also: (1) Samarel N, Fawcett J, Tulman L. The effects of coaching in breast cancer support groups: A pilot study. *Oncology Nursing Forum* 1993; 20:795–798. (2) Samarel N, Fawcett J. Enhancing adaptation to breast cancer: The addition of coaching to support groups. *Oncology Nursing Forum* 1992; 19:591–596.

<u>BOX B-13 Clinical Trials of Psychosocial Interventions in Breast Cancer</u>

Author(s):	Kolcaba K, Fox C.
Title:	The effects of guided imagery on comfort of women with early stage breast cancer undergoing radiation therapy.
Journal:	*Oncology Nursing Forum* 1999; 26:67–72.
Category:	( ) Education ( ) Individual Therapy (X) Relaxation/Hypnosis/Imagery ( ) Group Therapy ( ) Behavioral Therapy/CBT ( ) Other _____
Setting:	United States – mid-western radiation and oncology departments
Study Design:	RCT (1) Guided imagery audiotape (2) Control
Phase/Stage of Disease:	Stage I or II breast cancer patients about to begin radiation therapy
Number of Subjects:	53 _____ **Dropouts:** _3_____ **Compliance:** _?_____
Intervention:	• Audiotape – 20 minutes of verbal guided imagery focusing on comfort – psychospiritual, environmental, social - plus 20 minutes of soft jazz music **# Sessions:** _Not stated_____ **Duration:** _Daily during XRT and for 3 weeks after
Measures:	(1) State-Trait Anxiety Inventory – baseline only (2) Radiation Therapy Comfort Questionnaire (RTCQ)
Time of Administration:	Baseline, 3 weeks later, 3 weeks after radiation completed
Analysis:	Repeated measures ANOVA
Results:	Intervention significantly improved comfort across all three time periods.
Comments:	See also: Kolcaba KY. A taxonomic structure for the comfort concept. *Image: Journal of Nursing Scholarship* 1991; 23 237–240.

BOX B-14 Clinical Trials of Psychosocial Interventions in Breast Cancer

Author(s):	Walker LG, Walker MB, Ogston K, Heys SD, Ah-See AK, Miller ID, Hutcheon AW, Sarkar TK, Eremin O.
Title:	Psychological, clinical and pathological effects of relaxation training and guided imagery during primary chemotherapy.
Journal:	*British Journal of Cancer* 1999; 80:262–268.
Category:	( ) Education ( ) Individual Therapy (X) Relaxation/Hypnosis/Imagery ( ) Group Therapy ( ) Behavioral Therapy/CBT ( ) Other
Setting:	United Kingdom – Aberdeen Royal Infirmary
Study Design:	RCT (1) Relaxation training and guided imagery. (2) Standard care
Phase/Stage of Disease:	Newly diagnosed locally advanced breast cancer (T2 > 4 cm, T3, T4 or N2, M0)
Number of Subjects:	96 **Dropouts:** 10 (death progression) **Compliance:** 56% ≥ 1/day
Intervention:	• Progressive muscular relaxation and cue-controlled relaxation • Audiocassettes and cartoon images of host defenses destroying cancer cells (the first 40 women also received "live" training) – daily use **# Sessions:** — **Duration:** Daily x 6 chemotherapy cycles
Measures:	(1) Courtauld Emotional Control Scale (2) Eysenck Personality Questionnaire (3) Rotterdam Symptom Checklist (4) Global Self-rated Quality of Life (5) Mood Rating Scale (6) Tumor size measurements Using calipers (7) Histological response
Time of Administration:	Variable – all before chemotherapy cycle 1, 6; MRS and RSCL before each cycle
Analysis:	MANCOVA
Results:	• Intervention reduced emotional repression (overall, unhappiness). • Intervention enhanced overall quality of life (RSCL, Global Self-rated QOL). • No effect on mood.
Comments:	• No effect on tumor size or histological response to chemotherapy.

<u>BOX B-15 Clinical Trials of Psychosocial Interventions in Breast Cancer</u>

Author(s):	Wengström Y, Häggmark C, Strander H, Forsberg C.
Title:	Effects of a nursing intervention on subjective distress, side effects and quality of life of breast cancer patients receiving curative radiation therapy. A randomized study.
Journal:	*Acta Oncologica* 1999; 38:763–770.
Category:	( ) Education (X) Individual Therapy ( ) Relaxation/Hypnosis/Imagery ( ) Group Therapy ( ) Behavioral Therapy/CBT ( ) Other _____
Setting:	Stockholm, Sweden – University Hospital
Study Design:	RCT (1) Intervention (2) Standard care
Phase/Stage of Disease:	Adjuvant – radiation therapy
Number of Subjects:	134 **Dropouts:** 1 (control) **Compliance:** ?
Intervention:	Nursing intervention based on Orem's model for self-care – individual contact – education, support and guidance re: self-care, psychological support and coping strategies + body image + treatment **# Sessions:** 5 x 30 minutes **Duration:** Weekly x 5 weeks
Measures:	(1) Impact of Events Scale (2) Cancer Rehabilitation Evaluation System (CARES-sf) (3) Oncology Treatment Toxicity Assessment Tool (4) Wheel Questionnaire
Time of Administration:	(1) prior to XRT (2) 3 weeks into XRT (3) 2 weeks post XRT (4) 3 months post XRT
Analysis:	Repeated measures ANOVA, t-tests
Results:	• Intervention group had fewer distress reactions (IES) – there were no effects on QOL (CARES) or toxicity (OTTAT). • Intervention resulted in "stronger motivation to be emotionally involved" in women >59 years old.
Comments:	See also: Wengström Y, Häggmark C, Forsberg C. Coping with radiation therapy: Effects of a nursing intervention coping ability for women with breast cancer. *International Journal of Nursing Practice* 2001; 7:8–15.

BOX B-16 Clinical Trials of Psychosocial Interventions in Breast Cancer

Author(s):	Sandgren AK, McCaul KD, King B, O'Donnell S, Foreman G.
Title:	Telephone Therapy for Patients with Breast Cancer.
Journal:	*Oncology Nursing Forum* 2000; 4:683–688
Category:	( ) Education ( ) Individual Therapy ( ) Relaxation/Hypnosis/Imagery ( ) Group Therapy (X) Behavioral Therapy/CBT ( ) Other
Setting:	United States – Tertiary cancer center
Study Design:	RCT (1) Telephone based cognitive–behavioral therapy (individual) (2) Assessment only
Phase/Stage of Disease:	Stage I, II – within 3-4 months of diagnosis.
Number of Subjects:	62 **Dropouts:** 5 **Compliance:** 90% (17 randomized women declined participation)
Intervention:	Telephone support, coping skills, managing anxiety and stress, solving patient-generated problems – using cognitive restructuring – encouragement of emotional expression, diaphragmatic breathing. **# Sessions:** weekly x 4 q 2 weekly x 6 **Duration:** ≤ 30 minutes (average 20-25)
Measures:	(1) Profile of Mood States (2) Medical Outcome Scales SF 36 (3) Perceived Stress (4) Satisfaction with therapy (5) Coping Response Indices - Revised
Time of Administration:	Baseline, 4 and 10 months follow-up
Analysis:	ANOVA, t-tests
Results:	• No consistent effects of intervention over time. • Some borderline effect of interaction for stress (early benefit, late detriment) anxiety and confusion (benefit), physical role functioning (early detriment), mental health (early benefit) • Intervention subjects used oncology nursing telephone line more.
Comments:	? Pre-consent randomization

BOX B-17 Clinical Trials of Psychosocial Interventions in Breast Cancer

Author(s):	Bultz BD, Speca M, Brasher PM, Geggie PHS, Page SA.
Title:	A randomized controlled trial of a brief psychoeducational support group for partners of early stage breast cancer patients.
Journal:	*Psycho-Oncology* 2000; 9:303–313.
Category:	( ) Education ( ) Individual Therapy ( ) Relaxation/Hypnosis/Imagery (X) Group Therapy ( ) Behavioral Therapy/CBT ( ) Other _____
Setting:	Canada – University affiliated Regional Cancer Center
Study Design:	RCT (1) Psychoeducational group for breast cancer partners (2) Control
Phase/Stage of Disease:	Stage I or II diagnosed within the past year.
Number of Subjects:	36 couples **Dropouts:** 2 couples **Compliance:** 31/34 – 100% attendance
Intervention:	•Psycho-education – first 2 sessions educational, last 4 unstructured •Focus on feelings, fears, strengthening relationships # Sessions: 6 **Duration:** Weekly x 1.5 to 2 hours
Measures:	(1) Profile of Mood States (2) Index of Marital Satisfaction (3) Duke – UNC Functional Social Support Scale (4) Mental Adjustment to Cancer Scale.
Time of Administration:	Pre and post-intervention, 3 months later
Analysis:	ANCOVA
Results:	• No statistically significant effects. • Author states intervention improved mood in partners at 3 months (p = 0.07) [wives' mood also improved (p = 0.06)].
Comments:	

BOX B-18 Clinical Trials of Psychosocial Interventions in Breast Cancer

Author(s):	Ritz LJ, Nissen MJ, Swenson KK, Farrell JB, Sperduto PW, Sladek ML, Lally RM, Schroeder, LM.
Title:	Effects of advanced nursing care on quality of life and cost outcomes of women diagnosed with breast cancer.
Journal:	*Oncology Nursing Forum* 2000; 6:923–932.
Category:	( ) Education (X) Individual Therapy ( ) Relaxation/Hypnosis/Imagery ( ) Group Therapy ( ) Behavioral Therapy/CBT ( ) Other _____
Setting:	United States – Health care setting not described
Study Design:	RCT (1) Advanced Practice Nursing Interventions (2) Control
Phase/Stage of Disease:	Within 2 weeks of diagnosis (invasive, and non-invasive breast cancer)
Number of Subjects:	210 Dropouts: ? Compliance: ?
Intervention:	•Written and verbal information about breast cancer; what to expect in consultation with physicians' decision, making support, answering questions, continuity of care (in person, by telephone, during home visits) **# Sessions:** Not specified **Duration:** Not specified
Measures:	(1) Functional Assessment of Cancer Therapy – Breast (2) Mishel Uncertainty in Illness Scale (3) Profile of Mood States
Time of Administration:	Baseline and 1, 3, 6, 12, 24 months later
Analysis:	Multiple regression models for repeated measures
Results:	•Intervention reduced uncertainty at 1, 3, 6 months (greatest effect in unmarried women) – overall and complexity, inconsistency and unpredictability subscales. •No effect on mood overall benefit at 1, 3 months and in women without a family history. •No effect on QOL.
Comments:	No effect on health-care costs.

APPENDIX B

BOX B-19 Clinical Trials of Psychosocial Interventions in Breast Cancer

Author(s):	Fukui S, Kugaya A, Okamura H, Kamiya M, Koike M, Nakanishi T, Imoto S, Kanagawa K, Uchitomi Y.
Title:	A psychosocial group intervention for Japanese women with primary breast carcinoma. A randomized controlled trial.
Journal:	*Cancer* 2000; 89:1026–1036.
Category:	( ) Education ( ) Individual Therapy ( ) Relaxation/Hypnosis/Imagery (X) Group Therapy ( ) Behavioral Therapy/CBT ( ) Other _____
Setting:	Japan – National Cancer Center
Study Design:	RCT (1) Cognitive–behavioral Group Therapy (2) Wait list controls
Phase/Stage of Disease:	High risk invasive breast cancer diagnosed 4-18 months before – no chemotherapy
Number of Subjects:	50 **Dropouts:** 4 **Compliance:** _____
Intervention:	•Group cognitive behavioral therapy – education, coping skills training, stress management (including muscle relaxation and guided imagery), psychosocial support •6 to 10 patients, 2 therapists – structured. **# Sessions:** 6 x 90 minutes **Duration:** Weekly x 6
Measures:	(1) Hospital Anxiety and Depression Scale (2) Mental Adjustment to Cancer Scale (3) Profile of Mood States
Time of Administration:	Baseline, 6 weeks (end of intervention), 6 months
Analysis:	ANCOVA
Results:	• Intervention significantly improved vigor and overall mood at the end of the intervention; effect marginal 6 months later. • Intervention significantly enhanced Fighting Spirit Coping at the end of the intervention; effect marginal 6 months later. • No significant effect on depression or anxiety.
Comments:	

BOX B-20 Clinical Trials of Psychosocial Interventions in Breast Cancer

Author(s):	Helgeson VS, Cohen S.
Title:	Long-term effects of educational and peer discussion group interventions on adjustment to breast cancer.
Journal:	*Health Psychology* 2001;20:387-392.
Category:	(X) **Education** ( ) **Individual Therapy** ( ) **Relaxation/Hypnosis/Imagery** ( ) **Group Therapy** ( ) **Behavioral Therapy/CBT** (X) **Other** Peer discussion
Setting:	United States (Pittsburgh) – oncology offices
Study Design:	RCT (1) Control (2) Education (3) Peer Discussion (4) Education and peer discussion (Factorial design)
Phase/Stage of Disease:	Prior to or early into adjuvant chemotherapy (Stage I to III)
Number of Subjects:	312 **Dropouts:** 2% **Compliance:** 62.5%
Intervention:	(1) Education – group – lecture + questions/answers; expert presenter and oncology RN/MSW – interaction inhibited (2) Peer Discussion – group – MSW/RN facilitation (did not direct) – focus on expression of feelings/self disclosure **# Sessions:** 8 x 60 minutes **Duration:** Weekly x 8
Measures:	(1) MOS SF-36 (2) Positive and Negative Affect Scale (3) Impact of Events Scale (4) Rosenberg Self-Esteem Scale (5) CARES (6) Interview
Time of Administration:	Pre-R; 1-2 weeks post interview; 6, 12, 24, 48 months post
Analysis:	• Intent to treat – Repeated measures ANOVA • Excluded 54 women who recurred before last measurement.
Results:	• Education vs. control: enhanced vitality, social function, mental health, reduced bodily pain; short term enhanced role functioning. • Education vs. peer discussion – enhanced vitality, mental health, social functioning. • No benefits for peer discussion (early or late). • Effects of intervention "dissipated over time".
Comments:	See also: (1) Helgeson VS, Cohen S, Schulz R, Yasko J. Education and peer discussion group interventions and adjustment to breast cancer. *Archives of General Psychiatry* 1999; 56:340–347. (2) Helgeson VS, Cohen S, Schulz R, Yasko J. Group support interventions for women with breast cancer: Who benefits from what? *Health Psychology* 2000; 19:107–114.

APPENDIX B

BOX B-21 Clinical Trials of Psychosocial Interventions in Breast Cancer

Author(s):	Simpson JSA, Carlson LE, Trew ME.
Title:	The effect of group therapy for breast cancer on healthcare utilization.
Journal:	*Cancer Practice* 2001; 9:19–26.
Category:	( ) Education ( ) Relaxation/Hypnosis/Imagery ( ) Behavioral Therapy/CBT ( ) Individual Therapy (X) Group Therapy ( ) Other
Setting:	Alberta (Canada)
Study Design:	RCT (1) Group Intervention (2) Control – "Self-initiated studies"
Phase/Stage of Disease:	Stage 0-2; treatment completed up to 2 years before study entry
Number of Subjects:	89 Dropouts: ? Compliance: ?
Intervention:	(1) Intervention – structured group psychotherapy with weekly themes – one therapist, 2 "survivor" leaders and 7 to 10 subjects (2) Control – self-study, "Helping Yourself – A Workbook for People Living with Cancer" **# Sessions:** 6 x 90 minutes **Duration:** Weekly x 6 weeks
Measures:	(1) Profile of Mood States (2) Mental Adjustment to Cancer (3) Beck Depression Inventory (4) Symptom Checklist – SCL 90R (5) Dealing with Illness Inventory (6) DS MIII R SCI D (structured clinical interview).
Time of Administration:	Baseline; post-intervention, 1 and 2 years (except SCID)
Analysis:	•t-tests at each timepoint •Repeated measures GLM
Results:	•Reduced depression, enhanced mood, QOL post-intervention and at 2 years follow-up (but not at one year) in intervention subjects. •Lower severity of psychiatric symptoms at 2 years in intervention subjects (results similar using repeated measures and t-tests).
Comments:	•Health care billing $147 less in intervention subjects (23.5% reduction) compared to controls.

BOX B-22   Clinical Trials of Psychosocial Interventions in Breast Cancer

Author(s):	Lev EL, Daley KM, Conner NE, Reith M, Fernandez C, Owens SV.
Title:	An intervention to increase quality of life and self-care self-efficacy and decrease symptoms in breast cancer patients.
Journal:	*Scholarly Inquiry for Nursing Practice: An International Journal* 2001; 15:277–294.
Category:	( ) Education (X) **Individual Therapy** ( ) **Relaxation/Hypnosis/Imagery** ( ) **Group Therapy** ( ) **Behavioral Therapy/CBT** (X) **Other** _Self–efficacy intervention_
Setting:	United States
Study Design:	RCT (1) Efficacy enhancing intervention (2) Control – Educational booklet on cancer chemotherapy
Phase/Stage of Disease:	Stage I or II – within first cycle of chemotherapy
Number of Subjects:	53 **Dropouts:** 27 **Compliance:**
Intervention:	(1) 5 minute videotape (2) Self-care behavior booklet (3) 5 efficacy-enhancing counseling interventions at one month intervals (individual) **# Sessions:** 5 x ? minutes **Duration:** Monthly x 5 months
Measures:	(1) Functional Assessment of Cancer Treatment - Breast (2) Symptom Distress Scale (3) Strategies Used by Patients to Promote Health (SUPPH)
Time of Administration:	Baseline, 4 and 8 months
Analysis:	No formal tests of statistical significance – reported effect sizes only
Results:	•Small (functional concerns) to large (social concerns) effect sizes for FACT-B. •Large effect sizes for SDS. •Small (Enjoying Life, Stress Reduction) to large (Making Decisions) effect sizes for SUPPH.
Comments:	Interpretation of results difficult because of high dropout rate and lack of statistical significance testing.

APPENDIX B

<u>BOX B-23 Clinical Trials of Psychosocial Interventions in Breast Cancer</u>

Author(s):	Antoni MH, Lehman JM, Kilbourn KM, Boyers AE, Culver JL, Alferi SM, Yount SE, McGregor BA, Arena PL, Harris SD, Price AS, Carver CS.
Title:	Cognitive–behavioral stress management intervention decreases the prevalence of depression and enhances benefit finding among women under treatment for early-stage breast cancer.
Journal:	*Health Psychology* 2001; 20:20–32.
Category:	( ) Education ( ) Individual Therapy ( ) Relaxation/Hypnosis/Imagery (X) Group Therapy (X) Behavioral Therapy/CBT ( ) Other _____
Setting:	United States Miami – several hospitals and medical practices
Study Design:	RCT (only the 73.5% who completed all assessments were included in the analysis) (1) Intervention (2) Control
Phase/Stage of Disease:	Stage 0-2; within 8 weeks of surgery
Number of Subjects:	100 **Dropouts:** 26.5% **Compliance:** 86.5% (Intervention) 75.5% (Control)

Intervention:	(1) Cognitive–behavioral stress management
	    - structured group intervention weekly for 2 hours x 10 weeks
	    - didactic/experiential exercises + homework
	    - several areas of emphasis
	(2) Control – 1 day seminar 16-18 weeks post operatively
	
	# Sessions: 10 x 2 hours **Duration:** Weekly x 10 weeks

Measures:	(1) Profile of Mood States – SF (2) Center for Epidemiologic Studies – Depression (3) Impact of Events Scale (4) Life Orientation Test – Revised (5) Novel Measures of Perceived Benefits and Emotional Processing
Time of Administration:	Baseline, post intervention, 3 and 9 months post intervention
Analysis:	Multiple techniques
Results:	•No overall effects. •Intervention reduced the prevalence of moderate depression, increased benefit finding and optimism (maximum effect in women with low baseline optimism scores).
Comments:	•Many secondary analyses presented. •Only the 100 women who completed all assessments were included in the analysis.

BOX B-24 Clinical Trials of Psychosocial Interventions in Breast Cancer

Author(s):	Molassiotis A, Yung HP, Yam BMC, Chan FYS, Mok TSK.
Title:	The effectiveness of progressive muscle relaxation training in managing chemotherapy-induced nausea and vomiting in Chinese breast cancer patients: A randomised controlled trial.
Journal:	*Support Care Cancer* 2002; 10:237–246.
Category:	( ) Education ( ) Individual Therapy (X) Relaxation/Hypnosis/Imagery ( ) Group Therapy ( ) Behavioral Therapy/CBT ( ) Other _____
Setting:	Hong Kong – outpatient oncology department of university hospital
Study Design:	RCT (1) Intervention (2) Control
Phase/Stage of Disease:	Stage I-III; first cycle of AC chemotherapy
Number of Subjects:	71 **Dropouts:** 0 **Compliance:** 100%
Intervention:	Progressive muscle relaxation training – 6 standardized sessions (25 minutes relaxation, 5 minutes imagery) with therapist (1 hour before chemo, days 1 to 5 post chemo) + individual audiocassettes + 30 minute video teaching program. **# Sessions:** 6 x 30 minutes **Duration:** Daily x 6 days
Measures:	(1) Profile of Mood States (2) State-Trait Anxiety Inventory (3) Morrow Assessment of Nausea and Vomiting Scale (MANV)
Time of Administration:	(1) and (2) Baseline, 7 and 14 days post chemotherapy; (3) daily x 7
Analysis:	Repeated measures ANOVA
Results:	• POMS – significant decrease in total mood disturbance (not anxiety) with intervention. • MANV – significant decrease in duration of nausea and vomiting with intervention – trend to lower frequency of nausea and vomiting with intervention (no effect on intensity of nausea and vomiting).
Comments:	

APPENDIX B

<u>**BOX B-25 Clinical Trials of Psychosocial Interventions in Breast Cancer**</u>

Author(s):	Allen SM, Shah AC, Nezu AM, Nezu CM, Ciambrone D, Hogan J, Mor V.
Title:	A problem-solving approach to stress reduction among younger women with breast carcinoma.
Journal:	*Cancer* 2002; 94:3089–3100.
Category:	( ) Education (X) **Individual Therapy** ( ) Relaxation/Hypnosis/Imagery ( ) **Group Therapy** ( ) Behavioral Therapy/CBT ( ) **Other** _____
Setting:	United States – 31 private oncology practices, 4 hospitals departments
Study Design:	RCT (1) Intervention (2) Control
Phase/Stage of Disease:	Adjuvant Chemotherapy Stage I-IIIA
Number of Subjects:	164 (<50 years old) **Dropouts:** 9% **Compliance:** Not stated
Intervention:	Problem-solving skills training based on "Home Care Guide for Women with Breast Cancer" • 5 interactive components • individualized worksheets • focus on problem-solving. **# Sessions:** 6 (2 in person x 2 hours each; 4 telephone calls **Duration:** Approximately 3 months
Measures:	(1) Cancer Rehabilitation Evaluation System (2) MH 1-5 (Mental Health Inventory) (3) Impact of Events Scale, Social Problem-Solving Inventory (Revised) (4) Unmet Needs for Assistance
Time of Administration:	Baseline; 4 and 8 months post baseline
Analysis:	ANOVA; multivariate analyses
Results:	• No overall significant differences (univariate or multivariate). • <u>Subgroups</u>: Good baseline problem-solving ability – significant decrease in number and severity of difficulties experienced. • Poor baseline problem-solving ability – no effect.
Comments:	• Effect of intervention differed according to baseline problem-solving ability in post-hoc analyses.

BOX B-26 Clinical Trials of Psychosocial Interventions in Breast Cancer

Author(s):	Spiegel D, Bloom JR, Yalom I.
Title:	Group support for patients with metastatic breast cancer. A randomized prospective outcome study.
Journal:	*Archives of General Psychiatry* 1981; 38:527–533.
Category:	( ) Education ( ) Individual Therapy ( ) Relaxation/Hypnosis/Imagery (X) Group Therapy ( ) Behavioral Therapy/CBT ( ) Other
Setting:	United States – University affiliated medical center
Study Design:	RCT (1) Support Group (2) Control
Phase/Stage of Disease:	Metastatic
Number of Subjects:	86 **Dropouts:** 28 **Compliance:** ?
Intervention:	Supportive–expressive group therapy: 7-10 women and 2 leaders – primary supportive – focus on content (death, dying, family problems, treatment, communication, living richly in face of terminal illness). **# Sessions:** Weekly x 90 minutes **Duration:** Weekly x 1 year (or longer)
Measures:	(1) Profile of Mood States (2) Health Locus of Control (3) Janis-Field Self-Esteem Scale (4) Maladaptive Coping Response (5) Phobia Checklist (6) Denial measure
Time of Administration:	Baseline, 4, 8, 12 months
Analysis:	Slopes analysis (psychological measures), Cox proportional hazards model (survival)
Results:	Intervention improved mood, reduced maladaptive coping responses, reduced phobias and prolonged survival (mean 36.6 months in intervention group, 18.9 months in controls).
Comments:	See also: (1) Spiegel D, Bloom JR. Pain in metastatic breast cancer. *Cancer* 1983; 52:341–345 . (2) Spiegel D, Bloom, JR, Kraemer H, Gottheil E. Effects of psychosocial treatment on survival of patients with metastatic breast cancer. *Lancet* 1989; 2:888–891.

APPENDIX B

Author(s):	Arathuzik D.
Title:	Effects of cognitive–behavioral strategies on pain in cancer patients.
Journal:	*Cancer Nursing* 1994; 17:207–214.
Category:	( ) Education ( ) Individual Therapy (X) Relaxation/Hypnosis/Imagery ( ) Group Therapy (X) Behavioral Therapy/CBT ( ) Other
Setting:	United States Boston – community and university hospitals
Study Design:	RCT (pilot) (1) relaxation/visualization (2) relaxation/visualization + cognitive–behavioral (3) control
Phase/Stage of Disease:	Metastatic breast cancer.
Number of Subjects:	24 **Dropouts:** 0 **Compliance:** 100%
Intervention:	(1) Structured relaxation and visualization – individual sessions, progressive relaxation/visualization (2) CBT – individual – pain distraction – written handout describing 23 methods of distraction **# Sessions:** 1 **Duration:** Relaxation/visualization – 75 minutes Relaxation/visualization + CBT – 120 minutes
Measures:	(1) Profile of Mood States - B (2) Johnson Pain Intensity Distress Scale
Time of Administration:	Pre/post intervention; 2 consecutive days controls
Analysis:	ANOVA, t-tests
Results:	• No between group differences in pain intensity, distress, control or ability to decrease pain or in mood. • Both treatment groups increased perceived ability to decrease pain. • Multiple within-group pre/post change identified.
Comments:	

BOX B-28 Clinical Trials of Psychosocial Interventions in Breast Cancer

Author(s):	Edelman S, Bell DR, Kidman AD.
Title:	A group cognitive behaviour therapy programme with metastatic breast cancer patients.
Journal:	*Psycho-Oncology* 1999; 8:295–305.
Category:	( ) **Education** ( ) **Individual Therapy** ( ) **Relaxation/Hypnosis/Imagery** (X) **Group Therapy** (X) **Behavioral Therapy/CBT** ( ) **Other** _____
Setting:	Australia – University associated hospital
Study Design:	RCT (1) CBT x 12 sessions (group) (2) Control
Phase/Stage of Disease:	Metastatic breast cancer
Number of Subjects:	121 **Dropouts:** 28 **Compliance:** ?
Intervention:	• Structured manual based homework exercises. • Specific themes – cognitive restructuring, relaxation, communication and coping strategies, group interaction and support, relationships, self-image. **# Sessions:** 12 x ? 2 hours **Duration:** Weekly x 8, monthly x 3, one family session
Measures:	(1) Profile of Mood States (2) Coopersmith Self-Esteem Inventory – Adult Form (3) Survival
Time of Administration:	Baseline, completion of therapy; 3, 6, 12 months post intervention (12 month data not analysed)
Analysis:	• Change scores – t-tests • Cox Proportional Hazards Model (Survival)
Results:	• No survival effects. • Intervention improved mood (depression, total mood disturbance) and enhanced self-esteem at completion of therapy. • No benefits at 3, 6 months.
Comments:	See also: Edelman S, Lemon J, Bell DR, Kidman AD. Effects of group CBT on the survival time of patients with metastatic breast cancer. *Psycho-Oncology* 1999; 8:474–481.

<u>BOX B-29 Clinical Trials of Psychosocial Interventions in Breast Cancer</u>

Author(s):	Edmonds CVI, Lockwood GA, Cunningham AJ.
Title:	Psychological response to long term group therapy: A randomized trial with metastatic breast cancer patients.
Journal:	*Psycho-Oncology* 1999; 8:74–91.
Category:	( ) **Education** ( ) **Individual Therapy** ( ) **Relaxation/Hypnosis/Imagery** (X) **Group Therapy** (X) **Behavioral Therapy/CBT** ( ) **Other** _____
Setting:	Canada – University associated cancer center
Study Design:	RCT (1) Group intervention – supportive + CBT (2) Home cognitive – behavioral study package
Phase/Stage of Disease:	Metastatic breast cancer
Number of Subjects:	66 ____ **Dropouts:** 8 _____ **Compliance:** 62.6% _____
Intervention:	(1) Group discussion, CBT assignments (20), coping skills weekend, relaxation (2) Home package – CBT/coping skills workbook, relaxation tapes, phone call at 2, 4, 5, 10, 12 months - supportive **# Sessions:** 35 x 2 hours ____ **Duration:** Weekly x 35 weeks + one weekend ____
Measures:	(1) Survival (2) Profile of Mood States (3) Functional Living Index for Cancer (4) Duke UNC Functional Social Support Questionnaire (5) Mental Adjustment to Cancer Scale (6) Rationality/Emotional Defensiveness Scale (7) Marlow Crowne Social Desirability Scale (8) Defensive Repression
Time of Administration:	Baseline, 4, 8, 12 months
Analysis:	• Change scores – t-tests/Mann-Whitney Tests (psychological) • Cox Proportional Hazards analysis (Survival)
Results:	• No survival effects. • "Little" psychometric effects – intervention subjects experienced more anxious-preoccupation and less helplessness.
Comments:	See also: Cunningham AJ, Edmonds CVI, Jenkins GP, Pollack H, Lockwood GA, Warr D. A randomized controlled trial of the effects of group psychological therapy on survival in women with metastatic breast cancer. *Psycho-Oncology* 1998; 7:508–517.

BOX B-30 Clinical Trials of Psychosocial Interventions in Breast Cancer

Author(s):	Classen C, Butler LD, Koopman C, Miller E, DiMiceli S, Giese-Davis J, Fobair P, Carlson RW, Kraemer HC, Spiegel D.
Title:	Supportive–expressive group therapy and distress in patients with metastatic breast cancer.
Journal:	*Archives of General Psychiatry* 2001; 58:494–501.
Category:	( ) Education ( ) Individual Therapy ( ) Relaxation/Hypnosis/Imagery (X) Group Therapy ( ) Behavioral Therapy/CBT ( ) Other
Setting:	United States – University associated hospitals
Study Design:	RCT (1) Supportive–expressive group therapy (2) Control (educational materials offered)
Phase/Stage of Disease:	Metastatic breast cancer (2 had local breast recurrences only)
Number of Subjects:	125 **Dropouts:** 11 **Compliance:** 82% questionnaires
Intervention:	Supportive–expressive group therapy: 2 therapists – supportive environment in which participants encouraged to confront problems, strengthen relationships, find enhanced meaning in life – unstructured. **# Sessions:** Variable x 90 minutes **Duration:** Weekly to end of life
Measures:	(1) Profile of Mood States (2) Impact of Events
Time of Administration:	Baseline, every 4 months x 1 year, every 6 months thereafter
Analysis:	Slopes analysis
Results:	• Intervention significantly reduced traumatic stress symptoms but had no significant impact on overall mood (effect enhanced if final assessment during the year before death excluded). • Intervention significantly improved mood if final assessments performed during the year before death excluded.
Comments:	Survival data not yet mature.

BOX B-31 Clinical Trials of Psychosocial Interventions in Breast Cancer

Author(s):	Goodwin PJ, Leszcz M, Ennis M, Koopmans J, Vincent L, Guther H, Drysdale E, Hundleby M, Chochinov H, Navarro M, Speca M, Hunter J et al.
Title:	The effect of group psychosocial support on survival in metastatic breast cancer.
Journal:	*New England Journal of Medicine* 2002; 345:1719–1726.
Category:	( ) Education　　　　　　　　　　　　　( ) Individual Therapy ( ) Relaxation/Hypnosis/Imagery　　　(X) Group Therapy ( ) Behavioral Therapy/CBT　　　　　　( ) Other _____
Setting:	Canada – University associated cancer centers
Study Design:	RCT (1) Supportive–expressive Group Therapy (2) Usual Care
Phase/Stage of Disease:	Metastatic breast cancer
Number of Subjects:	235 _____ **Dropouts:** 19.0% _____ **Compliance:** 66.7%
Intervention:	• Supportive–expressive group therapy: 8-12 women, 2 leaders foster support, encourage emotional expressiveness, confront effects of illness, change in self-image, roles, relationships, life altering nature of illness, coping and communication. • Monthly family sessions. **# Sessions:** Weekly sessions to death **Duration:** Weekly x 90 minutes
Measures:	(1) Profile of Mood States (2) Pain LASAs (3) European Organization for Research and Treatment of Cancer Quality of Life Questionnaire (EORTC QLQ-C30) (4) Survival
Time of Administration:	Baseline, 4, 8, 12 months
Analysis:	•Intervention to treat ANCOVA (psychological) •Cox Proportional Hazards Model (survival)
Results:	•No survival effects, no HRQOL effects. •Enhanced mood (total mood, anger, anxiety, depression, confusion) in intervention subjects. •Reduced experience of pain in intervention subjects.
Comments:	See also: Bordeleau L, Szalai JP, Ennis M, Leszcz M, Speca M, Sela R, Doll R, Chochinov HM, Navarro M, Arnold A, Pritchard KI, Bezjak A, Llewellyn-Thomas H, Sawka CA, Goodwin PJ. Quality of life in a randomized trial of group psychosocial support in metastatic breast cancer: overall effects of the intervention and an exploration of missing data. 2003. *J Clin Oncol* 21(10)1944:1951.

BOX B-32 Clinical Trials of Psychosocial Interventions in Breast Cancer

Author(s):	Fogarty LA, Curbow BA, Wingard JR, McDonnell K, Somerfield MR.
Title:	Can 40 Seconds of Compassion Reduce Patient Anxiety?
Journal:	*Journal of Clinical Oncology* 1999; 17:371–379.
Category:	( ) Education ( ) Individual Therapy ( ) Relaxation/Hypnosis/Imagery ( ) Group Therapy ( ) Behavioral Therapy/CBT (X) Other Videotape
Setting:	United States – University Centres, local support groups
Study Design:	RCT (1) Enhanced compassion videotape (2) Standard videotape
Phase/Stage of Disease:	Healthy breast cancer survivors (> 6 months post diagnosis, no recurrence)
Number of Subjects:	_____123_____ **Dropouts:** _____ **Compliance:** _____
Intervention:	Dramatized videotapes of a treatment consultation that did or did not enhance compassion – verbal acknowledgement of psychologic concern, offer of support and partnership – touching of hand **# Sessions:** 1 **Duration:** 18 minutes
Measures:	(1) State Trait Anxiety Index (2) Physician compassion (3) Treatment information recall and (4)Hypothetical discussion (5) Perceptions of physicians attributes
Time of Administration:	Pre/post intervention
Analysis:	Multiple techniques
Results:	• Reduced anxiety in Enhanced Compassion Group • Reduced information recall in Enhanced Compassion Group. • Differences in perception of compassion and physician attributes in expected direction.
Comments:	• Women with no history of breast cancer participated, as a second randomized group results were similar to those in breast cancer survivors.

BOX B-33 Clinical Trials of Psychosocial Interventions in Breast Cancer

Author(s):	McArdle JM, George WD, McArdle CS, Smith DC, Moodie AR, Hughson AVM, Murray GD.
Title:	Psychological support for patients undergoing breast cancer surgery: a randomised study
Journal:	*British Medical Journal* 1996; 312:813–817.
Category:	( ) Education (X) **Individual Therapy** ( ) **Relaxation/Hypnosis/Imagery** (X) **Group Therapy** ( ) **Behavioral Therapy/CBT** ( ) **Other** _____
Setting:	United Kingdom (Scotland)
Study Design:	RCT (1) Control (2) Support from breast cancer nurse (3) Support from voluntary organization (4) Support from nurse and organization
Phase/Stage of Disease:	At diagnosis – early stage breast cancer.
Number of Subjects:	272 **Dropouts:** 50/272 **Compliance:** variable
Intervention:	• Support from breast cancer nurse – individual support, education, encouragement of emotional expression; optional joint meeting with relatives • Support from voluntary organization – individual and group counseling (transactional analysis), education **# Sessions:** Variable **Duration:** Not stated
Measures:	(1) General Health Questionnaire (2) Hospital Anxiety and Depression Scale
Time of Administration:	First postoperative visit; 3, 6, 12, months later
Analysis:	Intent to treat; Kruskal-Wallis, Mann-Whitney tests
Results:	• Support from breast cancer nurse resulted in improved somatic symptoms, social dysfunction and depression. • Support from nurse significantly better than voluntary organization for above on all measures.
Comments:	

BOX B-34 Clinical Trials of Psychosocial Interventions in Breast Cancer

Author(s):	Targ EF, Levine EG.
Title:	The efficacy of a mind-body-spirit group for women with breast cancer: a randomized controlled clinical trial.
Journal:	*General Hospital Psychiatry* 2002; 24:238–248.
Category:	( ) Education ( ) Individual Therapy ( ) Relaxation/Hypnosis/Imagery (X) Group Therapy ( ) Behavioral Therapy/CBT ( ) Other _____
Setting:	United States (San Francisco)
Study Design:	RCT (1) Mind-body-spirit (complementary and alternative medicine) support group (CAM) (2) Standard cognitive–behavioral therapy group
Phase/Stage of Disease:	Within 18 months of diagnosis; 10 had metastatic disease.
Number of Subjects:	181 **Dropouts:** ___51___ **Compliance:** __?__ **(dropouts greater in standard arm)**
Intervention:	• <u>CAM</u> – Group support with emphasis on psychospiritual issues and inner process with education and dance that taught meditations, affirmation, imagery and ritual • <u>Standard</u> – Psychoeducational – coping, communication, problem-solving, emotional expression **# Sessions:** CAM 24/12 weeks **Duration:** CAM 2½ hours STD 12/12 weeks STD 1½ hours
Measures:	(1) Functional Assessment of Chronic Illness Therapy (2) Profile of Mood States (3) Principles of Living Survey
Time of Administration:	Pre, post
Analysis:	- MANOVA - Repeated Measures Analysis of Variance - Intent to Treat
Results:	- Both interventions improved many aspects of HRQOL and psychosocial functioning. - CAM resulted in enhanced spiritual integration, higher satisfaction and fewer dropouts. - Equivalence was seen for "most psychosocial outcomes."
Comments:	